# THE·COMPLETE·GUIDE·TO

# Homeopathy

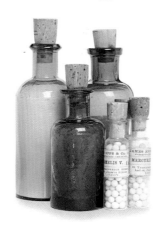

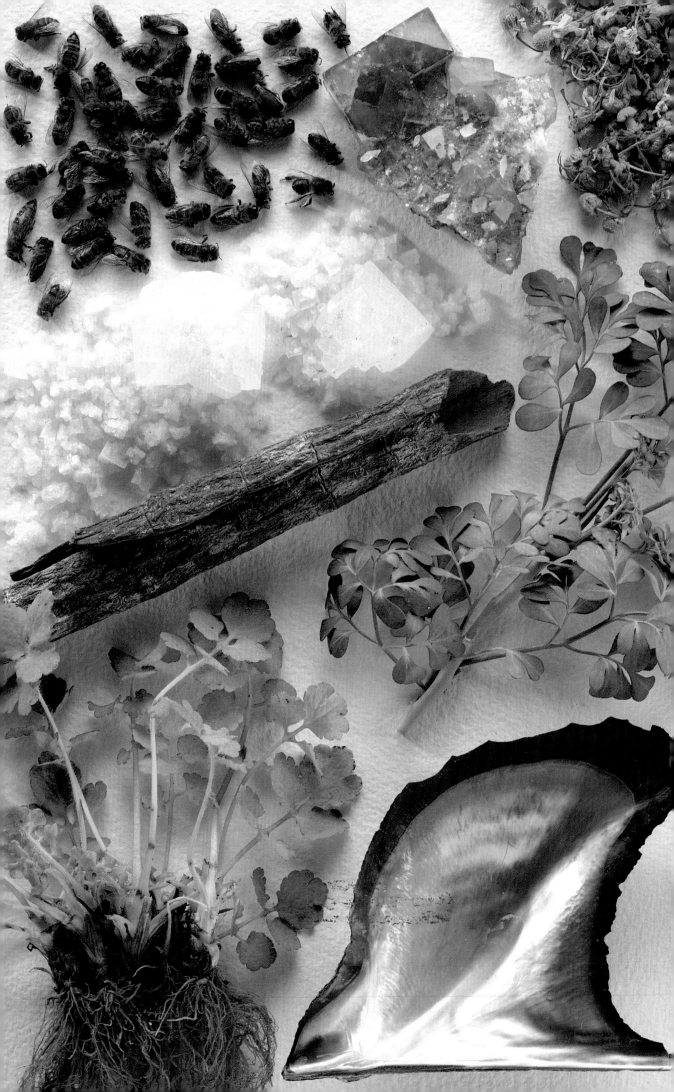

# THE·COMPLETE·GUIDE·TO

# Homeopathy

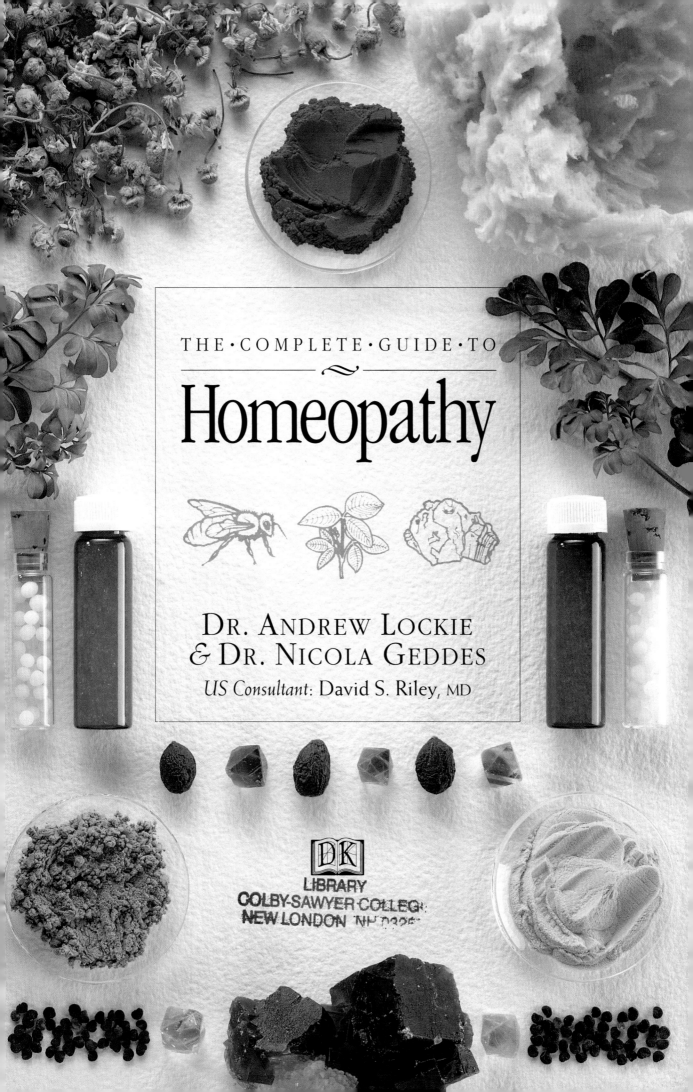

# DR. ANDREW LOCKIE
# & DR. NICOLA GEDDES

*US Consultant:* David S. Riley, MD

## A DK PUBLISHING BOOK

**Project Editor** Blanche Sibbald
**Art Editor** Robyn Tomlinson
**Senior Art Editor** Tracy Timson
**Design Assistant** Deborah Swallow
**DTP Designer** Karen Ruane

**Managing Editor** Rosie Pearson
**Senior Managing Art Editor** Carole Ash
**Production Manager** Maryann Rogers
**Main Photographers** Andy Crawford and Steve Gorton

*Dr. Lockie dedicates this book to M for teaching him that:
'that which you are looking for is inside you.'*

*Dr. Geddes dedicates this book to M and D for their lifelong
gifts of love, support, and humor.*

### IMPORTANT NOTICE

Do not try self-diagnosis or attempt self-treatment without consulting a
medical professional. Do not undertake any self-treatment while you are
undergoing a prescribed course of medical treatment. Always seek medical
advice if symptoms persist. Do not exceed any dosages recommended.
Before taking any remedy or supplement, refer to pp. 152–3, pp. 208–9,
p. 224 and check the precautions in *Remedies for Common Ailments*
(pp. 154–223). Homeopathic indications must be used in accordance with
all state and national regulations. If in doubt, consult your physician.

### Authors' note

Homeopathic remedy names are usually used in abbreviated form.
Commonly accepted abbreviations are used throughout the book.
Constitutional types have the same names as the remedies.

First American edition, 1995
2 4 6 8 10 9 7 5 3

Published in the United States by DK Publishing, Inc.
95 Madison Avenue, New York, NY 10016

Published in Great Britain by Dorling Kindersley Limited.

Distributed by Houghton Mifflin Company, Boston.

LIBRARY OF CONGRESS CATALOGING-IN-PUBLICATION DATA
Lockie, Andrew
  The complete guide to homeopathy : the principles and practice of
treatment with a comprehensive range of self-help remedies for
common ailments / by Andrew Lockie & Nicola Geddes. --
1st American ed.
             p.              cm.
Includes bibliographical references and index.
ISBN 0-7894-0148-7 hardback
ISBN 0-7894-0406-0 paperback
  1. Homeopathy--Popular works.   I. Geddes, Nicola.   II. Title.
RX76.L78   1995
615.5'32--dc20                           95–6746
                                           CIP

Reproduced in Italy by GRB Editrice, Verona
Printed and bound in Italy by A. Mondadori Editore, Verona

# CONTENTS

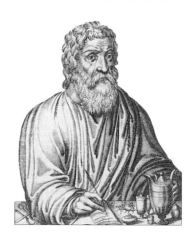

## INTRODUCTION 6

## 8

## HOMEOPATHY PAST & PRESENT

## 22

## ASSESSING YOUR HEALTH

How to determine which constitutional
type you most resemble

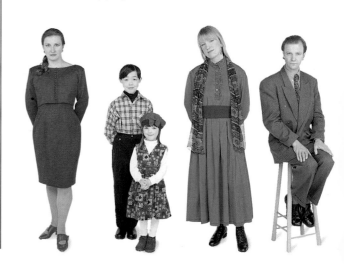

## 48
## INDEX OF HOMEOPATHIC REMEDIES

A visual index of 150 remedies
arranged by Latin name

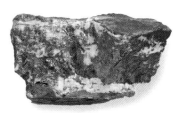

### Key Remedies 48

Fifteen of the most important remedies,
used for minor and long-term complaints

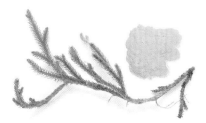

### Common Remedies 80

Thirty common remedies – most are used
for minor ailments; some are also suitable
for long-term conditions

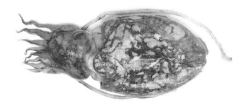

### Minor Remedies 112

105 less commonly used remedies

## 150
## REMEDIES FOR COMMON AILMENTS

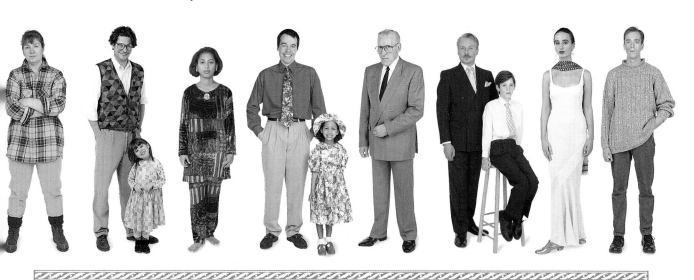

# INTRODUCTION

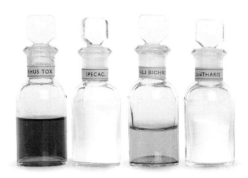

DURING THE LAST TWENTY YEARS the number of people using homeopathy has increased enormously. Nonetheless, there are still many misunderstandings about homeopathy and the way in which it works. We have written this book to explain, in easy-to-follow terms, what homeopathy is and how it can be used safely and effectively to treat common, everyday complaints.

A flexible system of medicine, homeopathy can be used by lay people and medical professionals alike. Minor ailments can be successfully treated at home using homeopathy. More serious complaints require a visit to a medical professional. For example, treat a cold with homeopathic remedies, but always see a doctor if it develops into a secondary infection. If you find that you are getting colds on a regular basis, this probably means that your immune system has been weakened and that you need homeopathic treatment to address the underlying causes. A doctor should be visited for any complaint that would ordinarily be referred to one, or for anything that requires conventional medical tests.

Homeopathy is a holistic form of medicine. In treating an illness, it takes into account the unique emotional and physical traits of the individual concerned. In orthodox medicine, several people suffering from stomach flu would receive the same diagnosis and the same type of treatment even though they do not necessarily have exactly the same symptoms, nor react to them in the same way. One person may be irritable, for example, and another tearful, while another finds it difficult to concentrate. In homeopathy the remedy is chosen to match the symptoms as closely as possible, so that each person might be given a different remedy.

Homeopathic remedies work by helping the body's defense system help itself. Obviously, anything that prevents the body from functioning properly, for example, a poor diet, lack of exercise, destructive emotions, or environmental stresses, gives remedies an uphill struggle and requires attention. Although homeopathy works very quickly in common, everyday complaints, it is not a treatment for those in search of an instant cure. It requires careful self-observation and the willpower to stick to a plan of action. The reward for this is a greater sense of well-being, energy, and resistance to disease.

The increased popularity of homeopathy is in part a reaction to orthodox medicine. Although few people would deny that orthodox medicine has greatly improved general health, many have come to realize that it does not cure all diseases and that many of its treatments have unacceptable side effects. The cost of medicine continues to increase, and many countries are having to reduce expenditure on health care. Holistic systems of medicine, such as homeopathy, take into account more than just the physical symptoms of an illness; they emphasize prevention and the involvement of individuals in their own cure. The holistic approach is best expressed by the words of the doctor and philosopher Albert Schweitzer (1875–1965), who said: "Within every patient there resides a doctor and we as physicians are at our best when we put our patients in touch with the doctor inside themselves."

Andrew H. Lockie    Nicola A. Geddes

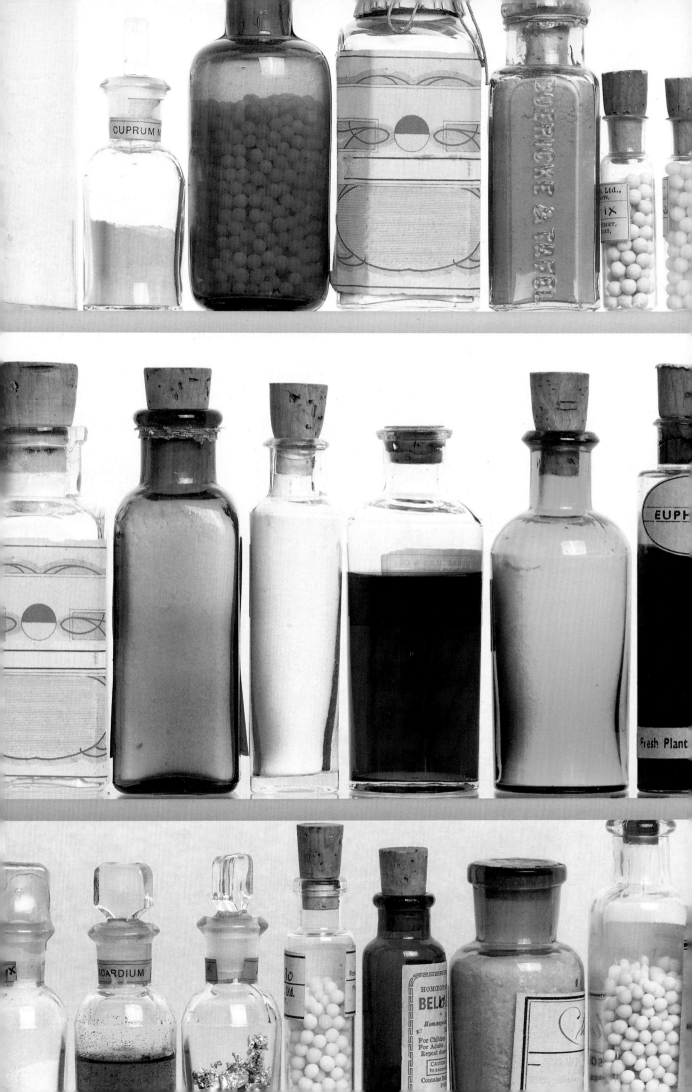

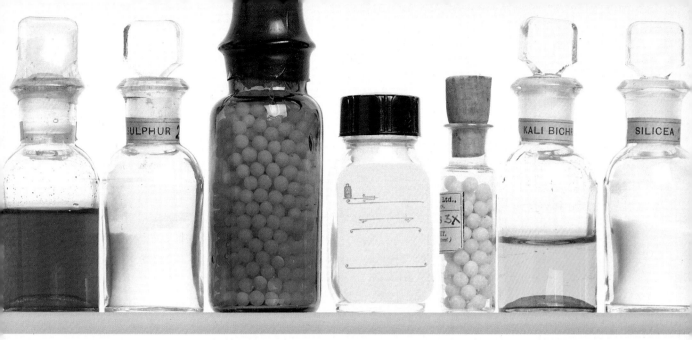

# HOMEOPATHY PAST & PRESENT

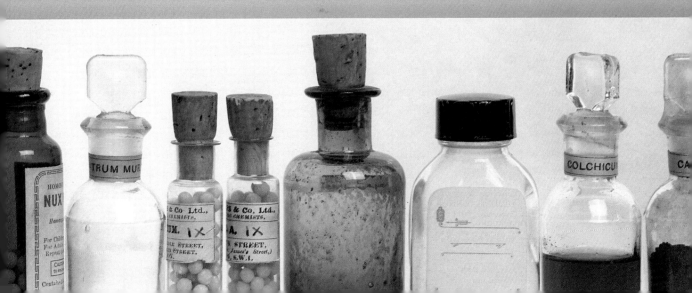

*The principles and practice of homeopathy
have remained largely unchanged since their
introduction some 200 years ago. This section
looks at the history of homeopathy and shows
how the remedies are made. It also explains
the key concepts of homeopathy, which are
central to understanding how it works.*

# THE ORIGINS OF HOMEOPATHY

The principle of "like can cure like" – that is, an illness can be treated by a substance capable of producing similar symptoms to those being suffered by the patient – is the basis of homeopathy. This principle dates back to the Greek physician Hippocrates in the 5th century BC. He is considered the seminal figure in the history of medicine because he was the first person to think that disease is the result of natural forces, not divine influences. Central to his beliefs was the idea that careful observation of the symptoms specific to an individual and of that person's reaction to disease should be taken into account before reaching a diagnosis. He also believed that the patient's own powers of healing are essential to choosing an appropriate cure and should be encouraged.

Hippocrates had a collection of several hundred remedies. One of the best examples of like curing like that he proved was the use of the root of *Veratrum album* (white hellebore) in the treatment of cholera. In large doses this highly poisonous root causes violent purging that leads to severe dehydration, mirroring the symptoms of cholera.

Most medical treatment in Hippocrates' time was based on the Law of Contraries, which held that an illness should be treated by a substance capable of producing opposite symptoms in a healthy person. Treating diarrhea with a substance such as aluminum hydroxide, which constipates, is an example of treating an illness according to the Law of Contraries.

## ROMAN INFLUENCES

During the 1st to 5th centuries AD the Romans made great advances in medicine. They introduced more herbs into the pharmacopoeias and placed greater emphasis on the importance of preventive health care by improving public hygiene. Roman physicians, especially Celsus, Galen, and Dioscorides, increased the knowledge and understanding of the structure and function of the human body. Hippocrates' theory that "like can cure like" and his idea of an individual prescription for an individual patient, however, were largely ignored.

During the Dark Ages in Europe, after the decline of the Roman Empire, there was little medical advancement. Although Greek and Roman medical traditions survived in Persia and throughout the Muslim world it was not until the 16th century that European medical study resumed and progressed.

**Hippocrates** (460–370 BC) *Known as the Father of Medicine, Hippocrates believed that disease came from external forces and not from the gods. He considered that the individual's specific symptoms were the key to choosing a remedy and that the body had the power to heal itself.*

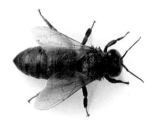

**Honeybee** *In homeopathy, like can cure like. Insect stings are treated with a remedy made from honeybees.*

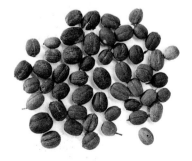

**Unroasted coffee beans** *Coffee causes insomnia: the homeopathic remedy Coffea, made from unroasted coffee beans, is used for sleeplessness and restlessness.*

## NEW IDEAS

Despite an improved understanding of the workings of the human body, knowledge about the nature of disease, in particular what causes it, remained firmly tied to the notion of a mystical force. It was not until the early 16th century and the work of the Swiss doctor Paracelsus (1493–1541) that the causes of disease were linked to external forces, such as contaminated food and drink.

Theophrastus Bombastus von Hohenheim changed his name to Paracelsus as a mark of respect for the Roman doctor, Celsus, and also to imply that he had surpassed Celsus in his abilities. One of Paracelsus's greatest achievements was laying down the foundations for modern chemistry by concentrating on practical experimentation rather than alchemy and its quest to transform base metals into valuable ones. He believed that plants and metals contained active ingredients that could be prescribed to match an illness. This belief was based in part on the notion that the external appearance of a plant gave an indication of the ailments it would cure, a theory that became known as the Doctrine of Signatures. For example, *Chelidonium majus* (celandine) was used to treat the liver and gallbladder because the yellow juice of the plant looked like bile. Paracelsus also believed that a poisonous substance that causes disease could also cure the disease, if given in very small doses, and that physicians should take into account the body's own natural ability to heal itself. Again, the "like can cure like" principle was advocated but it was ignored by Paracelsus's fellow physicians. It did not gain popularity for another 300 years, when homeopathy was founded.

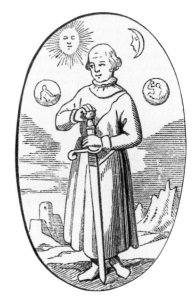

**Paracelsus** *This alchemist and physician changed attitudes about health care, advocating the use of natural medicines.*

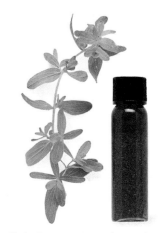

**St.-John's-wort** *According to the Doctrine of Signatures, this was a good wound herb because its oil is blood-red.*

## MEDICAL PRACTICES

From the 16th to the 19th centuries, medical knowledge in Europe increased unabated. The great herbals, namely *The Herball or Generall Historie of Plantes*, by John Gerard (1545–1612), and *The Pharmacopoeia of Herbal Medicine*, by Nicholas Culpeper (1616–54), were published and translated from Latin into English, allowing ordinary people to understand them. Many of the most important healing herbs and other remedies were later used in homeopathy.

Despite the growth of medical knowledge, the general health of the population slowly deteriorated as more people moved to crowded, dirty industrial cities, and standards of public hygiene declined. Medical practice became increasingly invasive, with many physicians using bloodletting and purging as means of cure. Treatments with extremely toxic materials, such as arsenic, lead, and bismuth, which often shortened a patient's life or so weakened it that the afflicted were no longer capable of complaining, became more widespread. It was against this background that homeopathy was born.

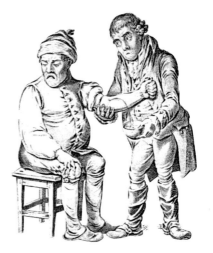

**Bloodletting** *Venesection, either by cupping or leeches, was considered indispensable to healing and became a widespread medical practice.*

# THE WORK OF HAHNEMANN

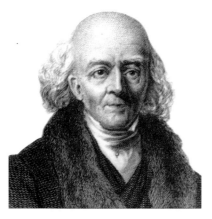

**Samuel Hahnemann** (1755–1843)
*This German doctor and chemist devised homeopathy, a new system of medicine, which literally means "treatment by the same." It is based on the key principle that a drug taken in small amounts will cure the same symptoms it causes in large amounts.*

The founder of homeopathy, Samuel Christian Hahnemann, was born in Dresden, Germany, in 1755. Despite an impoverished background, he acquired a good education and studied chemistry and medicine at the universities of Leipzig, Erlangen, and Vienna. After qualifying as a doctor in 1779, he set up in practice.

Although Hahnemann worked mainly as a doctor, he supplemented his income by writing articles and books on medicine and chemistry. In these writings he protested against the harsh medical practices of the time, especially bloodletting, purging, and the massive doses of medicines that were administered to patients, often with terrible side effects. He argued for better public hygiene and advocated the importance of sensible eating, fresh air, exercise, and less cramped housing conditions. At a time when overcrowding was common and standards of hygiene were poor, he advised regular bathing and cleanliness of bed linen.

By the late 18th century, Europe began a period of enormous upheaval and social change. With the Industrial Revolution came widespread technological advances and many new scientific discoveries. In medicine, considerable work was done to identify and extract the active ingredients of herbs and other plants. The first important breakthrough occurred in 1803 in Germany when Friedrich Serturner isolated morphine from the opium poppy.

## THE FIRST PROVING

Hahnemann became increasingly disillusioned with conventional medical practice and eventually gave up being a doctor to work as a translator. In 1790, while translating *A Treatise on Materia Medica*, by Dr. William Cullen, Hahnemann came across a passage about Peruvian bark, or cinchona, which was to change his life as well as the lives of many people throughout the world. In his book, Cullen stated that quinine, which is a substance purified from the bark of the cinchona tree, was a good treatment for malaria because of its astringent qualities. This made no sense to Hahnemann who, as a chemist, was aware that there were other much more powerful astringents that had no effect whatsoever on malaria. He decided to investigate further. For several days he dosed himself with quinine and recorded his reactions in great detail. To his astonishment, he began to develop the symptoms of malaria one after another, despite the fact that he did not actually have the disease. The symptoms

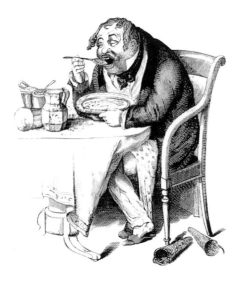

**Overindulgence** *Hahnemann was a great believer in the curative powers of a healthy diet and good hygiene. He railed against gluttonous eating and excessive drinking of alcohol and coffee.*

recurred every time he took a dose of quinine and lasted for several hours. If he did not take any quinine, he had no symptoms. Was this, he wondered, why malaria was also cured by quinine? To test out his theory, he repeated the doses of quinine, which he called "provings," on people he knew well, again noting the reactions in great detail. He then went on to repeat the process using other substances that were in use as medicines, such as arsenic and belladonna. These provings were carried out under strict conditions, and the provers were not allowed to drink or eat anything that might confuse the results, such as alcohol, tea, coffee, and salty or spicy foods.

## UNDERSTANDING SYMPTOMS

Hahnemann found that the provers' responses varied; some showed a few mild symptoms in response to a substance, whereas others experienced vigorous reactions with a variety of symptoms. The symptoms that were most commonly found for each substance he called first-line, or keynote, symptoms. Second-line symptoms were less common and third-line symptoms were rare or idiosyncratic. The combination of symptoms made up a "drug picture" for each substance being tested.

Hahnemann continued to carry out his experiments and provings, testing a wide range of natural sources. He had rediscovered the principle of "like can cure like," and his work would bring about the establishment of a new system of medicine.

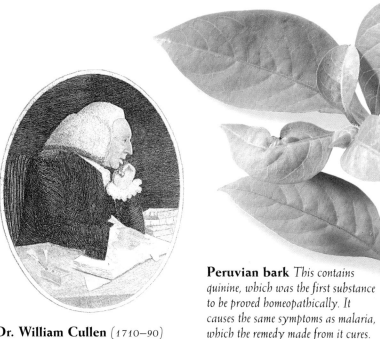

**Dr. William Cullen** (1710–90)
*This leading Scottish chemist and physician was considered an expert on medicinal substances.*

**Peruvian bark** *This contains quinine, which was the first substance to be proved homeopathically. It causes the same symptoms as malaria, which the remedy made from it cures.*

**Belladonna** *In 1801 Hahnemann published results of using this herb (deadly nightshade) to cure scarlet fever.*

# THE DEVELOPMENT OF HOMEOPATHY

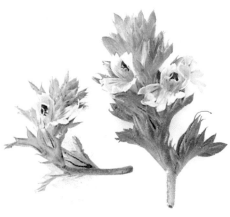

**Eyebright** Euphrasia officinalis *was one of the first herbs to be proved by Hahnemann. In large doses it irritates the eyes; in small ones it has a healing effect.*

After six years of conducting provings of many different substances, Hahnemann had accumulated a great deal of information about their effects. From this careful research and the "drug pictures" he had compiled, Hahnemann embarked on the next stage of his work, which was to test each substance on the sick to see whether they benefited or not. Before he did so, however, he gave his patients a physical examination and questioned them thoroughly about their symptoms, what factors made them better or worse, their general health, the way they lived, and their outlook on life. By taking note of all these details Hahnemann was able to build up a "symptoms picture" of each patient. He would then match an individual's symptoms picture to the drug picture of various substances. Only when he had established the closest match would he prescribe a remedy. He found that the closer the match, the more successful the treatment.

## NEW MEDICAL PRINCIPLES

Hahnemann surmised from this that he had indeed discovered a new system of medicine, in which a drug and a disease that produce similar symptoms cancel each other out in some way, thereby restoring the patient to health. He described this phenomenon as *similia similibus curentur*, or "like can cure like," which is the first and foremost rule of homeopathy.

In 1796 Hahnemann's first work on this new medical system, *A New Principle for Ascertaining the Curative Powers of Drugs and Some Examination of Previous Principles*, was published. In it he stated: "One should imitate Nature which at times heals the chronic illness by another additional one. One should apply in the disease to be healed, particularly if it is chronic, that remedy which is able to stimulate another artificially produced disease as similar as possible and the former will be healed." He called this "homeopathy," from the Greek, *homeo*, meaning "similar," and *pathos*, meaning "suffering." In 1810 he set out his principals in *The Organon of Rationale Medicine*, and two years later began teaching homeopathy at the University of Leipzig.

**Remedy carrying case** *There have been homeopathic practitioners since 1812. Most carried a number of important remedies with them at all times.*

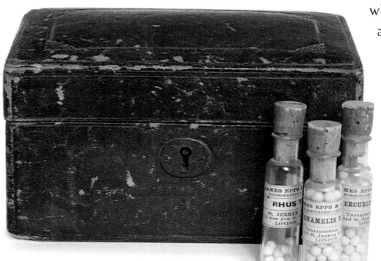

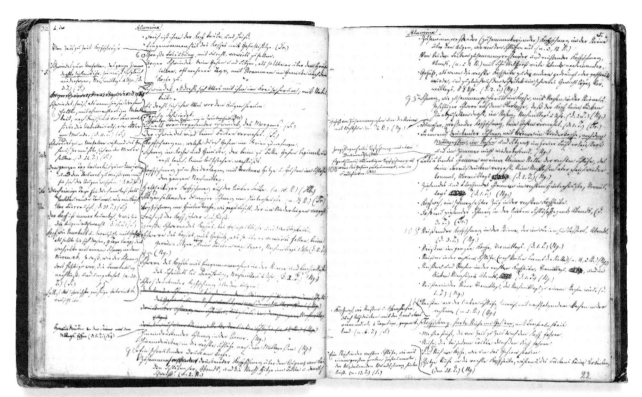

## DILUTED REMEDIES

Some of the medicines administered by Hahnemann were poisonous, so he gave them to patients in very small, dilute doses. He was disturbed to learn, however, that some of his patients' symptoms worsened before becoming better. In order to prevent these "aggravations," as he called them, he changed the method of dilution. He devised a two-step process whereby he diluted each remedy by "succussing," or shaking it vigorously, and banging it down on a hard surface, at each stage of the dilution. He believed that by vigorously shaking a remedy the energy of a substance was released. To Hahnemann's surprise, not only did the diluted medicines cease to produce such strong aggravations, but they also seemed to act faster and more effectively than more concentrated solutions. Although they were weaker, they were actually more potent. For this reason Hahnemann called his new homeopathic remedies "potentizations." In homeopathy, "potency" is used to describe the dilution, or strength, of a remedy.

Hahnemann continued to experiment with diluting remedies throughout his life, using gradually weaker and weaker solutions, which paradoxically became increasingly potent. The remedies became so dilute that they no longer contained a single molecule of the original substance used to make them, yet they remained extremely effective. During his lifetime, Hahnemann proved the efficacy of about 100 homeopathic remedies. He believed that only a single remedy dose should be given, for the shortest period of time necessary, to stimulate the body's healing power.

**Research writings** *A page from Hahnemann's original manuscript,* The Chronic Diseases, Their Nature and Their Cure, *published in 1828, in which the results of his own and his collaborators' provings were written up.*

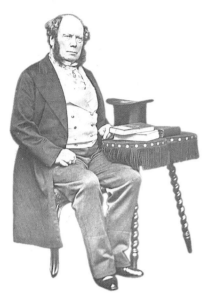

**Dr. Quin** (1799–1878) *The establishment of homeopathy in Great Britain was mainly due to the work he did after he cured himself of cholera with the homeopathic remedy* Camphor, *in 1831.*

**London Homeopathic Hospital**
*In 1849, the first homeopathic hospital was founded by Dr. Quin.*

## HAHNEMANN'S FOLLOWERS

During the 19th century, Hahnemann's philosophy spread rapidly from Germany across Europe, and to Asia and the Americas. Although there were many in the medical profession who disputed Hahnemann's ideas, homeopathy became established in many countries and its reputation grew steadily.

In 1831 there was a cholera outbreak in central Europe. To treat the disease Hahnemann gave the remedy *Camphor.* Where this homeopathic treatment was used the results were very successful. Hahnemann also advised that those infected should be quarantined. Again, he proved himself to be ahead of his time.

One of Hahnemann's followers, Dr. Frederick Foster Hervey Quin, was one of many people cured of cholera by *Camphor.* He had been interested in homeopathy for some time, but the success of his treatment so enhanced his respect for it that in 1832 he set up a homeopathic practice in London and founded the first homeopathic hospital there in 1850. The cholera epidemic of 1854 allowed Dr. Quin the chance to prove the success of homeopathy once again. The death rate from cholera at the London Homeopathic Hospital was about 30 percent less than in other hospitals. These results, however, were suppressed and published only after Parliamentary intervention. The author of the official report concluded by saying, "If it should please the Lord to visit me with cholera I would wish to fall into the hands of a homeopathic physician."

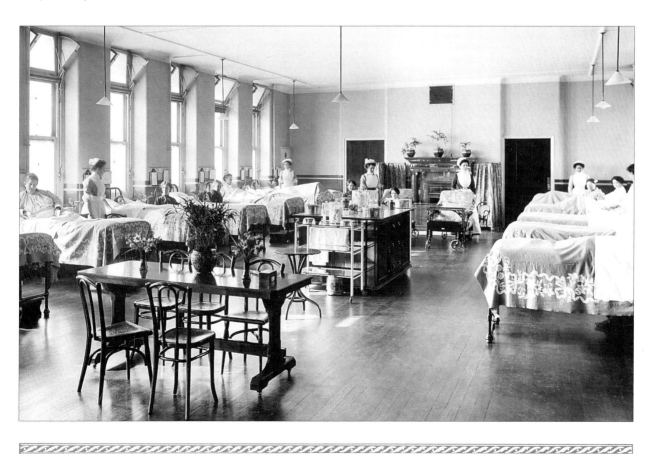

## THE INFLUENCE OF HERING AND KENT

Homeopathy was established in the US during the 1820s and quickly gained a widespread following. Dr. Constantine Hering (1800–80) and Dr. James Tyler Kent (1849–1916) were two important American homeopaths who continued Hahnemann's work in proving remedies and also introduced new ideas and practices to homeopathy.

The Laws of Cure, devised by Dr. Hering, explain how disease is cured in homeopathy. There are three basic Laws of Cure: symptoms move from the top of the body downward; from the inside out; and from the most important organs to the least important. Hering also believed that a cure occurred in reverse order to the onset of symptoms. For example, people generally feel better emotionally before the physical symptoms disappear.

Dr. Kent observed that different kinds of people reacted to certain remedies more strongly than to others. He maintained that people with similar body shapes and personalities tended to suffer from the same types of disease. This formed the basis of his theory that remedies should be prescribed according to an individual's emotional makeup and appearance, as well as his or her physical symptoms. He grouped people according to "constitutional types." For example, *Natrum mur.* types tend to be pear-shaped, have a dark complexion, be fastidious, keep to themselves, crave salt, and suffer from constipation. High-potency remedies were prescribed according to the patient's constitutional type and physical symptoms; this became known as classical homeopathy.

## HIGH VERSUS LOW POTENCIES

Toward the end of the 19th century, the English homeopath Richard Hughes (1836–1902) had begun to question the use of higher potencies prescribed constitutionally and insisted that pathological information only should form the basis of diagnosis. He also advocated using lower potencies. This division between the followers of Kent, who used high potencies and believed that a person's emotional characteristics should be taken into account as well as physical symptoms, and those of Hughes, who used low potencies based on physical symptoms, led to a split in homeopathy. Because of this internal split in practice, homeopathy, despite having become a strong rival of the orthodox medical establishment, was in a weak position in the face of orthodox medicine, and by the 1920s had been almost totally suppressed. Since that time, homeopathy has experienced a resurgence throughout the world and the practice of classical homeopathy, in particular, has gained widespread recognition from homeopaths and orthodox doctors alike.

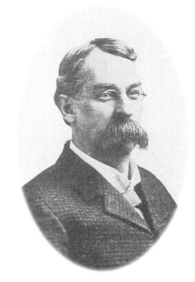

**Dr. James Tyler Kent** (1849–1916) *Classical homeopathy is based on the work of Kent, an American homeopath. He introduced the concept of constitutional types and constitutional prescribing, in which both the physical symptoms of an illness and the distinct emotional characteristics of an individual are taken into account before a remedy is prescribed.*

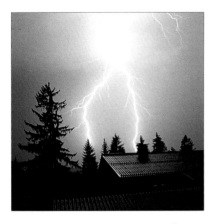

**The effects of weather** *In order to build up a symptoms picture, a homeopath considers how general factors, for example, the weather, seasons, and times of day, may worsen or improve the physical symptoms of a patient.*

# THE PRINCIPLE OF THE VITAL FORCE

Hahnemann had difficulty understanding how remedies worked. He had discovered that the higher the dilution level, or potency, of a remedy the more effective its cure would be. He reasoned that there must be some kind of subtle energy within the body that responded to the tiny provocations of the remedies and enabled the body to heal itself.

Hahnemann called this energy the body's "vital force." This is the force or energy responsible for the healthy running of the body, coordinating its defenses against disease. If this force is disturbed by stress, a poor diet, lack of exercise, hereditary problems, or environmental changes, illness results. The symptoms of illness are the outward manifestation of the vital force's attempt to redress the imbalance and restore order. The concept of the vital force is also recognized in orthodox medicine as the body's own healing power. In orthodox medicine, however, it is attributed less importance than in homeopathy, in which it is central to understanding how the remedies work and how people recover from illness.

## ACUTE AND CHRONIC ILLNESSES

Homeopaths classify illnesses as acute or chronic. In an acute, self-limiting illness, such as a cold, a person becomes ill rapidly, the illness runs its course, and then clears up on its own, with or without treatment. By contrast, in chronic illnesses, a person

**The vital force** *These two diagrams illustrate the difference between a strong and weak vital force. Imagine the vital force as a trampoline and the stresses that assail it as balls bounced onto the trampoline from a great height. Homeopathic remedies strengthen the vital force.*

### HOW THE VITAL FORCE WORKS

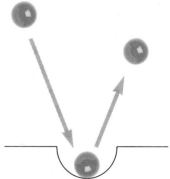

**Strong vital force** If the vital force is strong, the stresses that beset it from time to time, even serious ones, are flung off quickly The body recuperates quickly and good health is maintained.

**Weak vital force** If the vital force is weak, the body does not have the energy to fight illness, which may set in and further weaken the vital force.

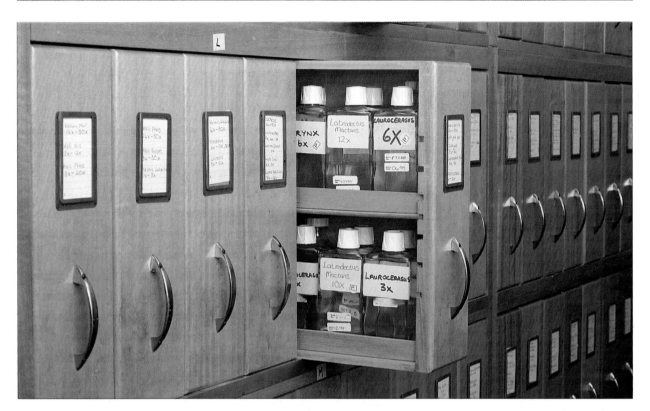

**Remedy potencies** *The greater the dilution of the remedy, the higher the potency. Low potency remedies are generally used to treat acute illnesses, whereas higher potencies are used in constitutional prescribing for chronic complaints.*

suffers from continual or recurrent illness, for example, recurrent infections or degenerative diseases, such as arthritis. Although there are a series of minor victories and defeats on the part of the vital force, and relapses may be followed by remission, the general trend of health is downward.

Homeopathic remedies help to hasten recovery by stimulating the vital force, which although temporarily depressed is more than capable of bouncing back. The remedies energize the vital force to rid the body of disease, helping it return to its healthy state. To ensure that the vital force responds in the most effective manner, homeopaths must choose a remedy that matches as accurately as possible the symptoms picture. This is why a homeopathic assessment takes into account a person's character, stress levels, lifestyle, level of exercise, diet, food preferences, family medical history, and the effects of general factors, such as the weather, to provide a unique symptoms picture. Pinpointing the strengths and weaknesses of an individual enables a homeopath to prescribe the best remedy and to decide which potency is suitable.

## MIASMS

Hahnemann observed that some people prone to frequent, acute complaints always seemed to acquire new symptoms and were never totally healthy. He concluded that there must be a deep-seated weakness, or "miasm," that blocked the remedy. In home-opathy, a miasm is the chronic effect of an underlying disease that has been present in previous generations or in an individual.

# HOW REMEDIES ARE MADE

Homeopathic remedies are made from plant, animal, and mineral extracts and diluted in varying degrees in order to avoid unpleasant side effects. Paradoxically, the more dilute the remedies are, the more effectively they work.

The process of making remedies is very precise. For remedies derived from soluble substances, such as animal or plant extracts, the raw material is dissolved in an alcohol/water mixture that contains approximately 90 percent pure alcohol and 10 percent distilled water (this ratio may vary depending on the substance). This mixture is left to stand for 2–4 weeks, shaken occasionally, then strained through a press. The resulting liquid is known as the mother tincture or tincture. Insoluble substances, such as gold, calcium carbonate, and graphites, must first be made soluble by a process known as trituration, in which they are ground continually until they become soluble. They are then diluted and used in the same way as naturally soluble substances.

## REMEDY POTENCIES

To produce different remedy potencies, the mother tincture is diluted in an alcohol/water mixture according to one of two scales, the decimal (x) and centesimal (c). Between every stage of dilution the diluted tincture is succussed (shaken vigorously). In the decimal scale, the dilution factor is 1:10; and in the centesimal, it is 1:100. To produce a 1c potency of the *Allium* remedy, for example, one drop of the mother tincture is added to 99 drops of an alcohol/water mixture and succussed. To produce a 2c potency, one drop of the 1c mixture is added to 99 drops of

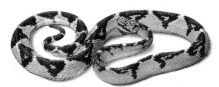

**Siberian rhododendron**

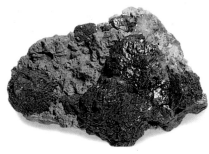

**Bushmaster snake**

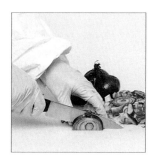

**Zinc**

**Remedy sources** *Homeopathic remedies are made from plant, animal, and mineral extracts, ranging from toxic substances such as snake venom and mercury to common foods such as oats and onions.*

## MAKING THE *ALLIUM* REMEDY

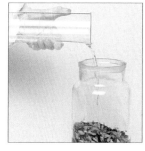

1 *Fresh onions are washed and some of the outer skin removed, before being coarsely chopped.*

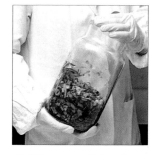

2 *The chopped onions are put in a large glass jar. An alcohol/water mixture is poured onto the onions.*

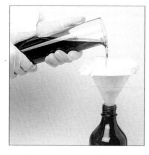

3 *The jar is sealed with an airtight lid, and the mixture is left to stand for 2–4 weeks. It is shaken occasionally.*

4 *The mixture is strained through a large press, and the resulting brown mother tincture is strained into a dark glass bottle.*

an alcohol/water mixture and succussed. The number of a homeopathic remedy shows how many times it has been diluted and succussed; for example, *Allium* 6c has been diluted and succussed six times.

## PROOF OF HOMEOPATHY

Once a homeopathic remedy has been diluted beyond a 12c potency, it is unlikely that a molecule of the original substance still remains. This is the main reason why homeopathy is viewed with such skepticism by many orthodox medical practitioners and scientists. Despite the successful practical experience of homeopaths and their patients, scientific proof is needed before a wider acceptance of homeopathy is possible. There are three main areas of proof to be considered: first, clinical trials must show homeopathy to work; second, proof must be obtained that highly diluted remedies have a measurable effect on living organisms; and third, the potentization effect must be explained scientifically.

Although homeopathy was effective in treating cholera in the 19th century and was also used successfully to treat mustard gas burns during World War II, the main breakthrough did not occur until 1986, when it was shown, in controlled trials, that homeopathy was helpful in preventing hay fever. In 1995 a team from Glasgow University succeeded in proving, in controlled trials, that 30c potencies of pollen and house dust mite were more effective than placebos in treating hay fever and asthma, respectively. Nonetheless, much more work needs to be done.

As yet no theory has been put forward to explain convincingly how potentized remedies work on the body. This is largely because of a limitation of medical science at the present time, and doubtless in the future the potentization phenomenon will be fully understood.

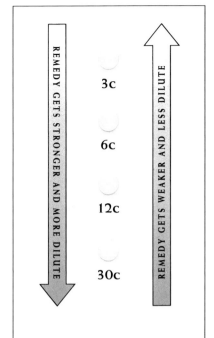

**Remedy strengths** The more dilute a remedy, the stronger it is and the higher the number or potency. A less dilute remedy is not as strong and has a lower number, or potency.

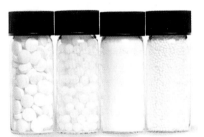

**Remedies** *These are available as lactose tablets, pillules, powder, and granules.*

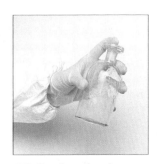

5 One drop of mother tincture is added to 99 drops of an alcohol/water mixture. This is succussed (shaken vigorously).

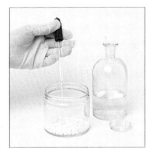

6 The mixture is succussed and diluted repeatedly. A few drops of the potentized remedy are added to lactose (milk sugar) tablets.

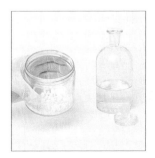

7 The lactose tablets are swirled around to ensure that each one is impregnated by the potentized remedy.

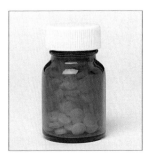

8 The tablets are then placed in an airtight, dark glass bottle and stored away from direct sunlight.

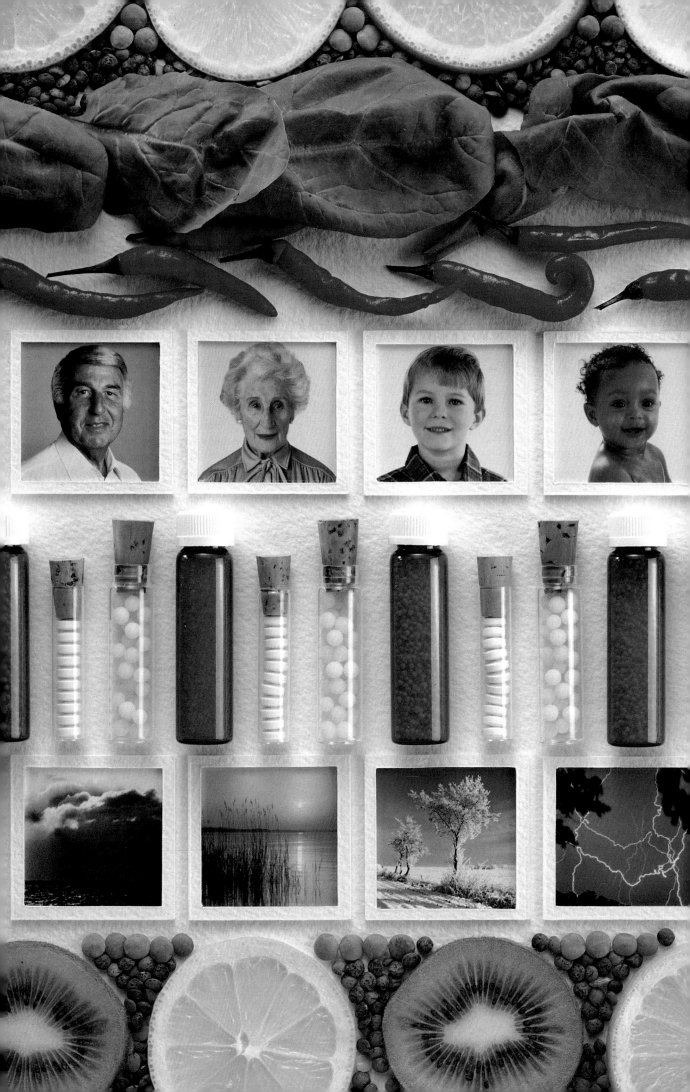

# ASSESSING
# YOUR
# HEALTH

*Good health is not simply the absence of disease but complete physical and emotional well-being. In homeopathy, maintaining a healthy lifestyle, coping well with stress and adopting a strong emotional outlook all play an important part in the prevention of illness.*

# CONSTITUTIONAL TYPES

*In homeopathic terms, a person's constitution is his or her inherited and acquired physical, emotional, and intellectual makeup. A closely fitting constitutional remedy selected according to these* *criteria acts preventatively and curatively. For example, someone with a Pulsatilla constitution will respond well to the Pulsatilla remedy almost regardless of his or her illness.*

## WHAT DO HOMEOPATHS ASSESS?

Homeopaths categorize people into constitutional types. In addition to examining the symptoms of an illness, they look at fears, food preferences, and responses to general factors, such as the weather. They also take into account a person's physical appearance and weak areas of the body. The homeopath then selects a remedy that closely matches a person's constitutional type.

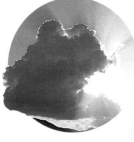

**General factors**
*The weather, seasons, temperature, and time of day may worsen or improve physical conditions.*

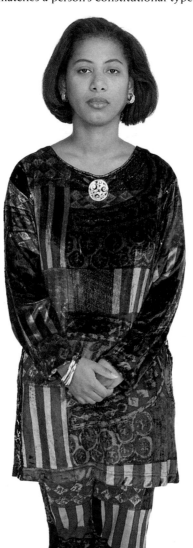

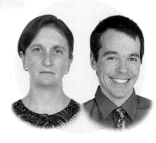

**Food preferences**
*Some people are inclined to crave sweet foods, whereas others cannot tolerate them. Food likes and dislikes are an important part of assessing constitutional types.*

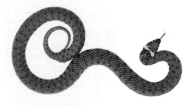

**Fears** *Before prescribing a remedy, homeopaths take into account tangible fears, for example, insects and snakes, and emotional fears, such as fear of death, failure, and insanity.*

**Personality & temperament** *Some people are optimistic and cheerful by nature, while others are negative and irritable. Homeopaths categorize people according to their emotional characteristics.*

# CONSTITUTIONAL PRESCRIBING

In homeopathy, when an illness occurs, the symptoms are seen as an attempt by the body to readjust or eliminate an imbalance in its energy, or vital force (see pp. 18–19).

When a case history is taken by a homeopath, it is quite common to find that there is more than one remedy to treat the symptoms of the illness in question. Knowing a person's constitutional type helps the homeopath choose the most appropriate remedy.

In acute, self-limiting complaints, for example, colds or indigestion, homeopathic remedies work quickly and effectively. The choice of remedy does not depend on knowing the constitutional type and is relatively easy. By contrast, chronic illnesses, such as arthritis and other recurrent, long-term, degenerative conditions, are more difficult to treat. The choice of remedy is harder and depends on a person's constitutional type.

In both acute and chronic illnesses, the homeopath studies the whole person in order to discover the imbalance that has triggered the illness. This is especially important for chronic illnesses, where constitutional prescribing helps unravel the underlying causative factors of an illness.

Constitutional prescribing by a homeopath ensures that remedies act as efficiently as possible to heal on a very deep level.

# CASE HISTORY

Louise, aged 37, who has recently begun to suffer from rheumatoid arthritis, consults a homeopath. As in orthodox medicine, she is given a physical diagnosis. The homeopath, however, also asks questions about her food preferences and her response to general factors, such as the weather, and tries to find out more about the things that trigger stress.

As a result, the homeopath learns that Louise's mother died 18 months before the onset of the rheumatoid arthritis. As Louise talks about her mother, tears well up in her eyes, which she finds very embarrassing. In addition to the grief she feels for her mother's death, Louise also suffers much guilt because of an argument she had with her mother just before she died. She has suppressed these feelings, acting as if nothing had happened.

The homeopath discovers that Louise has a strong desire for chocolate and for salt, adding the latter copiously to her food and in cooking. She dislikes fatty foods, finds hot weather uncomfortable, and enjoys being near the sea.

To the homeopath, Louise's emotional state is critically important to curing her rheumatoid arthritis. It is likely that by suppressing her grief and its attendant guilt, Louise's vital force has been imbalanced, weakening her immune system. The rheumatoid arthritis is an attempt by her body to overcome this imbalance.

Although her food preferences and the way she is affected by weather have remained unchanged since her mother's death, they are an integral part of constitutional prescribing. After considering all the information, the homeopath decides that the

*Natrum mur.* remedy closely matches Louise's emotional and physical profile, and she is given one dose. After a month the homeopath sees her again and learns that the remedy has been successful. The grieving process has been facilitated and she has released much of her guilt. In turn, there has been a lessening of pain and the rheumatoid arthritis has been arrested.

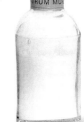

**Natrum mur.** *Many people who need this remedy, which is made from salt, either crave or dislike salt and salty foods.*

# COMMON QUESTIONS ANSWERED

**Q** Can a person who is completely healthy be a constitutional type or does this become apparent only when he or she is ill?

**A** Yes, a healthy person may be a constitutional type without showing any signs of illness or imbalance until the body's energy and vitality, or vital force, are disturbed. When this happens, the characteristics that point to his or her constitutional type become more marked as the symptoms of an illness develop.

**Q** Once someone is matched to a constitutional type will he or she remain that type throughout life or might the type change with age?

**A** People can either remain one type throughout life or change and resemble another type. For example, many babies correspond to the constitutional type *Calc. carb.*, but as they grow up some of them will remain *Calc. carb.* types while others may grow taller and thin out to become other types such as *Calc. phos.*, *Silica*, or *Phos.* The individuality of people, with their different sensitivities and emotions, is partly hereditary and partly conditioned by environment.

**Q** Can people be a mixture of types?

**A** Yes. Just as an onion comprises many layers, so people may reveal different constitutional characteristics as their treatment progresses.

**Q** Can more than one remedy be taken at once?

**A** It is best not to take more than one remedy at a time. If an illness is acute and there is no underlying cause, one remedy will be sufficient irrespective of the person's constitutional type. Recurrent, chronic illnesses, however, might require an acute remedy followed by a constitutional type remedy.

# LIFESTYLE & HEALTH

*Although genetic disposition plays a role in determining disease, the way in which we live can also prevent, cause, or aggravate illness. For this reason, homeopaths do not simply prescribe remedies. They take into account lifestyle factors such as diet, exercise, stress levels, and sleep.*

*A person's emotional outlook is also considered; a negative attitude to life limits emotional well-being and causes stress, which strains the vital force (see pp. 18–19). The smaller the load on the body and mind, the more likely it is that a homeopathic remedy will work and the longer its effect will last.*

## THE EFFECTS OF DIET

It is important to eat a healthy, balanced diet and to eat the correct proportions of certain types of food. Too much protein, saturated animal fat, sugar, and vegetable fat can cause sluggishness and sow the seeds of future chronic illness. Conditions such as diabetes, heart disease, obesity, gallbladder disease, and diverticular disease are linked to the overconsumption of certain foods, especially fatty, refined, and cholesterol-rich foods.

Many people are inclined to eat too many sweet or fatty foods but not enough fiber. Food preferences not only help the homeopath assess someone's overall health but tell them about that person's constitutional type.

**GROUP 1**
Meat and poultry are good sources of protein, but because they contain saturated animal fat they should not be eaten excessively.

**GROUP 2**
Fish should not be eaten more than twice a week. Choose oily fish, which provide essential fatty acids, in preference to other fish.

**Twice-a-week rule** *Designed to work as a memory aid, the twice-a-week rule helps simplify diet planning and ensure healthier eating. Foods in groups 1–5 should not be eaten more than twice a week. There is no limit to eating whole foods. This balanced diet puts less strain on the digestive system and meets your nutritional needs.*

*If you have any bad food habits try not to indulge in them more than twice a week, although preferably not at all. Use little or no salt, and if you have a sweet tooth, eat granola bars, dried fruit, carob candies, or whole-grain cakes and cookies made with unrefined sugars.*

**GROUP 3**
Eggs are an excellent source of protein, but because they are high in cholesterol they should be eaten in moderation.

**GROUP 5**
Sweet refined foods such as chocolate, cookies, cakes, and pastries are full of calories, but have little nutritional value.

**GROUP 4**
Among dairy products, cheese and butter are particularly high in saturated fat and salt, and should be eaten in moderation.

**WHOLE FOODS**
Whole-grain bread, flour, and cereals, whole-wheat pasta, nuts, seeds, legumes, fresh fruit, and vegetables are all important sources of essential nutrients and should form the bulk of a balanced diet.

## EXERCISE

Some people are energetic by nature and find it difficult to relax, whereas others lack stamina and are sluggish, less inclined to exercise, and more likely to gain weight. Homeopaths take into account the physical appearance of people and their levels of indoor and outdoor activity and use this information to help determine their constitutional type. Some constitutional types, for example *Natrum mur.*, are always restless and in a hurry, whereas *Sulfur* types are indolent and lazy and *Phos.* types feel generally burned-out and fatigued.

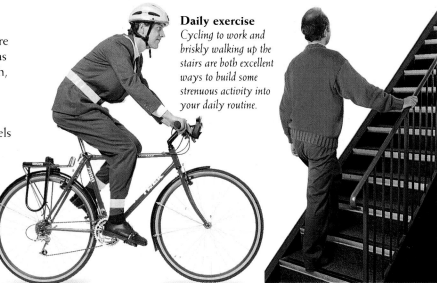

**Daily exercise**
*Cycling to work and briskly walking up the stairs are both excellent ways to build some strenuous activity into your daily routine.*

Homeopaths encourage fitness and regular exercise. For many people, strenuous exertion is increasingly rare and sitting behind a desk is common. The human body, however, is designed for muscular activity and does not function properly without it.

The easiest way to start exercising is to increase the amount of physical activity you do every day, for example, by walking energetically to the station or getting off the bus a few stops earlier. If you cannot do this, try to set aside a few minutes each day to work through an exercise routine. Always warm up before you begin and start with gentle exercises to tune up the body. Gradually increase the amount you do until you can exercise vigorously enough to make yourself breathe hard and sweat, which benefits the heart and cardiovascular system.

## ENVIRONMENTAL FACTORS

The weather, the seasons, the time of day, and temperature changes influence people in completely different ways. To the homeopath, the way in which environmental factors affect people generally, as well as how they affect the specific symptoms of an illness, is of great significance and can help ascertain a person's constitutional type. For example, sensitivity to the approach of a thunderstorm causes a headache in some people, whereas others find thunderstorms relaxing and soothing. Someone suffering pain in the knee may feel better from applying a warm compress to the affected part but feel worse generally from heat.

Information, such as whether a person is most energetic and creative on waking, or can hardly get out of bed but comes to life at night, adds to the homeopath's understanding of a person's constitutional type.

**Response to sea air** *Whereas some people find sea air very invigorating, others find it exhausting. Of greater interest to the homeopath is whether a particular complaint, such as asthma, is better or worse from sea air.*

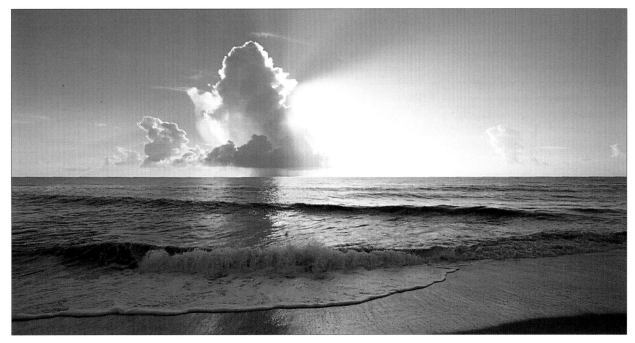

## SLEEP AND ITS IMPORTANCE

Lack of sleep is a significant contributory cause of stress and can also lead to illness. Many people are exhausted from inadequate rest and sleep, either due to physical stress or prolonged emotional stress. Paradoxically, the more exhausted you are, the more energy you may appear to have and the less able you are to sleep.

Sleep patterns, dream content, and the usual sleeping position may all be taken into account by a homeopath in the selection of a constitutional remedy.

## THE INFLUENCE OF STRESS

Anything that puts a load on the body's systems can be defined as stress. People are affected by stress in different ways. For example, some cope well with pressure at work and thrive on it, whereas others cannot cope, become irritable or sensitive, and may feel overwhelmed by stress.

Stress is not necessarily always a bad thing. Performance and efficiency both increase under a certain amount of stress. It is only when stress reaches too high a level that fatigue sets in. As with everything else, this breaking point varies from person to person. If the stress is not reduced and the resulting fatigue is not corrected, exhaustion and illness occur.

Stress produces an increase in hormones such as adrenaline, noradrenaline, and corticosteroids. In the short term, these cause an increase in breathing and heart rate, a queasy stomach, and tense muscles.

In the long term, stress can lead to a wide range of ailments. The following list is a sobering reminder of the importance of avoiding prolonged stress, which can lead to high blood pressure, hair loss, skin complaints, mouth ulcers, asthma, angina, gastritis, peptic ulcers, nervous twitching, irritable bowel syndrome, an irritable bladder, heart disease, cancer, lung ailments, accidental injuries, mental illness, and even suicide. Diseases such as multiple sclerosis, diabetes, and herpes may be aggravated by stress.

Some people become addicted to the "buzz" of adrenaline caused by stress and deliberately seek thrills. They may take to high-risk sports or drugs such as cocaine, and without help they, too, will become exhausted.

It is usually relatively easy to deal with short-term, or acute, stress. Often a trivial incident will cause the person under stress to snap and release tension. Long-term, or chronic, stress can be more difficult to deal with. It often produces feelings such as lack of purpose, helplessness, and alienation.

Stress is often seen in cases of poverty and unemployment. It is common in unhappy families and is often related to lack of communication. Factors such as not being close to one's family and parents, loneliness, or trying to achieve too much in too little time can all increase vulnerability to stress. Any areas of difficulty that cannot be discussed and resolved, for example, sexual problems or family tensions, will become stressful.

## RELIEVING STRESS

Any activity that you find relaxing and that calms your mind will help to dissipate stress. This varies according to individuals: exercise; a hot bath; taking a vacation; going to the movies; sexual intercourse – each helps someone to unwind. For many people, activities such as these are enough to keep balanced. For others, external sources of satisfaction are not enough and they need an internal technique to develop peace of mind. Yoga, t'ai chi, deep breathing, the Alexander technique (a special method of adjusting body posture), psychotherapy, and meditation can all be helpful.

A sound emotional outlook in the face of stressful situations is very important because it helps reduce vulnerability to stress in the first place and enables better management of it. On the whole, optimistic people ride out stressful periods better than pessimists. Pessimism makes it more difficult to keep calm in stressful situations so that they become overwhelming. A positive mental attitude helps to control stress and to confront it head on.

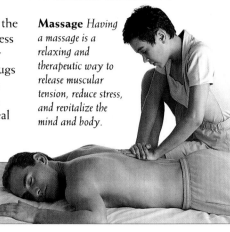

**Massage** *Having a massage is a relaxing and therapeutic way to release muscular tension, reduce stress, and revitalize the mind and body.*

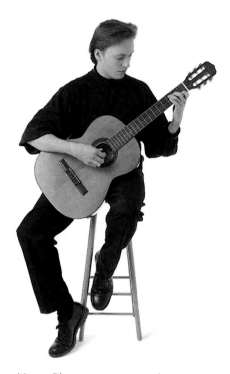

**Music** *Playing an instrument or listening to music are both excellent ways to unwind and help focus the mind away from stressful worries.*

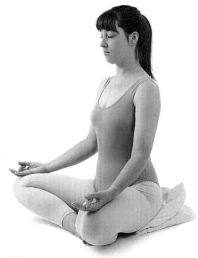

**Meditation** *Deep breathing and meditating calm the mind and reduce stress.*

# HOW TO MEASURE STRESS

The following questionnaire will give you some idea of the amount of stress in your life. The total score gives an indication of the degree of stress you have been exposed to and your likely vulnerability to stress-related illness. The questionnaire is only a guide, however; it does not take into consideration the different responses of individuals to stress.

| Score your answers: | |
|---|---|
| Yes/always | 1 |
| Probably/usually | 2 |
| I suppose/it depends | 3 |
| Rarely/not a lot | 4 |
| No/never | 5 |

Add up your score. If the total is less than 50 you probably cope well with stress. Higher scores indicate increasing vulnerability to stress.

## DO YOU:

1. Eat at least one hot, balanced meal a day?

2. Have seven hours of sleep at least four nights a week?

3. Give and receive affection frequently?

4. Have a relative within 50 miles (80 km) on whom you can rely?

5. Exercise to perspiration at least twice a week?

6. Smoke fewer than 10 cigarettes a day?

7. Drink alcohol less than five times a week?

8. Keep within the appropriate weight for your height?

9. Have an adequate income for your needs?

10. Get strength from religious, philosophical, or some other deeply held beliefs?

11. Regularly attend social gatherings?

12. Have a network of friends and acquaintances?

13. Have a close friend to confide in?

14. Have good health?

15. Express feelings of anger or worry?

16. Have regular domestic discussions with those you live with?

17. Do something for fun at least once a week?

18. Organize your time effectively and have some quiet time to yourself each day?

19. Drink fewer than three cups of caffeine (tea, coffee, or cola) a day?

20. Have an optimistic outlook on life?

*The Susceptibility Scale of the Stress Audit, devised by Lyle H. Miller, Alma Dell Smith, and Larry Rothstein, of Boston University Medical Center and reproduced with permission.*

**TOTAL**

# HOW TO COPE WITH STRESS

**Taking control of a situation relieves stress. Here are a few simple guidelines.**

- Deal only with things you can do something about
- Take one problem at a time
- Talk problems over with other people and listen to their advice
- Act positively, even if you make the wrong decision; remember, everyone makes mistakes
- Do not harbor grudges
- Relax daily
- Occupy yourself rather than just sitting in solitude
- Have routines for mealtimes, sleep, exercise, relaxation
- Do not dwell on problems after 8 p.m., if at all
- Admit to yourself if you become overwhelmed by problems and seek help from a relative, a trusted friend, or a professional.

# THE CONSTITUTIONAL TYPE QUESTIONNAIRE

*The questionnaire on pp. 32–45 is a simplified version of what a homeopath might ask at the first consultation. It will enable you to find out which of the 15 main constitutional types you most resemble and help you to learn more about yourself and how homeopathy works. The questionnaire will not enable you to self-prescribe constitutionally, as this takes years of experience and homeopaths ask many more questions. Nonetheless, it does demonstrate the importance homeopaths attach to personality and temperament, food preferences, fears, and general features.*

## FILLING IN THE QUESTIONNAIRE

The questionnaire is divided into four categories:
- **Personality & temperament**
- **Food preferences**
- **Fears**
- **General features**

1 Go through the entire questionnaire quickly, without dwelling on anything. It should take no more than 10 minutes to complete.

2 Check the boxes that best describe you. If a particular feature does not apply to you at all, leave the box blank.

Check the boxes that are applicable to you. Leave blank if they don't apply.

Remedy columns

Score 5 for each remedy listed in the "Very Strongly" column

Score 3 for each remedy listed in the "Strongly" column, unless a bonus score is indicated

Score 1 for each remedy listed in the "Slightly" column

**QUESTIONNAIRE**

32

| PERSONALITY & TEMPERAMENT | VERY STRONGLY Score 5 for each remedy | STRONGLY Score 3 for each remedy | SLIGHTLY Score 1 for each remedy |
|---|---|---|---|
| CRY READILY (for no obvious cause) | ☑ NM PULS SEP SULF | ☐ NM PULS SEP SULF | ☐ GRAPH LYC |
| CRY WHEN THANKED | ☐ LYC | ☑ LYC (score 5) | ☐ LYC |
| CRY FROM ANXIETY | ☐ GRAPH | ☐ GRAPH (score 5) | ☑ ARS NM |
| CRY FROM SELF-PITY | ☐ CALC PULS | ☑ CALC PULS | ☐ CALC PULS |
| MOVED TO TEARS BY MUSIC | ☐ GRAPH NM | ☐ GRAPH NM | ☑ NV |
| RELIEVED BY CRYING | ☐ LACH PULS | ☑ LACH PULS | ☐ GRAPH LYC |
| CRY PREMENSTRUALLY | ☐ PULS | ☐ PULS | ☑ LYC NM PHOS SEP |
| LIKE SYMPATHY | ☐ PHOS PULS | ☑ PHOS PULS | ☐ PHOS PULS |
| DISLIKE SYMPATHY | ☐ IGN NM SEP SIL | ☐ IGN NM SEP SIL | ☑ ARS |
| SYMPATHETIC | ☐ PHOS PULS | ☑ PHOS PULS | ☐ IGN NM NV |
| LACK SYMPATHY (especially toward own family) | ☐ PHOS SEP | ☐ PHOS SEP | ☑ LYC PHOS SEP |
| TEND TO SIGH FREQUENTLY | ☐ IGN | ☑ IGN (score 5) | ☐ GRAPH NM NV PULS SEP |

Finish the whole questionnaire, then fill in the score cards. Total the scores (*right*), then fill in the result cards on pp. 46–7.

**SCORE CARD 1**

| ARG | ARS | CALC | GRAPH | IGN | LACH | LYC | MERC | NM | NV | PHOS | PULS | SEP | SIL | SULF |
|---|---|---|---|---|---|---|---|---|---|---|---|---|---|---|
| | | | | | | | | 5 | | | 5 | 5 | | 5 |
| | | | | | | 5 | | | | | | | | |
| 1 | | | | | | | | 1 | | | | | | |
| | | 3 | | | | | | | | | 3 | | | |
| | | | | | | | | | 1 | | | | | |
| | | | | | 3 | | | | | | 3 | | | |
| | | | | | | 1 | | 1 | | 1 | | 1 | | |
| | | | | | | | | | | 3 | 3 | | | |
| 1 | | | | | | | | | | | | | | |
| | | | | | | | | | | 3 | 3 | | | |
| | | | | | | 1 | | 1 | | | | 1 | 1 | |
| | | | | 5 | | | | | | | | | | |
| **0** | **2** | **3** | **0** | **5** | **3** | **7** | **0** | **7** | **1** | **8** | **17** | **7** | **0** | **5** |

Score 3 for each remedy listed in the "Strongly" column, unless a bonus score is indicated

Score 1 for each remedy listed in the "Slightly" column

Abbreviated names of the 15 key remedies

Bonus scores are shown in brackets

Write the total for each remedy column in the box. Transfer these totals to the corresponding result cards

# SCORING

1 After completing the question-naire, fill in the score card. For each box checked in the "Very Strongly" column, score 5 for the remedies listed; for each box checked in the "Strongly" column, score 3 for the remedies listed; for each box checked in the "Slightly" column, score 1 for the remedies listed.

2 Write the scores in the matching remedy columns on the adjacent score card.

Some boxes in the "Strongly" column have a bonus score in brackets. If you checked one of these, fill in the bonus score and not the column score for each remedy.

# THE RESULT

The highest score on the final result card indicates which of the 15 key constitutional types you most resemble. If the highest score appears in more than one remedy column, you may be a mixture of types. In this instance compare several profiles to find the closest match.

## QUESTIONNAIRE

| VERY STRONGLY<br>Score 5 for each remedy | STRONGLY<br>Score 3 for each remedy | SLIGHTLY<br>Score 1 for each remedy |
|---|---|---|
| ☐ NM PULS SEP SULF | ☐ NM PULS SEP SULF | ☑ |
| ☐ LYC | ☑ LYC (score 5) | ☐ |

This remedy has a bonus score of 5; fill in 5 in the remedy column instead of 3

If there are no remedies listed next to the checked box, do not score

## SCORE CARD

| Argent. nit.<br>ARG | Arsen. alb.<br>ARS | Calc. carb.<br>CALC | Graphites<br>GRAPH | Ignatia<br>IGN | Lachesis<br>LACH | Lycopodium<br>LYC | Merc. sol.<br>MERC | Natrum mur.<br>NM | Nux vomica<br>NV | Phos.<br>PHOS | Pulsatilla<br>PULS | Sepia<br>SEP | Silica<br>SIL | Sulfur<br>SULF |
|---|---|---|---|---|---|---|---|---|---|---|---|---|---|---|
| | | | | 5 | | | | 5 | | | | | | |
| | | | | | | | | | | | | | | |

Fill in the appropriate score for all the remedies listed next to the checked box

# FINAL SCORE

1 Add up the numbers in each remedy column. Write the total in the box provided at the bottom of each column.

2 After completing all the score cards, transfer the totals to the result card for each category of the questionnaire. Add up the totals in each remedy column on the result cards (see pp. 46–7).

3 Transfer the totals from the result cards to the final result card. Add them up to work out your final score for each remedy column.

## SCORE CARD

| ARG | ARS | CALC | GRAPH | IGN | LACH | LYC | MERC | NM | NV | PHOS | PULS | SEP | SIL | SULF |
|---|---|---|---|---|---|---|---|---|---|---|---|---|---|---|
| 0 | 2 | 3 | 0 | 5 | 3 | 7 | 0 | 7 | 1 | 8 | 17 | 7 | 0 | 5 |

Add up the numbers for each remedy column and write the total at the bottom

Transfer the total score onto the result cards for each category of questions

## A CONSTITUTIONAL TYPE PROFILE FROM THE INDEX OF REMEDIES

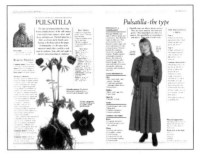

**Selecting a constitutional type** *The highest score indicates which of the 15 key constitutional types you most resemble. Consult the appropriate constitutional type profile and see how well it matches you.*

**ARGENT. NIT.**
*see pp. 50–1*

**ARSEN. ALB.**
*see pp. 52–3*

**CALC. CARB.**
*see pp. 54–5*

**GRAPHITES**
*see pp. 56–7*

**IGNATIA**
*see pp. 58–9*

**LACHESIS**
*see pp. 78–9*

**LYCOPODIUM**
*see pp. 60–1*

**MERC. SOL.**
*see pp. 62–3*

**NATRUM MUR.**
*see pp. 64–5*

**NUX VOMICA**
*see pp. 74–5*

**PHOS.**
*see pp. 66–7*

**PULSATILLA**
*see pp. 68–9*

**SEPIA**
*see pp. 70–1*

**SILICA**
*see pp. 72–3*

**SULFUR**
*see pp. 76–7*

## SCORE CARD 1

| | Sulfur SULF | Silica SIL | Sepia SEP | Pulsatilla PULS | Phos. PHOS | Nux vomica NV | Natrum mur. NM | Merc. sol. MERC | Lycopodium LYC | Lachesis LACH | Ignatia IGN | Graphites GRAPH | Calc. carb. CALC | Arsen. alb. ARS | Argent. nit. ARG |
|---|---|---|---|---|---|---|---|---|---|---|---|---|---|---|---|
| | | | | | | | | | | | | | | | |
| | | | | | | | | | | | | | | | |
| | | | | | | | | | | | | | | | |
| | | | | | | | | | | | | | | | |
| | | | | | | | | | | | | | | | |
| | | | | | | | | | | | | | | | |
| | | | | | | | | | | | | | | | |
| | | | | | | | | | | | | | | | |
| | | | | | | | | | | | | | | | |
| | | | | | | | | | | | | | | | |
| | | | | | | | | | | | | | | | |
| | | | | | | | | | | | | | | | |

SULF SIL SEP PULS PHOS NV NM MERC LYC LACH IGN GRAPH CALC ARS ARG

## PERSONALITY & TEMPERAMENT

| PERSONALITY & TEMPERAMENT | VERY STRONGLY Score 5 for each remedy | STRONGLY Score 3 for each remedy | SLIGHTLY Score 1 for each remedy |
|---|---|---|---|
| CRY READILY (for no obvious cause) | NM PULS SEP SULF | NM PULS SEP SULF | GRAPH LYC |
| CRY WHEN THANKED | LYC | LYC (score 5) | LYC |
| CRY FROM ANXIETY | GRAPH | GRAPH (score 5) | ARS NM |
| CRY FROM SELF-PITY | CALC PULS | CALC PULS | CALC PULS |
| MOVED TO TEARS BY MUSIC | GRAPH NM | GRAPH NM | NV |
| RELIEVED BY CRYING | LACH PULS | LACH PULS | GRAPH LYC |
| CRY PREMENSTRUALLY | PULS | PULS | LYC NM PHOS SEP |
| LIKE SYMPATHY | PHOS PULS | PHOS PULS | PHOS PULS |
| DISLIKE SYMPATHY | IGN NM SEP SIL | IGN NM SEP SIL | ARS |
| SYMPATHETIC | PHOS PULS | PHOS PULS | IGN NM NV |
| LACK SYMPATHY (especially toward own family) | PHOS SEP | PHOS SEP | LYC PHOS SEP |
| TEND TO SIGH FREQUENTLY | IGN | IGN (score 5) | GRAPH NM NV PULS SEP |

Finish the whole questionnaire, then fill in the score cards.
Total the scores (*right*), then fill in the result cards on pp. 46–7.

## SCORE CARD 2

| | | | | | | | | | | | | | | | | | |
|---|---|---|---|---|---|---|---|---|---|---|---|---|---|---|---|---|---|
| Sulfur **SULF** | | | | | | | | | | | | | | | SULF | | |
| Silica **SIL** | | | | | | | | | | | | | | | SIL | | |
| Sepia **SEP** | | | | | | | | | | | | | | | SEP | | |
| Pulsatilla **PULS** | | | | | | | | | | | | | | | PULS | | |
| Phos. **PHOS** | | | | | | | | | | | | | | | PHOS | | |
| Nux vomica **NV** | | | | | | | | | | | | | | | NV | | |
| Natrum mur. **NM** | | | | | | | | | | | | | | | NM | | |
| Merc. sol. **MERC** | | | | | | | | | | | | | | | MERC | | |
| Lycopodium **LYC** | | | | | | | | | | | | | | | LYC | | |
| Lachesis **LACH** | | | | | | | | | | | | | | | LACH | | |
| Ignatia **IGN** | | | | | | | | | | | | | | | IGN | | |
| Graphites **GRAPH** | | | | | | | | | | | | | | | GRAPH | | |
| Calc. carb. **CALC** | | | | | | | | | | | | | | | CALC | | |
| Arsen. alb. **ARS** | | | | | | | | | | | | | | | ARS | | |
| Argent. nit. **ARG** | | | | | | | | | | | | | | | ARG | | |

## PERSONALITY & TEMPERAMENT

| PERSONALITY & TEMPERAMENT | VERY STRONGLY Score 5 for each remedy | STRONGLY Score 3 for each remedy | SLIGHTLY Score 1 for each remedy |
|---|---|---|---|
| TEND TO BROOD OR SULK | IGN NM | IGN NM | ARS |
| IRRITABLE (at the least thing) | NV | NV | ARS CALC NM PHOS |
| IRRITABLE PREMENSTRUALLY | SEP | SEP | LACH LYC NM NV PULS |
| EASILY ANGERED | LYC NV | LYC NV | PHOS |
| DICTATORIAL (especially at home) | LYC | LYC (score 5) | LYC |
| ANGRY WHEN CONTRADICTED | IGN LYC SEP | IGN LYC SEP | NV SIL |
| PRONE TO CONTRADICT | IGN LACH | IGN LACH | ARS LYC MERC SEP |
| COMPULSIVE | ARG IGN PULS | ARG IGN PULS | ARS |
| CHANGEABLE AND INCONSISTENT | IGN | IGN | GRAPH |
| JEALOUS | LACH NV | LACH NV | LYC PULS |
| SUSPICIOUS | ARS LACH LYC | ARS LACH LYC | MERC NV PHOS SULF |
| CRITICAL | ARS GRAPH SULF | ARS GRAPH SULF | LACH LYC MERC NV PHOS |

Finish the whole questionnaire, then fill in the score cards.
Total the scores (*right*), then fill in the result cards on pp. 46–7.

33

## SCORE CARD 3

| | Sulfur SULF | | | | | | | | | | | | | | |
|---|---|---|---|---|---|---|---|---|---|---|---|---|---|---|---|
| | Silica SIL | | | | | | | | | | | | | | |
| | Sepia SEP | | | | | | | | | | | | | | |
| | Pulsatilla PULS | | | | | | | | | | | | | | |
| | Phos. PHOS | | | | | | | | | | | | | | |
| | Nux vomica NV | | | | | | | | | | | | | | |
| | Natrum mur. NM | | | | | | | | | | | | | | |
| | Merc. sol. MERC | | | | | | | | | | | | | | |
| | Lycopodium LYC | | | | | | | | | | | | | | |
| | Lachesis LACH | | | | | | | | | | | | | | |
| | Ignatia IGN | | | | | | | | | | | | | | |
| | Graphites GRAPH | | | | | | | | | | | | | | |
| | Calc. carb. CALC | | | | | | | | | | | | | | |
| | Arsen. alb. ARS | | | | | | | | | | | | | | |
| | Argent. nit. ARG | | | | | | | | | | | | | | |

ARG ☐ | ARS ☐ | CALC ☐ | GRAPH ☐ | IGN ☐ | LACH ☐ | LYC ☐ | MERC ☐ | NM ☐ | NV ☐ | PHOS ☐ | PULS ☐ | SEP ☐ | SIL ☐ | SULF ☐

## PERSONALITY & TEMPERAMENT

| PERSONALITY & TEMPERAMENT | VERY STRONGLY Score 5 for each remedy | STRONGLY Score 3 for each remedy | SLIGHTLY Score 1 for each remedy |
|---|---|---|---|
| FASTIDIOUS | ARS NV PULS ☐ | ARS NV PULS ☐ | CALC GRAPH NM ☐ |
| CONCERNED WITH PRECISION/ACCURACY | ARS ☐ | ARS ☐ | PULS ☐ |
| CONSCIENTIOUS ABOUT TRIVIAL MATTERS | ARS IGN SIL SULF ☐ | ARS IGN SIL SULF ☐ | LYC NV PULS ☐ |
| VAIN | LYC SULF ☐ | LYC SULF ☐ | LYC PULS SULF ☐ |
| EGOTISTICAL | LYC SULF ☐ | LYC SULF ☐ | LACH PULS SIL ☐ |
| AMBITIOUS | NV ☐ | NV ☐ | ARS IGN LACH LYC SULF ☐ |
| TEND TO THEORIZE | SULF ☐ | SULF ☐ | LACH SEP ☐ |
| PESSIMISTIC | ARS ☐ | ARS ☐ | NV ☐ |
| TEND TO WORRY ABOUT EVERYTHING | ARS CALC IGN ☐ | ARS CALC IGN ☐ | LYC NM PULS SULF ☐ |
| ANXIOUS IN COMPANY | LYC ☐ | LYC (score 5) ☐ | LYC ☐ |
| ANXIOUS WHEN ANYTHING IS EXPECTED OF YOU | ARS LYC ☐ | ARS LYC ☐ | ARG IGN ☐ |
| ANXIOUS WITH A HURRIED FEELING | ARG NM ☐ | ARG NM ☐ | ARG NM ☐ |

Finish the whole questionnaire, then fill in the score cards.
Total the scores (right), then fill in the result cards on pages 46–7.

## SCORE CARD 4

| | | | | | | | | | | |
|---|---|---|---|---|---|---|---|---|---|---|
| Sulfur **SULF** | | | | | | | | | | |
| Silica **SIL** | | | | | | | | | | |
| Sepia **SEP** | | | | | | | | | | |
| Pulsatilla **PULS** | | | | | | | | | | |
| Phos. **PHOS** | | | | | | | | | | |
| Nux vomica **NV** | | | | | | | | | | |
| Natrum mur. **NM** | | | | | | | | | | |
| Merc. sol. **MERC** | | | | | | | | | | |
| Lycopodium **LYC** | | | | | | | | | | |
| Lachesis **LACH** | | | | | | | | | | |
| Ignatia **IGN** | | | | | | | | | | |
| Graphites **GRAPH** | | | | | | | | | | |
| Calc. carb. **CALC** | | | | | | | | | | |
| Arsen. alb. **ARS** | | | | | | | | | | |
| Argent. nit. **ARG** | | | | | | | | | | |

Result boxes: ARG · ARS · CALC · GRAPH · IGN · LACH · LYC · MERC · NM · NV · PHOS · PULS · SEP · SIL · SULF

## PERSONALITY & TEMPERAMENT

| PERSONALITY & TEMPERAMENT | VERY STRONGLY Score 5 for each remedy | STRONGLY Score 3 for each remedy | SLIGHTLY Score 1 for each remedy |
|---|---|---|---|
| ANXIOUS AND CAUTIOUS | ARS | ARS | IGN LYC PULS |
| ANXIOUS AND INDECISIVE | GRAPH | GRAPH (score 5) | GRAPH |
| YIELDING/PASSIVE | PULS SIL | PULS SIL | ARS IGN LYC NM NV PHOS |
| LACK CONFIDENCE | LYC SIL | LYC SIL | NM NV PULS |
| FEARFUL OF OTHERS' OPINIONS | NV PULS | NV PULS | LYC |
| AVOID UNDERTAKING NEW THINGS FOR FEAR OF FAILURE | ARG ARS LYC SIL | ARG ARS LYC SIL | ARG ARS LYC SIL |
| TIMID ABOUT PUBLIC SPEAKING (but capable) | LYC SIL | LYC SIL | LYC SIL |
| APPREHENSIVE (e.g., before a performance) | ARG LYC NM | ARG LYC NM | ARS SIL |
| INHIBITED | MERC | MERC | LYC NM PULS SIL |
| IMPRESSIONABLE | PHOS | PHOS | ARG |
| THINK RAPIDLY | IGN LACH PHOS | IGN LACH PHOS | NV SULF |
| THINK SLOWLY | ARS CALC PHOS PULS | ARS CALC PHOS PULS | GRAPH SEP SULF |

Finish the whole questionnaire, then fill in the score cards.
Total the scores (*right*), then fill in the result cards on pp. 46–7.

## SCORE CARD 5

| | Sulfur **SULF** | Silica **SIL** | Sepia **SEP** | Pulsatilla **PULS** | Phos. **PHOS** | Nux vomica **NV** | Natrum mur. **NM** | Merc. sol. **MERC** | Lycopodium **LYC** | Lachesis **LACH** | Ignatia **IGN** | Graphites **GRAPH** | Calc. carb. **CALC** | Arsen. alb. **ARS** | Argent. nit. **ARG** |
|---|---|---|---|---|---|---|---|---|---|---|---|---|---|---|---|
| | | | | | | | | | | | | | | | |
| | | | | | | | | | | | | | | | |
| | | | | | | | | | | | | | | | |
| | | | | | | | | | | | | | | | |
| | | | | | | | | | | | | | | | |
| | | | | | | | | | | | | | | | |
| | | | | | | | | | | | | | | | |
| | | | | | | | | | | | | | | | |
| **Totals** | SULF ☐ | SIL ☐ | SEP ☐ | PULS ☐ | PHOS ☐ | NV ☐ | NM ☐ | MERC ☐ | LYC ☐ | LACH ☐ | IGN ☐ | GRAPH ☐ | CALC ☐ | ARS ☐ | ARG ☐ |

## PERSONALITY & TEMPERAMENT

| PERSONALITY & TEMPERAMENT | VERY STRONGLY Score 5 for each remedy | STRONGLY Score 3 for each remedy | SLIGHTLY Score 1 for each remedy |
|---|---|---|---|
| TALKATIVE AND FREQUENTLY CHANGE SUBJECT | ☐ LACH | ☐ LACH (score 5) | ☐ LACH |
| TEND TO PROCRASTINATE | ☐ LYC | ☐ LYC (score 5) | ☐ SULF |
| RESTLESS WHILE AT WORK | ☐ GRAPH | ☐ GRAPH (score 5) | ☐ GRAPH |
| ANXIOUS ON WAKING IN THE MORNING | ☐ GRAPH LACH | ☐ GRAPH LACH | ☐ LYC NV PHOS |
| ANXIOUS ABOUT OWN HEALTH | ☐ ARG LYC PHOS | ☐ ARG LYC PHOS | ☐ CALC PULS SEP |
| SUPPRESS GRIEF FOLLOWING BEREAVEMENT | ☐ IGN NM | ☐ IGN NM | ☐ IGN NM |
| AFFECTIONATE | ☐ PHOS | ☐ PHOS PULS | ☐ ARS IGN NM |
| FEEL BETTER MENTALLY AFTER VIGOROUS EXERCISE | ☐ SEP | ☐ SEP | ☐ IGN |
| DISLIKE BEING TOUCHED | ☐ NM SEP | ☐ NM SEP | ☐ IGN LACH SIL |
| CLAIRVOYANT | ☐ PHOS | ☐ PHOS (score 5) | ☐ CALC LACH SIL |
| LOW SEX DRIVE (female) | ☐ NM SEP | ☐ NM SEP | ☐ GRAPH LACH LYC PHOS SULF |
| LOW SEX DRIVE (male) | ☐ GRAPH LYC | ☐ GRAPH LYC | ☐ IGN |

Finish the whole questionnaire, then fill in the score cards.
Total the scores (*right*), then fill in the result cards on pp. 46–7.

## SCORE CARD 1

| | SULF | SIL | SEP | PULS | PHOS | NV | NM | MERC | LYC | LACH | IGN | GRAPH | CALC | ARS | ARG |
|---|---|---|---|---|---|---|---|---|---|---|---|---|---|---|---|
| Sulfur **SULF** | | | | | | | | | | | | | | | |
| Silica **SIL** | | | | | | | | | | | | | | | |
| Sepia **SEP** | | | | | | | | | | | | | | | |
| Pulsatilla **PULS** | | | | | | | | | | | | | | | |
| Phos. **PHOS** | | | | | | | | | | | | | | | |
| Nux vomica **NV** | | | | | | | | | | | | | | | |
| Natrum mur. **NM** | | | | | | | | | | | | | | | |
| Merc. sol. **MERC** | | | | | | | | | | | | | | | |
| Lycopodium **LYC** | | | | | | | | | | | | | | | |
| Lachesis **LACH** | | | | | | | | | | | | | | | |
| Ignatia **IGN** | | | | | | | | | | | | | | | |
| Graphites **GRAPH** | | | | | | | | | | | | | | | |
| Calc. carb. **CALC** | | | | | | | | | | | | | | | |
| Arsen. alb. **ARS** | | | | | | | | | | | | | | | |
| Argent. nit. **ARG** | | | | | | | | | | | | | | | |

Totals row: SULF □ | SIL □ | SEP □ | PULS □ | PHOS □ | NV □ | NM □ | MERC □ | LYC □ | LACH □ | IGN □ | GRAPH □ | CALC □ | ARS □ | ARG □

## FOOD PREFERENCES

| FOOD PREFERENCES | VERY STRONGLY Score 5 for each remedy | STRONGLY Score 3 for each remedy | SLIGHTLY Score 1 for each remedy |
|---|---|---|---|
| LIKE WARM FOODS AND DRINKS | ARS | ARS (score 5) | LYC |
| DISLIKE WARM FOODS | GRAPH PHOS PULS | GRAPH PHOS PULS | CALC IGN LACH LYC SIL |
| LIKE RAW FOODS | SIL SULF | SIL SULF | CALC IGN |
| LOSE APPETITE DURING MENSTRUATION | IGN | IGN (score 5) | LYC PULS |
| MIXTURES OF FOODS DISAGREE | LYC | LYC | PULS SIL |
| EAT TO BURSTING POINT | LYC PULS | LYC PULS | CALC SULF |
| FRUIT DISAGREES | ARS PULS | ARS PULS | LYC SEP |
| DISLIKE FRUIT | IGN PHOS PULS | IGN PHOS PULS | ARS IGN PHOS PULS |
| LIKE EGGS (especially soft-boiled eggs) | CALC | CALC | PULS |
| DISLIKE EGGS | PULS SULF | PULS SULF | PHOS |
| BEANS/PEAS DISAGREE | LYC | LYC | CALC |
| LIKE STARCHY FOODS | LACH LYC | LACH LYC | CALC NM SULF |

Finish the whole questionnaire, then fill in the score cards.
Total the scores (*right*), then fill in the result cards on pp. 46–7.

## SCORE CARD 2

| | Sulfur SULF | Silica SIL | Sepia SEP | Pulsatilla PULS | Phos. PHOS | Nux vomica NV | Natrum mur. NM | Merc. sol. MERC | Lycopodium LYC | Lachesis LACH | Ignatia IGN | Graphites GRAPH | Calc. carb. CALC | Arsen. alb. ARS | Argent. nit. ARG |
|---|---|---|---|---|---|---|---|---|---|---|---|---|---|---|---|
| | | | | | | | | | | | | | | | |
| | | | | | | | | | | | | | | | |
| | | | | | | | | | | | | | | | |

Totals: SULF | SIL | SEP | PULS | PHOS | NV | NM | MERC | LYC | LACH | IGN | GRAPH | CALC | ARS | ARG

## FOOD PREFERENCES

| FOOD PREFERENCES | VERY STRONGLY Score 5 for each remedy | STRONGLY Score 3 for each remedy | SLIGHTLY Score 1 for each remedy |
|---|---|---|---|
| LIKE BREAD AND BUTTER | MERC | MERC (score 5) | IGN PULS |
| LIKE RICH, FATTY FOODS | NV SULF | NV SULF | ARS PHOS SIL |
| RICH, FATTY FOODS CAUSE DIGESTIVE UPSET | GRAPH PULS | GRAPH PULS | ARS LYC SEP SULF |
| LIKE ICE CREAM | PHOS | PHOS | CALC PULS SIL |
| LIKE PEANUT BUTTER | PULS | PULS (score 5) | PULS |
| LIKE CHEESE | ARG PHOS | ARG PHOS | CALC IGN PULS SEP |
| LIKE OLIVE OIL | ARS LYC | ARS LYC | CALC SULF |
| DISLIKE PORK | PULS | PULS | SEP |
| LIKE SWEET FOODS | ARG LYC SULF | ARG LYC SULF | ARS CALC PHOS PULS SEP |
| DISLIKE SWEET FOODS | GRAPH | GRAPH | ARG ARS LYC MERC PHOS SULF |
| LIKE SWEET FOODS BUT THEY DISAGREE | ARG LYC SULF | ARG LYC SULF | CALC PHOS PULS |
| LIKE SWEET FOODS BUT NOT UPSET BY THEM | ARS SEP | ARS SEP | ARS SEP |

Finish the whole questionnaire, then fill in the score cards.
Total the scores (*right*), then fill in the result cards on pp. 46–7.

## SCORE CARD 3

| | ARG | ARS | CALC | GRAPH | IGN | LACH | LYC | MERC | NM | NV | PHOS | PULS | SEP | SIL | SULF |
|---|---|---|---|---|---|---|---|---|---|---|---|---|---|---|---|
| Argent. nit. **ARG** | | | | | | | | | | | | | | | |
| Arsen. alb. **ARS** | | | | | | | | | | | | | | | |
| Calc. carb. **CALC** | | | | | | | | | | | | | | | |
| Graphites **GRAPH** | | | | | | | | | | | | | | | |
| Ignatia **IGN** | | | | | | | | | | | | | | | |
| Lachesis **LACH** | | | | | | | | | | | | | | | |
| Lycopodium **LYC** | | | | | | | | | | | | | | | |
| Merc. sol. **MERC** | | | | | | | | | | | | | | | |
| Natrum mur. **NM** | | | | | | | | | | | | | | | |
| Nux vomica **NV** | | | | | | | | | | | | | | | |
| Phos. **PHOS** | | | | | | | | | | | | | | | |
| Pulsatilla **PULS** | | | | | | | | | | | | | | | |
| Sepia **SEP** | | | | | | | | | | | | | | | |
| Silica **SIL** | | | | | | | | | | | | | | | |
| Sulfur **SULF** | | | | | | | | | | | | | | | |

## FOOD PREFERENCES

| FOOD PREFERENCES | VERY STRONGLY Score 5 for each remedy | STRONGLY Score 3 for each remedy | SLIGHTLY Score 1 for each remedy |
|---|---|---|---|
| PASTRIES DISAGREE | PULS | PULS | LYC PHOS |
| LIKE SALTY FOODS | ARG NM PHOS | ARG NM PHOS | CALC |
| DISLIKE SALTY FOODS | GRAPH | GRAPH | MERC NM SEP |
| LIKE OYSTERS | LACH | LACH | CALC LYC NM SULF |
| DISLIKE FISH | GRAPH | GRAPH | PHOS |
| SHELLFISH DISAGREE | LYC | LYC (score 5) | LYC |
| LIKE LEMONS | SEP | SEP | MERC NM PULS |
| LIKE PICKLES | SEP | SEP | ARS IGN LACH SULF |
| DISLIKE TOMATOES | PHOS | PHOS (score 5) | PHOS |
| LIKE SPICY FOODS | NV PHOS SULF | NV PHOS SULF | ARS |
| GARLIC DISAGREES | PHOS | PHOS (score 5) | PHOS |
| ONIONS DISAGREE | LYC | LYC | IGN PULS SULF |

Finish the whole questionnaire, then fill in the score cards.
Total the scores (*right*), then fill in the result cards on pp. 46–7.

## SCORE CARD 4

| | Sulfur SULF | Silica SIL | Sepia SEP | Pulsatilla PULS | Phos. PHOS | Nux vomica NV | Natrum mur. NM | Merc. sol. MERC | Lycopodium LYC | Lachesis LACH | Ignatia IGN | Graphites GRAPH | Calc. carb. CALC | Arsen. alb. ARS | Argent. nit. ARG |
|---|---|---|---|---|---|---|---|---|---|---|---|---|---|---|---|
| | | | | | | | | | | | | | | | |
| | | | | | | | | | | | | | | | |
| | | | | | | | | | | | | | | | |
| | | | | | | | | | | | | | | | |
| | | | | | | | | | | | | | | | |
| | | | | | | | | | | | | | | | |
| | | | | | | | | | | | | | | | |
| | | | | | | | | | | | | | | | |
| | | | | | | | | | | | | | | | |

| SULF | SIL | SEP | PULS | PHOS | NV | NM | MERC | LYC | LACH | IGN | GRAPH | CALC | ARS | ARG |
|---|---|---|---|---|---|---|---|---|---|---|---|---|---|---|
| ☐ | ☐ | ☐ | ☐ | ☐ | ☐ | ☐ | ☐ | ☐ | ☐ | ☐ | ☐ | ☐ | ☐ | ☐ |

## FOOD PREFERENCES

| FOOD PREFERENCES | VERY STRONGLY Score 5 for each remedy | STRONGLY Score 3 for each remedy | SLIGHTLY Score 1 for each remedy |
|---|---|---|---|
| LIKE MILK | ARS CALC MERC NM NV PHOS SIL | ARS CALC MERC NM NV PHOS SIL | ARS CALC MERC NM NV PHOS SIL |
| MILK DISAGREES | CALC SEP SULF | CALC SEP SULF | ARS LYC NM NV PHOS PULS |
| RELUCTANT TO TAKE BREAST MILK IN INFANCY | SIL | SIL | CALC MERC |
| HOT DRINKS DISAGREE | LACH PHOS PULS SULF | LACH PHOS PULS SULF | LACH PHOS PULS SULF |
| ICED DRINKS DISAGREE | ARS | ARS | NV PULS |
| LIKE CARBONATED DRINKS | PHOS | PHOS (score 5) | PHOS |
| LIKE ALCOHOL | ARS LACH NV SULF | ARS LACH NV SULF | CALC LYC PHOS PULS SEP |
| BEER DISAGREES | NV | NV (score 5) | LYC PULS SIL SULF |
| LITTLE THIRST | PULS | PULS (score 5) | ARG ARS LYC SEP |
| LIKE COFFEE | NV | NV (score 5) | ARS |
| DISLIKE COFFEE | CALC NV | CALC NV | MERC NM PHOS SULF |
| COFFEE DISAGREES | IGN NV | IGN NV | MERC PULS |

Finish the whole questionnaire, then fill in the score cards.
Total the scores (right), then fill in the result cards on pp. 46–7.

## SCORE CARD 1

| | | | | | | | | | | | | |
|---|---|---|---|---|---|---|---|---|---|---|---|---|
| Sulfur **SULF** | | | | | | | | | | | | SULF ☐ |
| Silica **SIL** | | | | | | | | | | | | SIL ☐ |
| Sepia **SEP** | | | | | | | | | | | | SEP ☐ |
| Pulsatilla **PULS** | | | | | | | | | | | | PULS ☐ |
| Phos. **PHOS** | | | | | | | | | | | | PHOS ☐ |
| Nux vomica **NV** | | | | | | | | | | | | NV ☐ |
| Natrum mur. **NM** | | | | | | | | | | | | NM ☐ |
| Merc. sol. **MERC** | | | | | | | | | | | | MERC ☐ |
| Lycopodium **LYC** | | | | | | | | | | | | LYC ☐ |
| Lachesis **LACH** | | | | | | | | | | | | LACH ☐ |
| Ignatia **IGN** | | | | | | | | | | | | IGN ☐ |
| Graphites **GRAPH** | | | | | | | | | | | | GRAPH ☐ |
| Calc. carb. **CALC** | | | | | | | | | | | | CALC ☐ |
| Arsen. alb. **ARS** | | | | | | | | | | | | ARS ☐ |
| Argent. nit. **ARG** | | | | | | | | | | | | ARG ☐ |

## FEARS

| FEARS | VERY STRONGLY Score 5 for each remedy | STRONGLY Score 3 for each remedy | SLIGHTLY Score 1 for each remedy |
|---|---|---|---|
| HEIGHTS | ARG ☐ | ARG ☐ | SULF ☐ |
| ENCLOSED SPACES | ARG LYC NM PULS ☐ | ARG LYC NM PULS ☐ | CALC IGN ☐ |
| CROWDS/PUBLIC PLACES | ARG LYC NM NV PULS ☐ | ARG LYC NM NV PULS ☐ | ARG LYC NM NV PULS ☐ |
| MICE | CALC ☐ | CALC (score 5) ☐ | CALC ☐ |
| SNAKES | LACH ☐ | LACH (score 5) ☐ | CALC ☐ |
| WATER | LACH PHOS ☐ | LACH PHOS ☐ | LACH PHOS ☐ |
| THUNDERSTORMS | PHOS ☐ | PHOS ☐ | CALC GRAPH MERC NM SEP ☐ |
| SHARP POINTED OBJECTS (e.g., hypodermic needles) | SIL ☐ | SIL (score 5) ☐ | ARS MERC NM ☐ |
| GHOSTS | ARS LYC PHOS PULS SULF ☐ | ARS LYC PHOS PULS SULF ☐ | CALC SEP ☐ |
| DARKNESS | PHOS ☐ | PHOS ☐ | ARS CALC LYC NM PULS ☐ |
| BURGLARS | ARS NM ☐ | ARS NM ☐ | ARG IGN LACH MERC PHOS ☐ |
| BEING ALONE | ARG ARS LYC PHOS ☐ | ARG ARS LYC PHOS ☐ | PULS SEP ☐ |

Finish the whole questionnaire, then fill in the score cards.
Total the scores (*right*), then fill in the result cards on pp. 46–7.

41

## SCORE CARD 2

| | SULF | SIL | SEP | PULS | PHOS | NV | NM | MERC | LYC | LACH | IGN | GRAPH | CALC | ARS | ARG |
|---|---|---|---|---|---|---|---|---|---|---|---|---|---|---|---|
| Sulfur **SULF** | | | | | | | | | | | | | | | |
| Silica **SIL** | | | | | | | | | | | | | | | |
| Sepia **SEP** | | | | | | | | | | | | | | | |
| Pulsatilla **PULS** | | | | | | | | | | | | | | | |
| Phos. **PHOS** | | | | | | | | | | | | | | | |
| Nux vomica **NV** | | | | | | | | | | | | | | | |
| Natrum mur. **NM** | | | | | | | | | | | | | | | |
| Merc. sol. **MERC** | | | | | | | | | | | | | | | |
| Lycopodium **LYC** | | | | | | | | | | | | | | | |
| Lachesis **LACH** | | | | | | | | | | | | | | | |
| Ignatia **IGN** | | | | | | | | | | | | | | | |
| Graphites **GRAPH** | | | | | | | | | | | | | | | |
| Calc. carb. **CALC** | | | | | | | | | | | | | | | |
| Arsen. alb. **ARS** | | | | | | | | | | | | | | | |
| Argent. nit. **ARG** | | | | | | | | | | | | | | | |

## FEARS

| FEARS | VERY STRONGLY Score 5 for each remedy | STRONGLY Score 3 for each remedy | SLIGHTLY Score 1 for each remedy |
|---|---|---|---|
| BEING LATE | ARG | ARG | NM |
| BEING HURT EMOTIONALLY | NM | NM (score 5) | IGN |
| BEING POISONED (by bad food or pollution) | ARS LACH | ARS LACH | ARS LACH |
| ILLNESS | ARS PHOS | ARS PHOS | ARG CALC NV |
| INSANITY | CALC PULS | CALC PULS | ARG GRAPH MERC NM NV PHOS SEP |
| CANCER | ARS CALC PHOS | ARS CALC PHOS | ARS CALC PHOS |
| DEATH | ARS CALC GRAPH NV PHOS | ARS CALC GRAPH NV PHOS | ARG LACH LYC MERC NM PULS |
| FOR THE HEALTH OF YOUR FAMILY | MERC | MERC (score 5) | ARS PHOS |
| FAILURE IN BUSINESS | LYC NV | LYC NV | ARG NM PHOS SIL SULF |
| POVERTY | ARS | ARS | CALC SEP |
| LOSS OF SELF-CONTROL | ARG | ARG | IGN NM |
| PHYSICAL/MENTAL EXERTION (due to lack of stamina) | SIL | SIL (score 5) | PHOS |

Finish the whole questionnaire, then fill in the score cards.
Total the scores (*right*), then fill in the result cards on pp. 46–7.

## SCORE CARD 1

| | ARG | ARS | CALC | GRAPH | IGN | LACH | LYC | MERC | NM | NV | PHOS | PULS | SEP | SIL | SULF |
|---|---|---|---|---|---|---|---|---|---|---|---|---|---|---|---|
| Sulfur **SULF** | | | | | | | | | | | | | | | |
| Silica **SIL** | | | | | | | | | | | | | | | |
| Sepia **SEP** | | | | | | | | | | | | | | | |
| Pulsatilla **PULS** | | | | | | | | | | | | | | | |
| Phos. **PHOS** | | | | | | | | | | | | | | | |
| Nux vomica **NV** | | | | | | | | | | | | | | | |
| Natrum mur. **NM** | | | | | | | | | | | | | | | |
| Merc. sol. **MERC** | | | | | | | | | | | | | | | |
| Lycopodium **LYC** | | | | | | | | | | | | | | | |
| Lachesis **LACH** | | | | | | | | | | | | | | | |
| Ignatia **IGN** | | | | | | | | | | | | | | | |
| Graphites **GRAPH** | | | | | | | | | | | | | | | |
| Calc. carb. **CALC** | | | | | | | | | | | | | | | |
| Arsen. alb. **ARS** | | | | | | | | | | | | | | | |
| Argent. nit. **ARG** | | | | | | | | | | | | | | | |

## GENERAL FEATURES

| GENERAL FEATURES | VERY STRONGLY Score 5 for each remedy | STRONGLY Score 3 for each remedy | SLIGHTLY Score 1 for each remedy |
|---|---|---|---|
| WARM AND MADE WORSE BY HEAT | PULS SULF | ARG PULS SULF | ARG PULS SULF |
| AILMENTS ARE WORSE IN STUFFY ROOMS | GRAPH LYC PULS SULF | GRAPH LYC PULS SULF | ARG MERC |
| FEET ARE HOT IN BED (stick them out of bedclothes) | PULS SULF | PULS SULF | CALC PHOS |
| CHILLY BUT MADE WORSE BY HEAT | MERC PULS | MERC PULS | CALC GRAPH LACH LYC NM |
| CHILLY AND BETTER WITH HEAT | ARS NV | ARS NV | CALC IGN PHOS SEP SIL |
| FEET ARE SWEATY AND SMELLY | GRAPH LYC PULS SIL | GRAPH LYC PULS SIL | CALC PHOS SEP SULF |
| AILMENTS ARE WORSE AFTER SWEATING | MERC SEP | MERC SEP | CALC PHOS PULS SULF |
| HEAD IS SWEATY IN BED | CALC | CALC (score 5) | MERC SIL |
| AILMENTS ARE WORSE FROM PROLONGED STANDING | PULS SEP SULF | PULS SEP SULF | CALC SIL |
| AILMENTS ARE WORSE IN COLD, WET WEATHER | ARS CALC SIL | ARS CALC SIL | ARG GRAPH LACH LYC MERC PULS SULF |
| AILMENTS ARE WORSE IN COLD, DRY WEATHER | NV | NV | ARS SIL |
| AILMENTS ARE WORSE IN WINDY WEATHER | LYC NV PHOS PULS | LYC NV PHOS PULS | ARS LACH SIL |

Finish the whole questionnaire, then fill in the score cards.
Total the scores (*right*), then fill in the result cards on pp. 46–7.

## SCORE CARD 2

| | | | | | | | | | | | | | | |
|---|---|---|---|---|---|---|---|---|---|---|---|---|---|---|
| Sulfur **SULF** | | | | | | | | | | | | | | |
| Silica **SIL** | | | | | | | | | | | | | | |
| Sepia **SEP** | | | | | | | | | | | | | | |
| Pulsatilla **PULS** | | | | | | | | | | | | | | |
| Phos. **PHOS** | | | | | | | | | | | | | | |
| Nux vomica **NV** | | | | | | | | | | | | | | |
| Natrum mur. **NM** | | | | | | | | | | | | | | |
| Merc. sol. **MERC** | | | | | | | | | | | | | | |
| Lycopodium **LYC** | | | | | | | | | | | | | | |
| Lachesis **LACH** | | | | | | | | | | | | | | |
| Ignatia **IGN** | | | | | | | | | | | | | | |
| Graphites **GRAPH** | | | | | | | | | | | | | | |
| Calc. carb. **CALC** | | | | | | | | | | | | | | |
| Arsen. alb. **ARS** | | | | | | | | | | | | | | |
| Argent. nit. **ARG** | | | | | | | | | | | | | | |

Result boxes: ARG | ARS | CALC | GRAPH | IGN | LACH | LYC | MERC | NM | NV | PHOS | PULS | SEP | SIL | SULF

## GENERAL FEATURES

| GENERAL FEATURES | VERY STRONGLY Score 5 for each remedy | STRONGLY Score 3 for each remedy | SLIGHTLY Score 1 for each remedy |
|---|---|---|---|
| FEEL BETTER FROM SEA AIR | NM PULS | NM PULS | NM PULS |
| FEEL WORSE FROM SEA AIR | NM SEP | NM SEP | ARS |
| LOVE TO WATCH THUNDERSTORMS | SEP | SEP (score 5) | LYC |
| SUFFER A HEADACHE BEFORE THUNDERSTORMS | PHOS | PHOS | SEP SIL |
| SENSITIVE TO SMELLS | GRAPH IGN LYC NV PHOS SEP | GRAPH IGN LYC NV PHOS SEP | ARS CALC SULF |
| SENSITIVE TO THE SMELL OF TOBACCO | IGN | IGN | NV PULS SEP |
| EYES ARE SENSITIVE TO SUNLIGHT | GRAPH NM SULF | GRAPH NM SULF | ARS IGN MERC PHOS |
| SENSITIVE TO THE SLIGHTEST NOISE | NV SIL | NV SIL | LYC PHOS SEP |
| SUFFER A HEADACHE OR FEEL FAINT ON MISSING A MEAL | GRAPH LYC PHOS SIL SULF | GRAPH LYC PHOS SIL SULF | GRAPH LYC PHOS SIL SULF |
| FEEL BETTER WHEN FASTING | NM | NM (score 5) | SIL |
| FEEL BETTER AFTER A SHORT NAP | PHOS | PHOS (score 5) | NV |
| AILMENTS ARE RELIEVED BY ONSET OF MENSTRUATION | LACH | LACH (score 5) | CALC PHOS PULS SEP SULF |

Finish the whole questionnaire, then fill in the score cards.
Total the scores (*right*), then fill in the result cards on pp. 46–7.

## SCORE CARD 3

| Remedy | | | | | | | | | | | | | | Result |
|---|---|---|---|---|---|---|---|---|---|---|---|---|---|---|
| Sulfur **SULF** | | | | | | | | | | | | | | SULF ☐ |
| Silica **SIL** | | | | | | | | | | | | | | SIL ☐ |
| Sepia **SEP** | | | | | | | | | | | | | | SEP ☐ |
| Pulsatilla **PULS** | | | | | | | | | | | | | | PULS ☐ |
| Phos. **PHOS** | | | | | | | | | | | | | | PHOS ☐ |
| Nux vomica **NV** | | | | | | | | | | | | | | NV ☐ |
| Natrum mur. **NM** | | | | | | | | | | | | | | NM ☐ |
| Merc. sol. **MERC** | | | | | | | | | | | | | | MERC ☐ |
| Lycopodium **LYC** | | | | | | | | | | | | | | LYC ☐ |
| Lachesis **LACH** | | | | | | | | | | | | | | LACH ☐ |
| Ignatia **IGN** | | | | | | | | | | | | | | IGN ☐ |
| Graphites **GRAPH** | | | | | | | | | | | | | | GRAPH ☐ |
| Calc. carb. **CALC** | | | | | | | | | | | | | | CALC ☐ |
| Arsen. alb. **ARS** | | | | | | | | | | | | | | ARS ☐ |
| Argent. nit. **ARG** | | | | | | | | | | | | | | ARG ☐ |

## GENERAL FEATURES

| GENERAL FEATURES | VERY STRONGLY Score 5 for each remedy | STRONGLY Score 3 for each remedy | SLIGHTLY Score 1 for each remedy |
|---|---|---|---|
| AILMENTS SEEM WORSE BETWEEN 4–8 A.M./P.M. | LYC ☐ | LYC (score 5) ☐ | SULF ☐ |
| AILMENTS SEEM WORSE BETWEEN 4–6 A.M./P.M. | SEP ☐ | SEP (score 5) ☐ | LYC SULF ☐ |
| AILMENTS SEEM WORSE BETWEEN 1–2 A.M. | ARS ☐ | ARS (score 5) ☐ | ARS ☐ |
| AILMENTS SEEM WORSE BETWEEN 2–5 A.M. | NV ☐ | NV (score 5) ☐ | SULF ☐ |
| AILMENTS ARE WORSE IN THE SPRING | CALC LACH LYC ☐ | CALC LACH LYC ☐ | NM PULS SEP SIL SULF ☐ |
| AILMENTS ARE WORSE AROUND FULL MOON | ARG ARS CALC LYC PHOS PULS SIL ☐ | ARG ARS CALC LYC PHOS PULS SIL ☐ | GRAPH LACH MERC SEP SULF ☐ |
| AILMENTS ARE WORSE IN THE MORNING AND EVENING | SEP ☐ | SEP ☐ | CALC GRAPH LYC PHOS ☐ |
| AILMENTS ARE WORSE FROM SUNSET TO SUNRISE | MERC ☐ | MERC (score 5) ☐ | MERC ☐ |
| AVOID LYING ON THE LEFT SIDE OF THE BODY IN BED | PHOS PULS ☐ | PHOS PULS ☐ | ARG NM SEP SULF ☐ |
| AVOID LYING ON THE RIGHT SIDE OF THE BODY IN BED | MERC ☐ | MERC ☐ | NV PHOS ☐ |
| PRONE TO LEFT-SIDED COMPLAINTS | ARG GRAPH LACH PHOS SEP SULF ☐ | ARG GRAPH LACH PHOS SEP SULF ☐ | |
| PRONE TO RIGHT-SIDED COMPLAINTS | ARS CALC LYC NV PULS ☐ | ARS CALC LYC NV PULS ☐ | |

Finish the whole questionnaire, then fill in the score cards.
Total the scores (*right*), then fill in the result cards on pp. 46–7.

# QUESTIONNAIRE RESULTS

Transfer your total scores from the four result cards to the final result card. Your final score may indicate either one constitutional type that outweighs all the others or several types. Consult the appropriate constitutional profiles on pp. 50–79. Do not be concerned if you bear little resemblance to the model in the photograph. Each constitutional type has infinite variations and people can also change from one constitutional type to another at various points in life. Even experienced homeopaths require years of practice to pinpoint the closest possible match.

## THE RESULT CARDS

### PERSONALITY & TEMPERAMENT RESULT CARD

*Add up the totals in each remedy column below*

| | ARG | ARS | CALC | GRAPH | IGN | LACH | LYC | MERC | NM | NV | PHOS | PULS | SEP | SIL | SULF |
|---|---|---|---|---|---|---|---|---|---|---|---|---|---|---|---|
| SCORE CARD 1 | | | | | | | | | | | | | | | |
| SCORE CARD 2 | | | | | | | | | | | | | | | |
| SCORE CARD 3 | | | | | | | | | | | | | | | |
| SCORE CARD 4 | | | | | | | | | | | | | | | |
| SCORE CARD 5 | | | | | | | | | | | | | | | |
| TOTAL SCORE | | | | | | | | | | | | | | | |

*(Transfer the totals to the final result card)*

### FOOD PREFERENCES RESULT CARD

*Add up the totals in each remedy column below*

| | ARG | ARS | CALC | GRAPH | IGN | LACH | LYC | MERC | NM | NV | PHOS | PULS | SEP | SIL | SULF |
|---|---|---|---|---|---|---|---|---|---|---|---|---|---|---|---|
| SCORE CARD 1 | | | | | | | | | | | | | | | |
| SCORE CARD 2 | | | | | | | | | | | | | | | |
| SCORE CARD 3 | | | | | | | | | | | | | | | |
| SCORE CARD 4 | | | | | | | | | | | | | | | |
| TOTAL SCORE | | | | | | | | | | | | | | | |

*(Transfer the totals to the final result card)*

# FEARS RESULT CARD

*Add up the totals in each remedy column below*

| | ARG | ARS | CALC | GRAPH | IGN | LACH | LYC | MERC | NM | NV | PHOS | PULS | SEP | SIL | SULF |
|---|---|---|---|---|---|---|---|---|---|---|---|---|---|---|---|
| **SCORE CARD 1** | | | | | | | | | | | | | | | |
| **SCORE CARD 2** | | | | | | | | | | | | | | | |

| | ARG | ARS | CALC | GRAPH | IGN | LACH | LYC | MERC | NM | NV | PHOS | PULS | SEP | SIL | SULF |
|---|---|---|---|---|---|---|---|---|---|---|---|---|---|---|---|
| **TOTAL SCORE** | | | | | | | | | | | | | | | |

*(Transfer the totals to the final result card)*

# GENERAL FEATURES RESULT CARD

*Add up the totals in each remedy column below*

| | ARG | ARS | CALC | GRAPH | IGN | LACH | LYC | MERC | NM | NV | PHOS | PULS | SEP | SIL | SULF |
|---|---|---|---|---|---|---|---|---|---|---|---|---|---|---|---|
| **SCORE CARD 1** | | | | | | | | | | | | | | | |
| **SCORE CARD 2** | | | | | | | | | | | | | | | |
| **SCORE CARD 3** | | | | | | | | | | | | | | | |

| | ARG | ARS | CALC | GRAPH | IGN | LACH | LYC | MERC | NM | NV | PHOS | PULS | SEP | SIL | SULF |
|---|---|---|---|---|---|---|---|---|---|---|---|---|---|---|---|
| **TOTAL SCORE** | | | | | | | | | | | | | | | |

*(Transfer the totals to the final result card)*

# FINAL RESULT CARD

*Add up the totals in each remedy column below*

| | ARG | ARS | CALC | GRAPH | IGN | LACH | LYC | MERC | NM | NV | PHOS | PULS | SEP | SIL | SULF |
|---|---|---|---|---|---|---|---|---|---|---|---|---|---|---|---|
| **PERSONALITY & TEMPERAMENT** | | | | | | | | | | | | | | | |
| **FOOD PREFERENCES** | | | | | | | | | | | | | | | |
| **FEARS** | | | | | | | | | | | | | | | |
| **GENERAL FEATURES** | | | | | | | | | | | | | | | |

| | ARG | ARS | CALC | GRAPH | IGN | LACH | LYC | MERC | NM | NV | PHOS | PULS | SEP | SIL | SULF |
|---|---|---|---|---|---|---|---|---|---|---|---|---|---|---|---|
| **FINAL SCORE** | | | | | | | | | | | | | | | |

The highest score indicates which of the 15 key constitutional types you most resemble. If the
highest score appears in more than one remedy column, it may be that you are a mixture of types.

## THE CONSTITUTIONAL TYPES

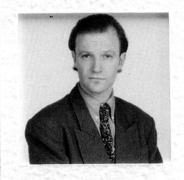
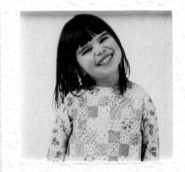
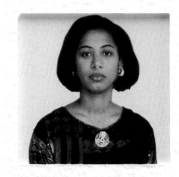

# INDEX

## OF

# HOMEOPATHIC
# REMEDIES

A photographic index featuring 150 key, common,
and minor remedies, with details of their source,
history, medicinal uses, and the factors that improve
or worsen the symptoms treated.

***Note*** *Remedies are arranged by Latin name within each section. For an explanation
of constitutional types see pp. 24–5 and homeopathic provings see pp. 12–15.*

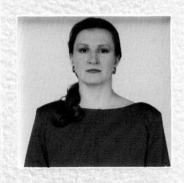
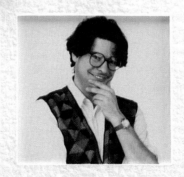
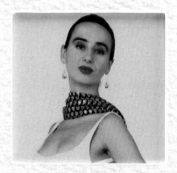

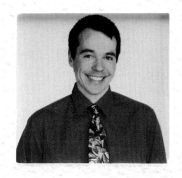
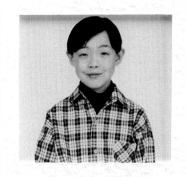
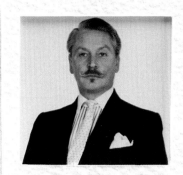

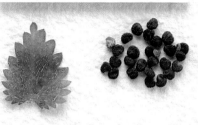
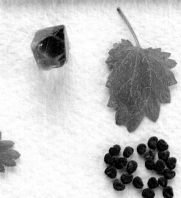

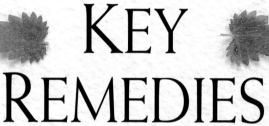

# KEY REMEDIES

The 15 key remedies have a wide range of self-help uses and
are regularly used by homeopaths because of their efficacy in
treating many common, everyday complaints as well as
long-term conditions. In addition, they correspond
to some of the most common constitutional types, which
are shown in a series of unique photographic profiles
of people who display emotional and physical
characteristics typical of these types.

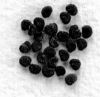
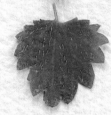

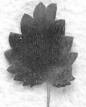
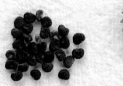
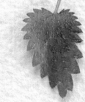

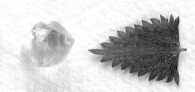

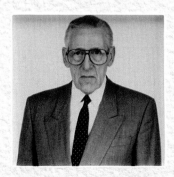
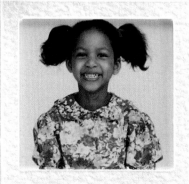
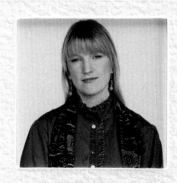
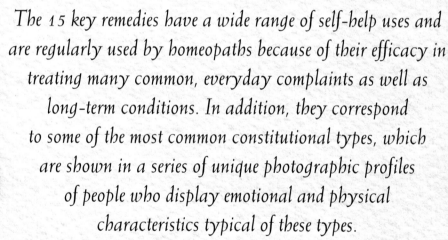

*ARGENTUM NITRICUM*

# ARGENT. NIT.

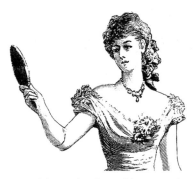

**Mirror backing** *Silver nitrate has been used for many years to make the backing of mirrors.*

*Silver nitrate (a compound of silver) is caustic and antibacterial and was once used medicinally to cauterize wounds and to treat warts, epilepsy, and eye infections in newborn infants. In large amounts silver nitrate is highly poisonous and causes severe breathing difficulties and damage to the skin, kidneys, liver, spleen, and aorta. The Argent. nit. remedy is mainly used for nervous and digestive problems.*

## KEY USES

- Anxieties, fears, and phobias
- Digestive complaints brought on by nervous excitement or from eating too much sweet food
- Ailments accompanied by a craving for sweet foods.

### SELF-HELP
*Diarrhea* – see pp. 184–5
*Fear* – see pp. 192–3
*Laryngitis* – see pp. 178–9.

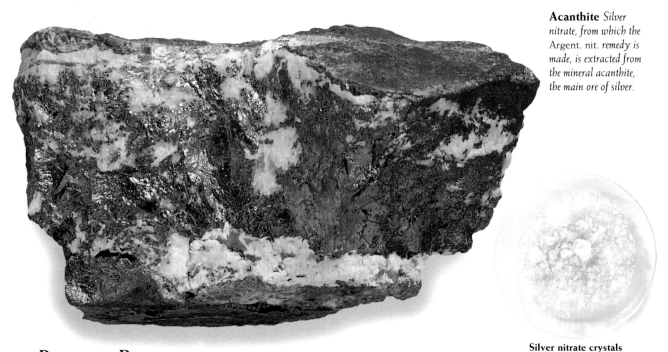

**Acanthite** *Silver nitrate, from which the Argent. nit. remedy is made, is extracted from the mineral acanthite, the main ore of silver.*

**Silver nitrate crystals**

## REMEDY PROFILE

**Common names** Hellstone, devil's stone, lunar caustic.
**Source** Acanthite, which is found in Norway, the US, and South America.
**Parts used** Silver nitrate.

### AILMENTS TREATED
This remedy is used for all types of fears and anxieties brought on by an overactive imagination. Stage fright, claustrophobia, and anxiety in the face of unexpected situations are all helped by *Argent. nit.* Often these fears and phobias are accompanied by a superstition that something awful is about to happen, for example, being crushed by a tall building.

Sometimes there is also a sense of great difficulty in resisting reckless behavior and dangerous impulses, such as jumping from a high window. Anxiety-induced sweats or palpitations are also helped by *Argent. nit.*

This remedy is given for digestive complaints, for example, diarrhea, gas, and vomiting, and pulsating headaches with a slow onset, which are caused by eating too many sweet foods or by nervous excitement.

*Argent. nit.* is also effective for pain that is better from pressure and fresh air but worse with movement or from talking; asthma; colicky pain during weaning; warts; laryngitis with

splinterlike pain and hoarseness; sore throats; epilepsy; and dizziness.

In women, this remedy is given for a bearing down sensation in the uterus due to prolapse or menstruation. It is also good for inflammation of the mucous membranes, especially in the eyes, and is used to treat conjunctivitis.

Complaints treated with *Argent. nit.* are usually left-sided.
**Symptoms better** From fresh air; from pressure; in cool surroundings.
**Symptoms worse** With warmth; at night; lying on the left side; from overwork or emotional stress; with movement or talking; in hot weather.

# Argent. nit.-the type

## PERSONALITY & TEMPERAMENT

These types are extroverted, cheerful, and impressionable. They find it difficult to control their far-ranging minds and emotions, and readily laugh, cry, or lose their tempers. This can make them perpetually agitated and apprehensive, and may intensify into fearful anticipation, for example, worry and fear about missing a train or forgetting lines in a forthcoming performance. Their constant anxiety and worry may lead to irrational fears, for example, being crushed by a tall building or impulsively jumping from a great height.

## FOOD PREFERENCES

### Likes
• Salty foods
• Sweet foods

### Upset by
• Cold foods

### Other
• Either love or loathe cheese
• Crave sweet foods but easily upset by them

## FEARS

• Heights and high buildings
• Enclosed spaces and crowds
• Failure in business
• Being late
• Being alone and burglars
• Losing self-control; insanity
• Incurable illness and death

## GENERAL FEATURES

### Better
• In cool surroundings
• From fresh air

### Worse
• With warmth
• At night
• Lying on the left side
• From emotional stress or overwork
• During menstruation

*Argent. nit.* types are often found in jobs that require quick thinking and a good memory, where the emphasis is on performance, for example, acting. They are driven individuals who think, talk, and act rapidly.

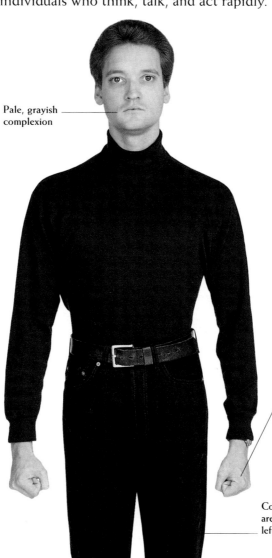

Pale, grayish complexion

Often appear tense, nervous, and agitated

Complaints are generally left-sided

## THE ARGENT. NIT. CHILD

• *Looks prematurely old.*

• *Hates stuffy rooms.*

• *Nervous, excitable, and apprehensive, and may be nauseated or may vomit at the thought of school.*

• *Prone to insomnia due to anticipatory anxiety.*

• *Craves salty and sweet foods, which may cause diarrhea. Breastfed babies have colic and diarrhea if the mother eats sweet foods.*

### Physical appearance
*Argent. nit.* types tend to have sunken features and develop early lines and wrinkles, which make them appear prematurely old and mentally overtaxed. They may be prone to sudden, profuse, nervous sweats.

### Weak areas of the body
• Nerves
• Mucous membranes, particularly in the stomach, the intestines, and the eyes
• Left side of the body

*ARSENICUM ALBUM*

# ARSEN. ALB.

*Historically, arsenic is well-known for its use as a poison. Because it is a metallic poison, it cannot be destroyed, even by fire. Acute poisoning causes burning pain in the digestive tract, with vomiting, convulsions, and even death. Medicinally, arsenic was once used to treat syphilis. The homeopathic remedy, made from a compound of arsenic, acts on the mucous membranes of the digestive tract and respiratory system.*

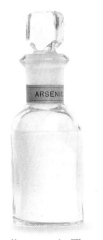

**Arsen. alb. remedy** *This remedy is good for symptoms ranging from burning pain to restlessness and fear.*

## KEY USES

• Anxiety and fear caused by deep-seated insecurity
• Digestive disorders and inflammation of the mucous membranes, especially in the digestive tract
• Ailments characterized by burning pain that is better for heat.

### SELF-HELP
*Anxiety* – see pp. 190–1
*Fever in children* – see pp. 218–9
*Gastroenteritis* – see pp. 182–3
*Mouth ulcers* – see pp. 164–5
*Tiredness* – see pp. 196–7.

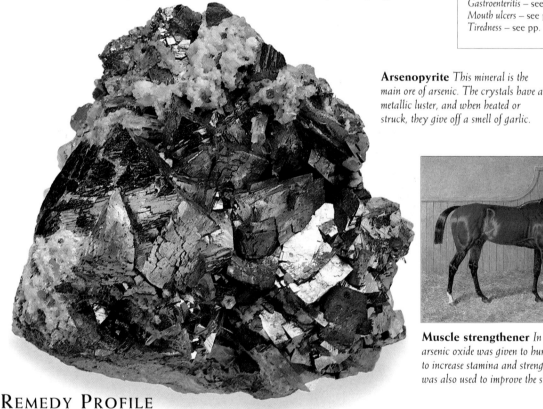

**Arsenopyrite** *This mineral is the main ore of arsenic. The crystals have a metallic luster, and when heated or struck, they give off a smell of garlic.*

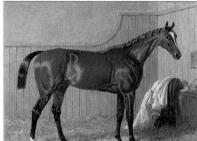

**Muscle strengthener** *In the past, white arsenic oxide was given to humans and animals to increase stamina and strengthen muscles. It was also used to improve the skin of animals.*

## REMEDY PROFILE

**Common name** Arsenic oxide.
**Source** Arsenopyrite, which is found in Sweden, Germany, Norway, England, and Canada.
**Parts used** Arsenic oxide.

### AILMENTS TREATED
*Arsen. alb.* is given for anxiety and fear caused by an underlying insecurity and oversensitivity.

This remedy is effective for a range of digestive disorders including: food poisoning that causes burning vomiting; indigestion; diarrhea; and gastroenteritis from eating too much ripe fruit and vegetables, iced foods, and drinking too much alcohol.

Children suffering from fever and diarrhea that causes severe dehydration are also helped by this remedy.

*Arsen. alb.* is effective for asthma with severe breathlessness; stinging mouth ulcers; cracked, dry lips from a burning nasal discharge; tiredness due to a physical illness, such as anemia or asthma, or mental strain; eye inflammation with watery, stinging eyes; headaches with dizziness and vomiting; and fluid retention, especially around the ankles.

When ill, those who need *Arsen. alb.* feel chilly, despite the burning pain that characterizes their symptoms. They are better with warmth but prefer their heads to be cool. This remedy is given for fever where the person is either hot to the touch but feels cold inside or is cold to the touch but feels burning hot inside.
**Symptoms better** With movement; from warm drinks; with warmth; lying down with the head raised.
**Symptoms worse** From cold foods and drinks; with cold; on the right side; between midnight and 2 a.m.

# Arsen. alb.-the type

*Arsen. alb.* types are tense, restless, ambitious individuals who worry about their own and their family's health. They are deeply pessimistic, with a constant need for reassurance. Elegance and finesse personified, they are particularly critical and intolerant of disorder and imprecision.

## PERSONALITY & TEMPERAMENT

The appearance, thoughts, and actions of *Arsen. alb.* types show meticulous attention to detail. To combat insecurity, they devise various contingency plans to cover most eventualities and may become hoarders in an attempt to protect against future misfortune. Their perfectionist tendencies result in an "all or nothing" attitude, and they may abandon their endeavors if they cannot achieve excellence. They express strong opinions and are intolerant of the ideas and beliefs of others.

## FOOD PREFERENCES

### Likes
- Warm foods and drinks (better from these), coffee
- Fatty foods; olive oil
- Sweet foods (tolerate these well)
- Sour foods: pickles, lemons, vinegar
- Alcohol

## FEARS

- Being alone and burglars
- Darkness and ghosts
- Poverty
- Incurable illness and death
- For the health of the family
- Poisoning from bad food or pollution

## GENERAL FEATURES

### Better
- With warmth
- With movement
- Lying down with the head raised

### Worse
- In cold, dry, windy weather
- With cold
- From cold foods and drinks
- Between midnight and 2 a.m.
- On the right side

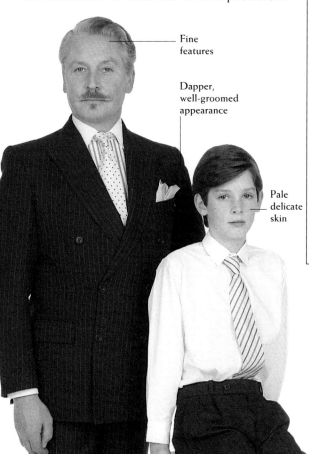

Fine features

Dapper, well-groomed appearance

Pale delicate skin

## THE ARSEN. ALB. CHILD

- *Thin and delicate with fine features, skin, and hair. Flushes easily despite pallor.*
- *High-strung, easily frightened, and oversensitive to smell, touch, and noise.*
- *Mentally and physically agile.*
- *Restless with sporadic bursts of activity, but tires quickly.*
- *Vivid imagination; may suffer from nightmares.*
- *Worries about everything, particularly parents' health.*
- *Neat and tidy, and hates to be sticky or messy.*

## Physical appearance
*Arsen. alb.* types are thin, stylish, well-groomed, and aristocratic looking, with fine features, pale, delicate skin, and worry lines. They are restless, with quick movements.

## Weak areas of the body
- Stomach and intestines
- Liver
- Respiratory tract
- Mucous membranes
- Skin
- Heart

*CALCAREA CARBONICA*

# CALC. CARB.

*The homeopathic remedy Calc. carb. is made from calcium carbonate, which is derived from oyster shells. Calcium carbonate is only one of several calcium salts that are widely used in homeopathy. Calc. carb. has many wide-ranging applications, but acts on the bones and teeth in particular. The remedy is especially good for backache, joint pain, fractured bones that are slow to heal, and painful teething in children.*

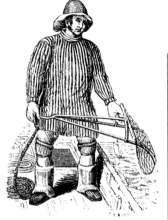

**Oyster dredger** *Just 10 grams of oyster shell powder yield 10 billion kilograms of Calc. carb. at 6c potency.*

## KEY USES
• Slow development of bones and teeth
• Joint and bone pain
• Ailments characterized by fears and anxieties, profuse, sour-smelling perspiration, and sensitivity to cold.

### SELF-HELP
Anxiety – see pp. 190–1
Candidiasis – see pp. 202–3
Glue ear – see pp. 218–9
Heavy menstruation – see pp. 204–5
Menopause – see pp. 206–7
Premenstrual syndrome – see pp. 204–5
Tiredness – see pp. 196–7.

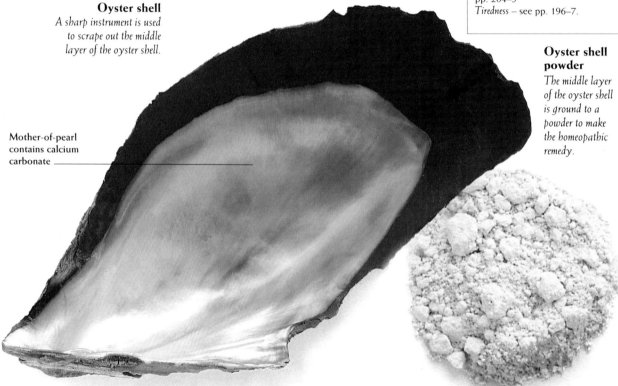

**Oyster shell**
*A sharp instrument is used to scrape out the middle layer of the oyster shell.*

Mother-of-pearl contains calcium carbonate

**Oyster shell powder**
*The middle layer of the oyster shell is ground to a powder to make the homeopathic remedy.*

## REMEDY PROFILE

**Common name** Calcium carbonate.
**Source** Mother-of-pearl from an oyster shell.
**Parts used** Calcium carbonate.

### AILMENTS TREATED

*Calc. carb.* is mainly used to treat slow development of bones and teeth, joint and bone pain, such as backache, slow-to-heal fractures, and painful teething in children. It is also effective for right-sided headaches.

Ear infections with a sour-smelling discharge, and eye infections where the white of the eye is red, especially in the right eye, are treated with *Calc. carb.* Other complaints helped by it include: eczema; candidiasis; PMS; heavy menstruation; menopausal symptoms; and digestive disorders.

People who require this remedy are anxious, tired, sensitive to cold, and tend to sweat copiously from the slightest physical exertion or when they sleep. Their sweat smells sour

and is profuse on the chest and the back of the head. They may have constipation but, curiously, feel better for it, and their urine has an offensive smell. Children who need this remedy tend to have glue ear and recurrent tonsillitis.
**Symptoms better** Lying on the affected side; in the late morning; from eating breakfast; in dry weather.
**Symptoms worse** In cold and damp; from physical exertion and sweating; on waking; premenstrually.

# Calc. carb.-the type

## PERSONALITY & TEMPERAMENT

These types are quiet, cautious, impressionable, and very sensitive. They often appear withdrawn and self-pitying, but this is because they do not wish to embarrass themselves in front of others and are frightened of failure. Anxious and worried, they become obsessive about things, which is irritating for those close to them, and they sleep poorly. They hate to see cruelty and poverty.

## FOOD PREFERENCES

### Likes
- Sweet foods: cookies, cakes, chocolate, pastries
- Sour foods: olives, pickles
- Starchy foods: bread, rice
- Cold drinks and ice cream
- Eggs
- Oysters

### Dislikes
- Milk and coffee, which may cause digestive upset

### Other
- May crave odd things, such as soil and chalk

## FEARS

- Darkness and ghosts
- Incurable illness and cancer
- Death
- Enclosed spaces
- Insanity
- Poverty
- Mice
- Thunderstorms

## GENERAL FEATURES

### Better
- In the late morning
- In dry weather

### Worse
- In cold and damp
- Premenstrually
- From sweating or exertion
- In spring
- With the full moon

Outwardly strong and stoical-looking, *Calc. carb.* types have a shy, contemplative nature. Generally very healthy, they are enthusiastic in their work and diligent. In contrast, when ill, they tend to be mildly depressed and introspective. Motivation becomes difficult and they need reassurance.

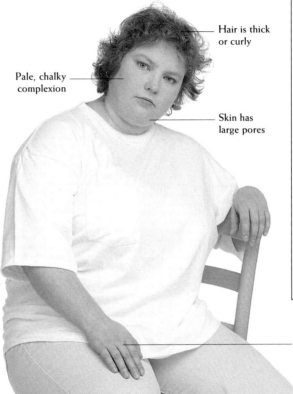

Hair is thick or curly

Pale, chalky complexion

Skin has large pores

Hands are cold and slightly clammy

Soles of the feet feel burning hot

## THE CALC. CARB. CHILD

- *Plump with strong features and a pale complexion.*
- *Large abdomen and head. Fontanel is slow to close.*
- *Slow to learn how to walk and talk, and teeth are slow to develop.*
- *Placid, calm, and sensitive; inclined to laziness.*
- *Extremely fearful of the dark and occasionally wakes up screaming from nightmares.*
- *Clumsy with a tendency to fall over easily; not very good at sports as a result.*
- *Hard-working at school but finds understanding difficult and gives up easily. Without encouragement, may fall behind and feel left out.*

### Physical appearance
Their hearty appetite can lead to excessive weight gain, general apathy, and sluggishness. *Calc. carb.* types often suffer head sweats and bone or joint abnormalities, such as scoliosis (curvature of the spine).

### Weak areas of the body
- Bones and teeth
- Bowels
- Ears, nose, and throat
- Glands
- Skin

*GRAPHITE*

# GRAPHITES

Graphite is a form of carbon and is the main constituent of pencils. The name graphite comes from the Greek word grapbein, meaning "to write." Graphite is also used in lubricants, polishes, batteries, and electric motors. The homeopathic remedy was proved by Hahnemann, who learned that workmen in a mirror factory were applying graphite to heal cold sores. Graphites is excellent for skin complaints and problems with the metabolism.

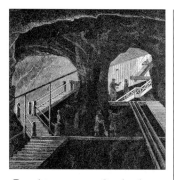

**Graphite mining** *Graphite has been mined extensively for many years. One of its uses is as pencil "lead."*

### KEY USES

• Skin complaints, especially eczema
• Metabolic imbalances that lead to skin problems, obesity, and abnormal nail formation
• Ulcers caused by a weakness in the stomach lining.

### SELF-HELP
*Eczema* – see pp. 186–7
*Phlegm* – see pp. 170–1.

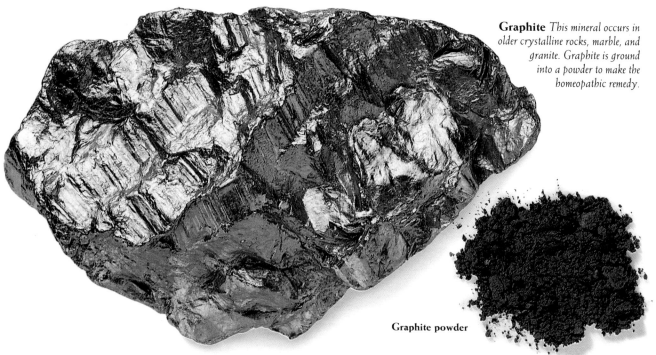

**Graphite** *This mineral occurs in older crystalline rocks, marble, and granite. Graphite is ground into a powder to make the homeopathic remedy.*

**Graphite powder**

## REMEDY PROFILE

**Common names** Graphite, plumbago.
**Source** Graphite, found in Sri Lanka, Mexico, Canada, and the US.
**Parts used** Graphite.

### AILMENTS TREATED
*Graphites* is a key remedy for skin complaints, especially weeping eczema with a honeylike discharge that often occurs behind the ears and the knees, on the palms of the hands, and on the nipples.

This remedy is good for people with a metabolic imbalance that may cause skin complaints, such as psoriasis and dry, cracked skin; cuts that easily become infected and pus-filled; scar tissue that hardens; keloids (raised, itchy scars); and abnormal nail formation where the nails are thick, cracked, and misshapen. Obesity may result due to an inability to absorb nutrients correctly.

*Graphites* is also used to treat the following conditions: ulcers caused by a weakness in the stomach lining (these are better when lying down and from eating hot food, and may alternate with skin complaints); cold sores; hair loss; cramps and numbness in the hands and feet; occasional hot sweats following nosebleeds; and swollen glands.

*Graphites* is also good for excess mucus production, especially if blowing the nose hurts because of cracks on the skin; eczema may accompany the condition.

In women, *Graphites* is given for infrequent, scanty, or absent menstruation; enlarged ovaries; swelling of the breasts; and late menstruation with constipation.
**Symptoms better** With warmth (but need fresh air); in the dark; with sleep; from eating.
**Symptoms worse** In cold air; from sweet foods and seafood; during menstruation; on the left side.

# Graphites - the type

*Graphites* types are anxious, timid, apprehensive, indecisive, and easily startled. Sustained mental effort is difficult for them, and they have a sense of being intellectually slow. They are attracted to manual work and outdoor jobs.

## PERSONALITY & TEMPERAMENT

Slow to react to external stimuli, *Graphites* types show little zest for anything involving concerted mental effort. Prone to frequent mood changes, these types tend to be lethargic and grumpy on waking, and become irritable, impatient, and agitated as the day wears on. They feel unlucky and readily become despondent, self-pitying, and tearful, particularly when listening to music.

## FOOD PREFERENCES

### Likes
• Sour and acidic cold drinks, such as beer

### Dislikes
• Sweet foods
• Salt and seafood

### Other factors
• Prone to headaches if a meal is missed
• Pork causes digestive upset

## FEARS

• Insanity
• Death
• Thunderstorms

## GENERAL FEATURES

### Better
• With warmth (but need fresh air)
• From eating
• With sleep
• In the dark

### Worse
• In cold, damp air and a draft (but dislike stuffiness)
• On the left side
• In the morning and evening
• From using steroids to suppress skin eruptions
• During menstruation
• From sweet foods and seafood

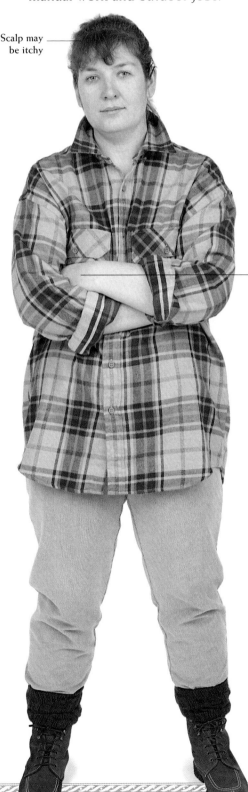

Scalp may be itchy

Skin is dry and cracks easily

## THE GRAPHITES CHILD

• *Heavily built or plump.*
• *Pale and chilly, but flushes easily.*
• *Rough, dry skin that tends to crack.*
• *Distended abdomen due to persistent constipation.*
• *Timid, anxious, and hesitant.*
• *Pessimistic.*
• *Is inclined to be lazy and low in stamina.*
• *Sensitive to movement and prone to motion sickness.*

### Physical appearance

*Graphites* types usually have dark hair, and may be coarse-featured, with pale, dry, rough skin. Their skin is particularly prone to cracking, especially behind the ears and knees, at the corners of the mouth, and on the fingertips. The scalp may be flaky and itchy with a yellow crust. They tend to be overweight and may even be obese, with large appetites. They flush or sweat easily and lack stamina.

### Weak areas of the body

• Skin and nails
• Metabolism
• Mucous membranes
• Left side of the body

*IGNATIA AMARA/STRYCHNOS IGNATII*

# IGNATIA

The homeopathic remedy, made from the seeds of Ignatia amara, is mainly given for emotional problems. Natives of the Philippine islands wore the seeds as amulets to prevent or cure all kinds of diseases. The Spanish Jesuits introduced the seeds into Europe in the 17th century. In orthodox medicine, the seeds were once used for gout, epilepsy, and cholera. The seeds contain strychnine, a powerful poison that acts on the nervous system.

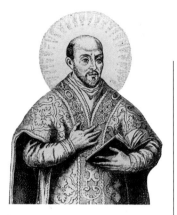

**Ignatius Loyola** *(1491–1556)*
*The Ignatia amara tree takes its name from Ignatius Loyola, a Catholic priest who founded the Jesuit order.*

## KEY USES

- Emotional problems
- Acute grief, for example, caused by bereavement or broken relationships
- Headaches
- Coughs and sore throats
- Ailments with changeable, contradictory symptoms.

### SELF-HELP
*Absent menstruation – see pp. 206–7*
*Bereavement – see pp. 192–3*
*Depression – see pp. 194–5*
*Headaches – see pp. 158–9*
*Insomnia – see pp. 194–5.*

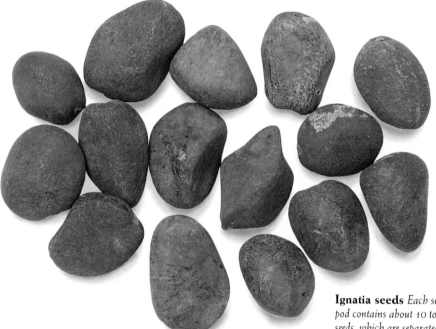

**Ignatia seeds** *Each seed pod contains about 10 to 20 seeds, which are separated from the pulp and powdered to make the homeopathic remedy.*

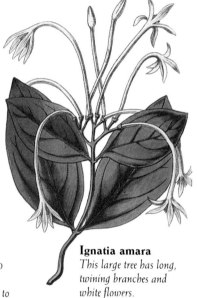

**Ignatia amara**
*This large tree has long, twining branches and white flowers.*

## REMEDY PROFILE

**Common name** St.-Ignatius's-bean.
**Source** Native to the East Indies, China, and the Philippines.
**Parts used** Seeds.

### AILMENTS TREATED
Complaints that benefit from *Ignatia* often arise as a result of extreme emotional stress, for example, grief, shock, anger, and the suppression of these feelings. This is a key remedy for bereavement with mood swings, hysteria, and insomnia.

Other emotional states helped by this remedy include: sudden tearfulness; self-pity; self-blame; a repressed response to anger or violence; fear of being thought forceful; depression; and worry.

*Ignatia* is effective for headaches that are worse lying on the painful side and that feel as if a nail had been driven into the head, nervous headaches due to emotional stress, and children's headaches that are worsened by caffeine and relieved by heat.

Ailments with changeable, contradictory symptoms are helped by *Ignatia*, for example, sore throats that are better from eating solids, and nausea and vomiting that are better from eating. Other conditions it is good for include: tickly coughs; fever with chills that induce thirst; fainting

in claustrophobic conditions; sensitivity to pain; craving for odd foods when ill; and upper abdominal pain.

In women, *Ignatia* is given for a prolapsed rectum with sharp, upward-shooting pain; painful uterine spasms during menstruation; hemorrhoids; emotionally-triggered constipation and absent menstruation.

**Symptoms better** Lying on the painful side; with a change of position; after urinating; from firm pressure; from eating; with warmth.
**Symptoms worse** In cold air; if touched; from emotional stress, such as grief or anger; from coffee and tobacco; near strong smells.

# Ignatia - the type

Most *Ignatia* types are women and are sensitive, artistic, cultured, and emotionally fragile. They are high-strung, with high ideals and expectations; when things go wrong, they are likely to blame themselves.

## PERSONALITY & TEMPERAMENT

Despite their extreme sensitivity, *Ignatia* women find it difficult to express their emotions, particularly if they are grieving. Often they will behave in a contradictory manner, for example, being perceptive but irrational. They expect those close to them to be perfect and as a result, have a tendency to hysterical overreaction. They are very sensitive to pain and being in crowded places. Frequently moody, with a brittle manner, they may laugh and cry simultaneously. They find it difficult to break the bond with a partner if disillusioned in love.

## FOOD PREFERENCES

### Likes
• Sour foods: pickles, vinegar
• Dairy foods: butter, cheese
• Bread

### Likes (and upset by)
• Coffee

### Upset by
• Sweet foods, alcohol, fruit

## FEARS

• Being hurt emotionally
• Losing self-control
• Enclosed spaces and crowds
• Burglars

## GENERAL FEATURES

### Better
• With warmth
• From eating
• After urinating
• From applying firm pressure
• With a change of position

### Worse
• In cold air
• From emotional stress, such as grief or anger
• If touched or stroked
• Near the smell of tobacco

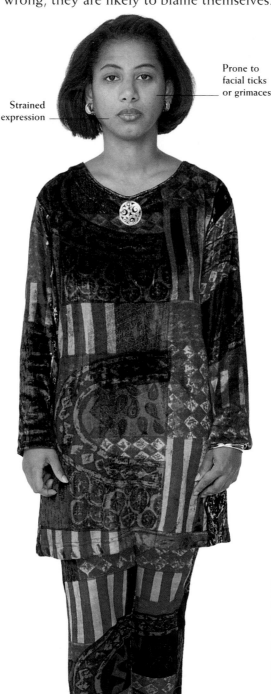

Strained expression

Prone to facial ticks or grimaces

## THE IGNATIA CHILD

• *Bright, excitable, sensitive, and precocious.*

• *High-strung with a rather strained expression. Extremely sensitive to noise and may grimace when speaking.*

• *Finds it difficult to cope with stress, which may lead to loss of concentration, crying, or anger.*

• *When stressed, may get scared of everything, even of going out alone.*

• *Prone to nervous headaches after school.*

• *Takes the blame for failures.*

• *Liable to faint in confined spaces.*

• *Prone to a nervous, dry cough and laryngitis.*

### Physical appearance
*Ignatia* types are generally thin, dark-haired women, possibly with a sunken face, cracked lips, bluish circles around the eyes, and a strained expression. They have a tendency to blink, sigh, or yawn repeatedly, which indicates that they find it difficult to release their deep emotions.

### Weak areas of the body
• Mind
• Nervous system

LYCOPODIUM CLAVATUM

# LYCOPODIUM

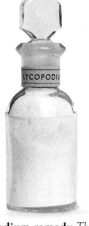

*Arabian physicians used this evergreen herb for stomach disorders and to disperse kidney stones. In the 17th century, the yellow powder, or pollen dust, from the spores was given on its own for gout and urine retention. The pollen dust, which is used to make the Lycopodium remedy, is both highly inflammable and water resistant. It was once used to make fireworks, and as a coating to keep pills from sticking together.*

**Lycopodium remedy** *This is a well-known remedy for digestive complaints, especially indigestion.*

## KEY USES
- Digestive disorders
- Prostate enlargement
- Kidney and bladder complaints
- Right-sided complaints with a desire for sweet foods
- Emotional problems caused by insecurity.

### SELF-HELP
*Anxiety* – see pp. 190–1
*Bloating & flatulence* – see pp. 184–5
*Hair loss* – see pp. 188–9
*Irritability & anger* – see pp. 192–3.

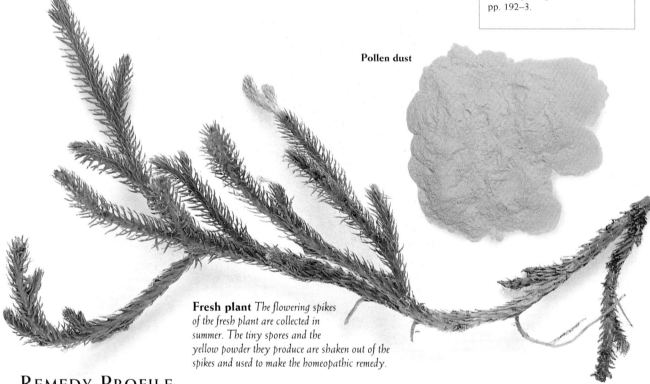

**Pollen dust**

**Fresh plant** *The flowering spikes of the fresh plant are collected in summer. The tiny spores and the yellow powder they produce are shaken out of the spikes and used to make the homeopathic remedy.*

## REMEDY PROFILE

**Common names** Wolfsclaw, club moss, running pine, stag's horn moss.
**Source** Native to mountains and forests in the Northern Hemisphere.
**Parts used** Spores and pollen dust.

### AILMENTS TREATED
*Lycopodium* alleviates digestive complaints, for example, indigestion caused by eating late at night; constant nausea; vomiting; ravenous hunger followed by discomfort after eating a small amount; a distended, bloated abdomen with gas; constipation; and bleeding hemorrhoids.

In men, *Lycopodium* is given for an enlarged prostate and reddish urine with a sandy sediment in it caused by kidney stones. It is also used to treat increased libido with an inability to achieve or sustain an erection.

Most ailments helped by this remedy tend to be right-sided and accompanied by a desire for sweet foods. *Lycopodium* is effective for neuralgia-type headaches; sore throats that are worse from cold drinks; persistent, dry coughs; tiredness from flu; chronic fatigue symdrome; hair loss; and psoriasis on the hands.

Emotional problems caused by insecurity, such as nervousness, anxiety, impatience, cowardice, fear of being alone, insomnia, talking and laughing during sleep, night fears, and fear on waking are all helped by this remedy.
**Symptoms better** From loosening the clothes; with movement; in cool air; from hot foods or drinks; at night.
**Symptoms worse** From tight clothing; after overeating; in stuffy rooms; on the right side; between 4 p.m. and 8 p.m., and 4 a.m. and 8 a.m.; in the spring.

# Lycopodium-the type

## PERSONALITY & TEMPERAMENT

Being deeply insecure, *Lycopodium* types may exaggerate the truth to bolster their low self-esteem. They resist change, since new challenges cause great apprehension. Although they seem self-disciplined and conscientious, they succumb easily to a weakness for sweet foods and are sexually promiscuous. Despite apparently enjoying company, they avoid commitment in close relationships. They are irritated by weakness and are intolerant of illness.

## FOOD PREFERENCES

### Likes
- Mixtures of foods
- Cabbage, onions, legumes
- Oysters and other shellfish
- Sweet foods: cookies, cakes, pastries, chocolate
- Olive oil
- Hot foods and drinks

### Other
- Feel full readily but disregard this sensation

## FEARS

- Being alone
- Darkness and ghosts
- Enclosed spaces and crowds
- Failure
- Death

## GENERAL FEATURES

### Better
- From cool, fresh air
- From being active
- From hot foods and drinks
- From loosening the clothes
- At night

### Worse
- From wearing tight clothing
- From fasting or overeating
- In stuffy rooms
- On the right side
- Between 4 a.m. and 8 a.m., and 4 p.m. and 8 p.m.

*Lycopodium* types have an air of quiet self-possession, stability, and detachment that inspires respect but belies a strong sense of inadequacy. They tend to be intellectual, with a conservative outlook, and often hold prestigious positions, for example, as diplomats, executives, lawyers, or doctors.

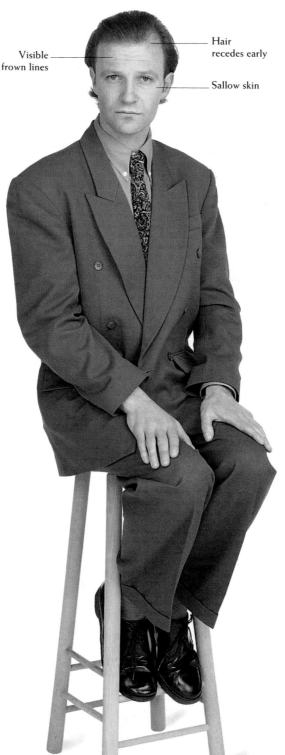

Visible frown lines

Hair recedes early

Sallow skin

## THE LYCOPODIUM CHILD

- *Thin with sallow skin.*
- *Abdomen is slightly distended.*
- *Shy and insecure.*
- *Prefers reading and quiet pursuits rather than being outdoors.*
- *Bossy and irritable at home if allowed to be, yet well-behaved and conscientious at school.*

### Physical appearance
Tall and sallow-skinned, *Lycopodium* types have a distinguished, almost haughty appearance. Their upper body is lean with poorly developed muscles, causing tremors after physical exertion. They usually have marked, vertical frown lines above the nose and may be prematurely gray or bald. The facial muscles twitch and the nostrils tend to flare.

### Weak areas of the body
- Right side of the body
- Digestive organs, particularly the bowels
- Liver
- Kidneys and bladder
- Prostate gland
- Brain
- Lungs
- Skin

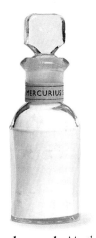

**Merc. sol. remedy** *Mouth and throat complaints with excessive salivation are helped by this remedy.*

*MERCURIUS SOLUBILIS HAHNEMANNI*

# MERC. SOL.

*Mercury was known to the ancient Chinese and Hindus and was found in an Egyptian tomb of 1500 BC. Although it is toxic, in the past mercury was given for syphilis and to promote bodily secretions. Today, it is used in thermometers and batteries. Symptoms of mercury poisoning include profuse salivation and vomiting. Illnesses characterized by excessive, strong-smelling secretions are helped by Merc. sol.*

## KEY USES

• Ailments accompanied by profuse, strong-smelling, burning bodily discharges, and a general sensitivity to heat and cold
• Throat and mouth complaints.

### SELF-HELP
*Bad breath* – see pp. 164–5
*Gingivitis* – see pp. 162–3
*Tonsillitis* – see pp. 178–9.

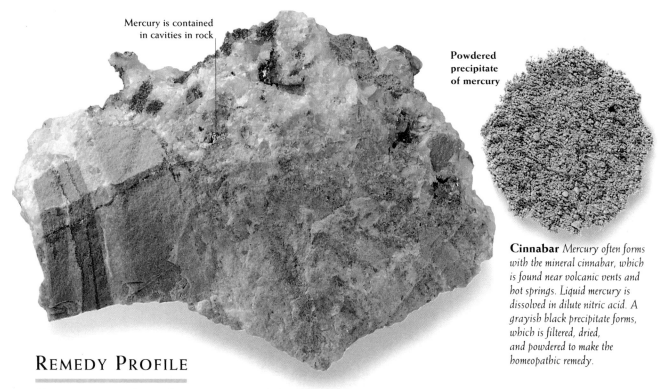

Mercury is contained in cavities in rock

**Powdered precipitate of mercury**

**Cinnabar** *Mercury often forms with the mineral cinnabar, which is found near volcanic vents and hot springs. Liquid mercury is dissolved in dilute nitric acid. A grayish black precipitate forms, which is filtered, dried, and powdered to make the homeopathic remedy.*

## REMEDY PROFILE

**Common names** Quicksilver, mercury.
**Source** Cinnabar, which is the most important ore of mercury, is found in Spain, Italy, the US, Peru, and China.
**Parts used** Mercury.

### AILMENTS TREATED
*Merc. sol.* is effective for a wide range of conditions that are accompanied by profuse, burning, strong-smelling secretions, and an associated sensitivity to heat and cold. It is used to treat mouth and throat complaints with a thirst for cold drinks. These include: excessive salivation; oral thrush; gingivitis (inflamed gums); bad

breath (halitosis); tonsillitis; loose teeth in infected gums; a swollen, dark, red throat; and painful throat ulcers.

Other conditions helped by this remedy are: spasmodic coughs; neuralgic pain; fever with drenching, oily, offensive-smelling sweat that chills the skin as it evaporates or aggravates other symptoms; swollen glands; a congestive, vicelike headache; aching joints; and earache with a smelly discharge.

*Merc. sol.* is good for eye complaints, for example, chronic conjunctivitis where the eyelids are red, swollen, and stuck together, or stinging, watery, aching eyes.

Nasal problems due to a cold or allergy, for example, watery, burning mucus, sneezing that makes the nose feel raw, or a burning nasal discharge, all respond well to *Merc. sol.*

This remedy also acts on the skin and is good for conditions such as encrusted lesions on the scalp with a smelly discharge, pus-filled eruptions or blisters on the skin, and open sores or ulcers that sting and itch.
**Symptoms better** With rest; in moderate temperatures.
**Symptoms worse** With changes in temperature; from being too hot in bed; in dampness; from sweating; lying on the right side; at night.

# Merc. sol. -the type

## PERSONALITY & TEMPERAMENT

Mentally restless and anxious, *Merc. sol.* types have a strong need for order and stability. Their deep insecurity makes them extremely conservative, cautious, and suspicious in their dealings with others. As a result, their actions and speech appear slow and deliberate. They are extremely sensitive to criticism and contradiction, sometimes exploding in rage, with a sudden impulse to kill whomever has offended them. When unwell, they are likely to become mentally dulled and muddled, hesitant in speech, and slow to comprehend, with poor memory and willpower.

## FOOD PREFERENCES

### Likes
- Cold drinks: milk, beer
- Bread and butter
- Lemons

### Dislikes
- Meat
- Sweet foods and coffee
- Alcohol (except beer)
- Salt

### Other factors
- Constantly hungry

## FEARS

- For the health of the family
- Burglars
- Insanity and death
- Thunderstorms

## GENERAL FEATURES

### Better
- In moderate temperatures
- With rest

### Worse
- At night
- From being too hot in bed
- Lying on the right side
- From sweating
- With temperature changes

*Merc. sol.* types are introverted and "closed," with a strong emotional undercurrent. They seem detached and arrogant, but in fact have an internal sense of haste, which they are at pains to restrain.

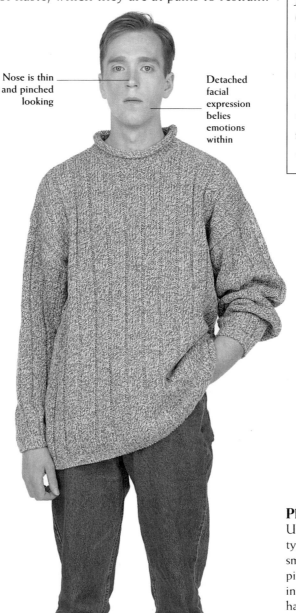

Nose is thin and pinched looking

Detached facial expression belies emotions within

## THE MERC. SOL. CHILD

- *Often precocious and flirtatious; has adultlike emotions.*
- *Cautious, sensitive, and irritable.*
- *Can be shy and withdrawn.*
- *Tends to stammer.*
- *Susceptible to recurrent ear, nose, and throat infections.*
- *Tends to drool when asleep.*

### Physical appearance
Usually fair-haired, *Merc. sol.* types have translucent, smooth, unlined skin with a pinched nose. Despite an inner feeling of agitation and haste, their facial expression is surprisingly untroubled and detached.

### Weak areas of the body
- Blood
- Mucous membranes in the respiratory system and bowels
- Salivary glands and tonsils
- Liver
- Bones and joints
- Skin

*NATRUM MURIATICUM*

# NATRUM MUR.

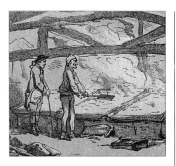

**Salt works** *Historically, salt was of great economic value in trade. To produce salt, brine was collected and evaporated in large boiling pans.*

*Salt, or sodium chloride, has long been a highly prized mineral resource. The word "salary" comes from the Latin salarium, which refers to the payment of salt to soldiers. Sodium and chlorine are essential trace elements; most people get more than enough from the salt in their diet. In orthodox medicine salt is used only in saline solution, but in homeopathy, the Natrum mur. remedy has a wide range of uses.*

## KEY USES

• Emotional problems caused by suppressed feelings, especially grief
• Ailments accompanied by discharges that look like the white of a raw egg
• Complaints that are generally worse for heat.

### SELF-HELP
Colds – see pp. 172–3
Cold sores – see pp. 164–5
Eyestrain – see pp. 166–7
Gingivitis – see pp. 162–3
Phlegm – see pp. 170–1.

**Rock salt** *The mineral rock salt, or halite, is formed by the evaporation of saline waters, usually lakes. A thick salt crust is left behind. Rock salt, the source of common table salt, is used to make the homeopathic remedy.*

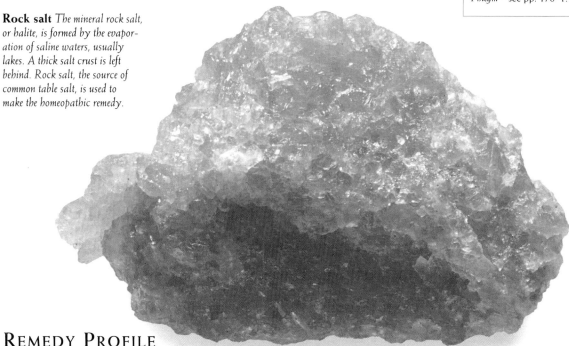

## REMEDY PROFILE

**Common names** Sodium chloride, rock salt.
**Source** Rock salt, which is found in the Dead Sea and in parts of the US, Europe, and India.
**Parts used** Sodium chloride.

### AILMENTS TREATED
Homeopaths give this remedy for emotional problems, such as anxiety and depression, that are caused by suppressed grief and other emotions.

*Natrum mur.* is also used to treat conditions with a watery discharge, such as colds, and phlegm or profuse, clear mucus. Complaints that are generally worse with heat and that are often brought on by stuffy heat

or exposure to hot sun are helped by this remedy. These include: migraines with zigzag lines in front of the eyes; eyestrain with aching eyes; headaches that come on after menstruation; and cold sores.

It is also good for mouth problems, for example, gingivitis (inflamed gums), dry, cracked lips, mouth ulcers, and bad breath (halitosis).

Skin complaints, for example, warts, dry cuticles, hangnails, boils, and painful acne are helped by *Natrum mur.* It is also effective for goiter; anemia; indigestion; constipation with dry, hard stools; bleeding anal fissures; backache; and delayed urine flow.

In women, *Natrum mur.* is given for absent menstruation induced by shock or grief; irregular menstruation; and a general feeling of being unwell both before and after menstruation. It is also good for a dry or sore vagina, vaginal discharge, and vaginismus (vaginal pain during sexual intercourse).

When ill, people who need this remedy are chilly but dislike heat.
**Symptoms better** From fresh air; from cold compresses; in a firm bed; from sweating; from fasting.
**Symptoms worse** In cold, thundery weather, hot sun, and sea air; in stuffy heat; from overexertion; from sympathy; between 9 a.m. and 11 a.m.

# Natrum mur. – the type

## PERSONALITY & TEMPERAMENT

*Natrum mur.* types are serious, conscientious people who can be moody and despondent, especially on waking. When self-absorbed they can be impatient and abrupt. Honest and idealistic, they are also inflexible and so tend to learn things the hard way. They cry or sulk over slights or insults, but abhor sympathy from others. Music notably can move them to tears.

## FOOD PREFERENCES

**Likes**
• Sour foods: sauerkraut
• Beer

**Likes (and upset by)**
• Milk
• Starchy foods: bread, rice

**Dislikes**
• Chicken
• Coffee

**Other**
• Either love or loathe salt and salty foods

## FEARS

• Being hurt emotionally
• Insanity; losing self-control
• Death
• Enclosed spaces and crowds
• Darkness and burglars
• Being late
• Failure in business
• Thunderstorms

## GENERAL FEATURES

**Better**
• From fresh air
• From sweating
• In a firm bed

**Worse**
• Between 9 a.m. and 11 a.m.
• In cold, thundery weather
• In stuffy heat, hot sun, and sea air
• From overexertion
• Lying on left side

Extremely sensitive and refined, *Natrum mur.* types are mostly women, and are easily wounded by criticism or insults. As a result they become introverted and appear stoical and self-reliant. They impose loneliness on themselves, although they actually desire the company of others.

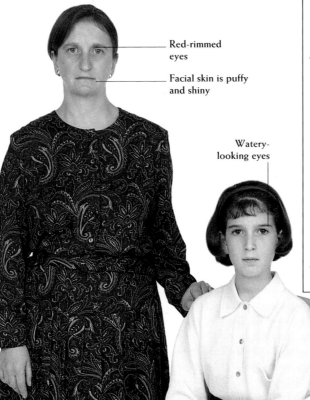

Red-rimmed eyes

Facial skin is puffy and shiny

Watery-looking eyes

### THE NATRUM MUR. CHILD

• *Small or underweight for his or her age.*

• *May be slow in learning to walk and talk.*

• *Relatively dark skin that perspires quickly, making the face flushed and shiny.*

• *Prone to hangnails.*

• *Well-behaved, responsible, and conscientious about doing schoolwork and looking after younger siblings.*

• *Sensitive to criticism and easily hurt; may become a difficult teenager*

• *Hates being fussed over.*

• *Tends to suffer headaches from the pressure of schoolwork.*

### Physical appearance

*Natrum mur.* types are pear-shaped or have a squarish build. Either sandy or dark haired, they have pale, puffy, slightly shiny facial skin. Their eyes may be watery and their eyelids appear reddened. There may be a crack in the center of the lower lip.

### Weak areas of the body

• Digestive tract
• Blood
• Muscles
• Skin
• Mind

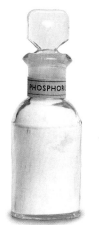

**Phos. remedy** *Profuse bleeding from the gums is one of the conditions helped by this remedy.*

*PHOSPHORUS*

# PHOS.

*Phosphorus is one of the most important minerals needed for life and is contained in the bones, teeth, DNA, and bodily fluids. It was discovered in the residue of evaporated urine. In orthodox medicine, phosphorus was once used for malaria, measles, pneumonia, rheumatism, headaches, and epilepsy. Homeopathically, it is given to people who are anxious and fearful and who suffer from nervous and digestive complaints.*

## KEY USES
- Anxiety and fear
- Bleeding and circulatory problems
- Digestive disorders
- Respiratory complaints
- Ailments characterized by burning pain.

### SELF-HELP
*Anxiety* – see pp. 190–1
*Laryngitis* – see pp. 202–3
*Nausea & vomiting* – see pp. 182–3
*Nosebleeds* – see p. 221.

**Phosphorus**
*This yellowish white solid is a nonmetallic element. It glows in the dark and is highly flammable.*

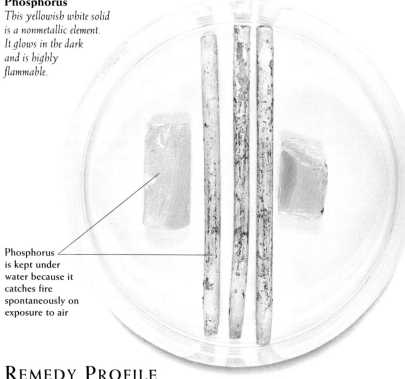

Phosphorus is kept under water because it catches fire spontaneously on exposure to air

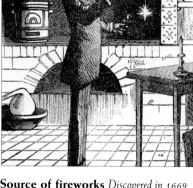

**Source of fireworks** *Discovered in 1669, ordinary white phosphorus ignites easily and was used to make fireworks and matches. Because it is highly toxic, it was replaced with red phosphorus in 1845, which is not toxic.*

## REMEDY PROFILE

**Common name** Phosphorus.
**Source** Phosphorus, which is found in phosphates and living matter.
**Parts used** Phosphorus.

### AILMENTS TREATED
*Phos.* is good for fear and anxiety that causes nervous tension, insomnia, and exhaustion. It is also used to treat circulatory problems, such as cold fingers and burning hot extremities. Profuse bleeding, for example, in nosebleeds, bleeding gums, heavy menstrual flow, and bleeding from the stomach lining is eased by *Phos.*

This remedy is good for digestive complaints, such as nausea and vomiting due to food poisoning or stress (in which ice-cold foods and drinks are craved and vomited as soon as they become warm in the stomach), stomach flu, stomach ulcers indicated by a saliva-filled mouth, and heartburn.

Respiratory problems, namely asthma, bronchitis, and pneumonia where there is tightness in the chest or breastbone, are alleviated by *Phos.* This remedy is also given for dry, tickly coughs that sometimes cause

retching and vomiting, and phlegm streaked with dark red blood. It is also helpful for headaches that are worse before a thunderstorm and laryngitis. Ailments helped by *Phos.* are characterized by burning pain.

When ill, people who require this remedy dislike being alone, need the company of others, and sympathy.
**Symptoms better** From fresh air; if touched or stroked; with sleep.
**Symptoms worse** From hot meals and drinks; lying on the left side; from overexertion; in the mornings and evenings; in thundery weather.

# Phos. -the type

Phos. people are open, expressive, and affectionate, and they often have artistic flair. They are very empathetic, giving readily of themselves. Their enthusiasm is relatively short-lived, however, and their energy is diffused; they may offer more than they can actually deliver.

## PERSONALITY & TEMPERAMENT

Phos. types need lots of stimuli to give their effervescent, imaginative natures full expression, and to avoid becoming irritable and apathetic. Generally optimistic, they love to be the center of attention. They may wilt under pressure, however, and can be surprisingly indifferent to family and close friends. When unwell or upset, they need lots of sympathy and adore being stroked.

## FOOD PREFERENCES

**Likes**
- Salty foods
- Spicy foods
- Cold, carbonated drinks
- Ice cream
- Wine
- Cheese
- Sweet foods

**Dislikes**
- Fish, fruit, tomatoes

**Upset by**
- Hot foods and drinks
- Milk

## FEARS

- Darkness and ghosts
- Burglars and being alone
- Thunderstorms and water
- Failure in business
- Illness, cancer, and death

## GENERAL FEATURES

**Better**
- From fresh air
- If stroked
- Lying on the right side
- With sleep

**Worse**
- In thundery weather
- In the mornings and evenings
- Lying on the left side
- From mental and physical exertion

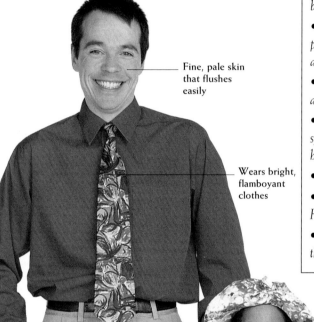

Fine, pale skin that flushes easily

Wears bright, flamboyant clothes

Delicate features and fine skin

## THE PHOS. CHILD

- *Tall and thin for his or her age and may have a reddish glint to the hair.*
- *Fine featured, with slender hands and a tendency to blush or flush readily.*
- *Fidgety, nervous, perceptive, excitable, and trusting.*
- *Likes to have company and feel popular.*
- *Very affectionate and sympathetic to others. Loves hugs and comforting.*
- *Imaginative and artistic.*
- *Dislikes sustained study. Hates exams and homework.*
- *Afraid of the dark and thunderstorms.*

**Physical appearance**
Phos. types are usually tall and slim and look well-proportioned. They have either dark or fair hair, often with a coppery tinge. Their skin is fine and pale and blushes or flushes easily. They dress with flair and flamboyance.

**Weak areas of the body**
- Left side of the body
- Lungs
- Digestive organs: stomach, bowels
- Liver
- Circulation
- Nervous system

*PULSATILLA NIGRICANS/ANEMONE PRATENSIS*

# PULSATILLA

*This delicate perennial plant has a long history of medicinal use. In the 18th century, it was used to treat cataracts, ulcers, tooth decay, and depression. The fresh plant has a bitter, acrid taste and if chewed causes burning in the throat and on the tongue. In homeopathy, it is the source of an important remedy that is used for a wide range of conditions, from colds and coughs to digestive and gynecological complaints.*

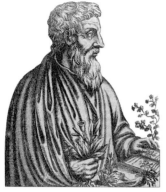

**Dioscorides** (AD 40–90) *This well-known Roman physician used pasqueflower for eye complaints.*

## REMEDY PROFILE

**Common names** Pasqueflower, wind flower, meadow anemone.
**Source** Native to Scandinavia, Denmark, Germany, and Russia.
**Parts used** Fresh plant in flower.

### AILMENTS TREATED

*Pulsatilla* is given for ailments with a profuse discharge of excess mucus, such as colds with either a runny or blocked nose, sinus congestion, and a loose cough with greenish yellow phlegm. Eye problems, for example, sties and conjunctivitis, and digestive complaints caused by eating rich, fatty foods, such as indigestion, gastroenteritis, nausea, and vomiting are helped by *Pulsatilla*.

An important remedy for gynecological complaints, *Pulsatilla* is effective for a range of menstrual and menopausal problems, which are often characterized by depression and tearfulness with a need for comfort and sympathy.

Other conditions that respond well to *Pulsatilla* include: depression; varicose veins; nosebleeds; toothache; osteoarthritis and rheumatism; low backache; chilblains; acne; migraines and headaches above the eyes; and fever without thirst.
**Symptoms better** From fresh air; with gentle exercise; from crying and sympathy.
**Symptoms worse** With heat; from rich or fatty foods; lying on the left side; in the evening.

### KEY USES

• Ailments accompanied by profuse, yellow or yellowish green discharges
• Digestive problems caused by rich, fatty foods
• Gynecological complaints
• Emotional problems, such as depression.

#### SELF-HELP

*Acne* – see pp. 188–9
*Chilblains* – see pp. 198–9
*Colds* – see pp. 172–3
*Coughs* – see pp. 174–5
*Depression* – see pp. 194–5
  *Frequent urination in pregnancy* – see pp. 212–3
  *Gastroenteritis* – see pp. 182–3
  *Indigestion* – see pp. 180–1
  *Labor pain* – see pp. 212–3
*Migraines* – see pp. 160–1
*Morning sickness* – see pp. 208–9
*Nausea & vomiting* – see pp. 182–3
*Osteoarthritis* – see pp. 154–5
*Painful menstruation* – see pp. 204–5
*Premenstrual syndrome* – see pp. 204–5
*Rheumatism* – see pp. 156–7
*Sinus congestion* – see pp. 170–1
*Sties* – see pp. 168–9.

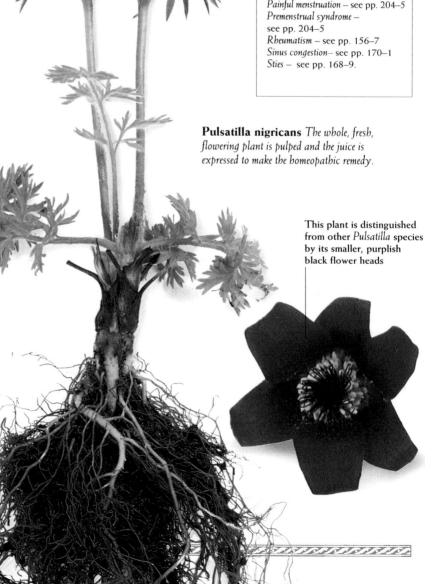

**Pulsatilla nigricans** *The whole, fresh, flowering plant is pulped and the juice is expressed to make the homeopathic remedy.*

This plant is distinguished from other *Pulsatilla* species by its smaller, purplish black flower heads

# Pulsatilla - the type

*Pulsatilla* types are almost always women. They are sweet-natured, shy, kind, and gentle. Often dependent on others for support, they gratefully accept guidance and advice. They make friends easily.

## PERSONALITY & TEMPERAMENT

Although *Pulsatilla* types adapt to different people and circumstances, their flexibility verges on indecision. They are not assertive, find it difficult to express anger, and avoid confrontation in order to keep the peace. Beneath this compliant exterior, however, lies considerable resilience. Readily empathetic with people or animals in distress, they tend to be swayed by emotion rather than by thought. They cry easily with little self-restraint, eliciting the comforting reassurance and consolation they need.

## FOOD PREFERENCES

### Likes
- Rich, sweet foods: cakes, pastries, chocolate
- Cold foods and drinks (although seldom thirsty)
- Peanut butter

### Dislikes
- Butter, pork, eggs, fruit
- Spicy foods

### Upset by
- Mixtures of foods

## FEARS

- Enclosed spaces and crowds
- Being alone
- Darkness and ghosts
- Insanity and death

## GENERAL FEATURES

### Better
- With gentle movement
- From fresh air and in cool, dry conditions

### Worse
- With heat and in stuffiness
- From sudden cooling
- In the evening
- Lying on the left side
- From prolonged standing
- Premenstrually

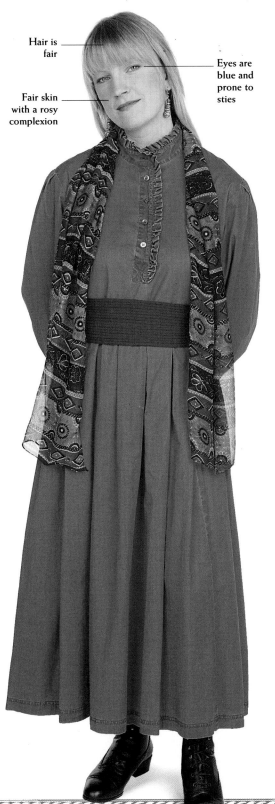

Hair is fair

Eyes are blue and prone to sties

Fair skin with a rosy complexion

## THE PULSATILLA CHILD

### Type 1
- *Small, fair, fine-boned, and inclined to blush. Bright, cheerful, and affectionate, yet shy and sensitive.*

### Type 2
- *Plump, with darker hair. More languid and tearful; craves reassurance and affection, but is slow to reciprocate.*

### Common characteristics
- *Become more lively as the day goes on, but they are nervous at bedtime and afraid of the dark.*
- *Sensitive to weather changes, particularly to cold. Even eating ice cream in hot weather can trigger stomach upsets and earache. Flag in hot weather and become irritable and tearful.*
- *Prone to stuffy colds with excessive mucus. Feel much better outdoors.*
- *Feel dizzy on looking up at anything high.*

### Physical appearance
*Pulsatilla* people tend to be plump with fair hair and blue eyes. They flush or blush easily.

### Weak areas of the body
- Veins
- Stomach
- Bowels
- Bladder
- Female reproductive organs

*SEPIA OFFICINALIS*

# SEPIA

*Cuttlefish ink has long been used as a pigment in artists' paints. Medicinally, it was used in ancient times to treat gonorrhea and kidney stones. Hahnemann published details about the homeopathic remedy in 1834. He proved the remedy after observing that an artist friend who licked his sepia-soaked paintbrush frequently developed an obscure illness, which was caused by the ink. It is an excellent remedy for gynecological complaints.*

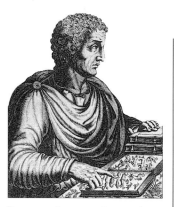

**Roman physician** *Dioscorides (AD 40–90) used the ink from cuttlefish for hair loss.*

## KEY USES
• Gynecological complaints, especially conditions related to a hormonal imbalance, such as premenstrual syndrome and menopause
• Ailments accompanied by exhaustion.

### SELF-HELP
*Candidiasis* – see pp. 202–3
*Heavy menstruation* – see pp. 204–5
*Menopause* – see pp. 206–7
*Painful menstruation* – see pp. 206–7
*Premenstrual syndrome* – see pp. 204–5.

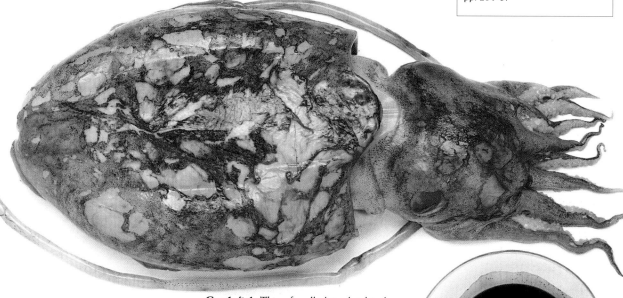

**Cuttlefish** *This soft mollusk is related to the octopus and squid. It frequently changes color to blend with its environment and squirts its brownish black ink for protection.*

**Cuttlefish ink**

## REMEDY PROFILE

**Common name** Cuttlefish.
**Source** Found mainly in the Mediterranean Sea.
**Parts used** Pure pigments in the ink.

### AILMENTS TREATED
*Sepia* acts on the uterus, ovaries, and vagina and is mainly used for gynecological complaints, for example, PMS, painful or heavy menstruation, hot flashes during menopause, emotional and physical symptoms during and after pregnancy, candidiasis, and a sagging or prolapsed uterus. It is an excellent remedy for women who are averse to, or suffer pain during sexual intercourse and feel exhausted afterward. Women who dislike being touched either premenstrually, during menopause, or as a result of emotional problems are also helped by this remedy.

*Sepia* is effective for complaints accompanied by exhaustion, such as an aching back and sides due to muscle weakness. It is also good for the following: indigestion from milk and fatty foods, with gas and tenderness in the abdomen; headaches with nausea; dizziness; hair loss; salty-tasting mucus due to a cold or allergy; brownish yellow, itchy, discolored patches of skin; profuse sweating; and sweaty feet.

This remedy is also good for circulatory problems, for example, hot and cold flashes, and varicose veins.
**Symptoms better** With warmth; from fresh air; from eating; with exercise; when occupied; with sleep.
**Symptoms worse** With mental and physical fatigue; premenstrually; in the early morning and evening; in thundery weather; on the left side.

# Sepia-the type

In the main, *Sepia* types are women. They tend to adopt a martyr's role in life and feel on the brink of being overwhelmed by their responsibilities. As a result, they harbor a deep-seated resentment.

## PERSONALITY & TEMPERAMENT

*Sepia* types are irritable at home yet extroverted in company, and transformed by dancing, which they love. They are strongly opinionated, hate to be contradicted and when unwell they detest sympathy and tend to withdraw. Although some men can be *Sepia* types, they are usually women who are either one, or a combination of two, distinct personae. The first is independent, career-minded, and seeks fulfilment from her work. She appears hard, yet disguises her vulnerability well. The second persona feels engulfed by her sense of duty as wife and mother and cannot assert her own needs.

## FOOD PREFERENCES

### Likes
- Sour foods and drinks: pickles, lemons, vinegar
- Sweet foods
- Alcohol

### Dislikes (and upset by)
- Milk and pork

## FEARS

- Being alone
- Poverty
- Insanity

## GENERAL FEATURES

### Better
- With warmth
- When occupied
- With vigorous exercise
- From fresh air

### Worse
- In dull, thundery weather, (but also loves thunderstorms)
- Premenstrually
- In the early morning and evening
- On the left side

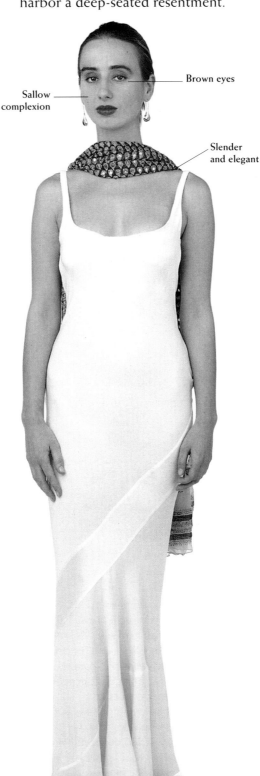

Sallow complexion

Brown eyes

Slender and elegant

## THE SEPIA CHILD
- *Sallow, sweaty skin.*
- *Chilly and sensitive to changes in the weather.*
- *Tires easily.*
- *Prone to fainting when standing.*
- *Nervous and dislikes being alone.*
- *Inclined to be negative, moody, and lazy.*
- *Dislikes parties, but if forced to make an effort will come alive, particularly if there is dancing.*
- *Greedy eater. Milk causes digestive upset.*
- *Tends to be constipated and to wet the bed in the early part of the night.*

### Physical appearance
*Sepia* types of both sexes are tall and lean with slim hips, dark hair, and brown eyes. Pigmentation across their nose and cheeks can result in a yellow-brown "saddle." *Sepia* women are attractive and elegant, with an angular, sightly masculine appearance. They may look downcast and sit with their legs crossed because of a weak feeling in the pelvic area.

### Weak areas of the body
- Left side of the body
- Skin
- Venous circulation
- Female reproductive organs

*SILICEA TERRA*

# SILICA

*Silica is found throughout nature. It is the main constituent of most rocks, and plants absorb it into their stems, which helps keep them strong. In the human body, silica is the constituent that strengthens the teeth, hair, and nails. Silica is also found in connective tissue, which is the material that holds together the various structures of the body. The homeopathic remedy is used for people who lack "grit" either physically or emotionally.*

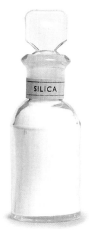

**Silica remedy** *Made from silica, this remedy is excellent for people who feel the cold intensely and tire easily.*

## KEY USES

• General undernourishment that leads to recurrent infections
• Skin and bone complaints
• Expelling foreign objects, such as splinters
• Nervous system problems.

### SELF-HELP
*Migraines – see pp. 160–1*
*Splinters – see p. 222.*

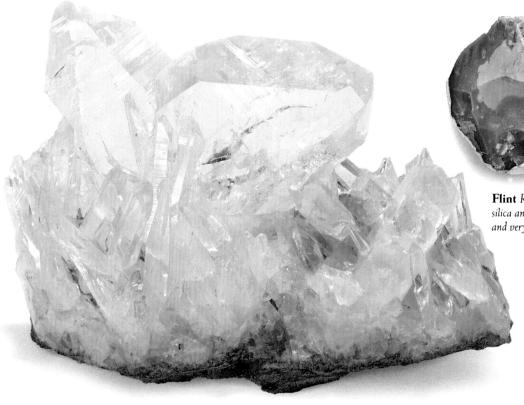

**Flint** *Rocks of flint consist of silica and are compact, hard, and very strong.*

**Rock crystal**
*Rock crystal is the colorless variety of quartz. Quartz is one of the most common minerals of the earth's crust and is found worldwide.*

## REMEDY PROFILE

**Common names** Silica, quartz, rock crystal, pure flint.
**Source** Formerly made from quartz or flint, now prepared chemically.
**Parts used** Silica.

### AILMENTS TREATED
*Silica* is mainly used for undernourishment that leads to a weakened immune system and recurrent infections, for example, colds, flu, and ear infections. It is also effective for skin and bone complaints, such as

an unhealthy complexion accompanied by acne, weak nails surrounded by hard skin, slow-to-heal fractures, slow bone growth, and fontanels that are slow to close in babies. It is also good for expelling splinters from the tissues.

Nervous system problems, for example, an inability to expel stools so that they slip back into the rectum, and migraines, where the pain starts at the back of the head and extends over one eye, are helped by *Silica*.

It is also given for glue ear (fluid in the middle ear); chronic phlegm; profuse sweating; and sleep that is disturbed by stress and overwork.
**Symptoms better** In hot, humid summer weather; from wrapping up warmly, especially the head.
**Symptoms worse** In the morning; in a draft; with cold and damp; for the new moon; from getting cold on undressing; if sweating is suppressed; from washing; from swimming; lying on the left side.

# Silica-the type

## PERSONALITY & TEMPERAMENT

*Silica* types lack physical and mental stamina and fear being overwhelmed, and yet they show great tenacity and determination once a challenge is accepted. When engrossed in a task, they are very conscientious and obsessive about small details, and overwork to the point of exhaustion or insomnia. Their outlook and aspirations are limited by fear of failure and a tendency to remain the eternal student. Since they are not assertive, they may feel pushed around, and in turn relieve their own frustrations on subordinates. In relationships, they may remain uncommitted for fear of giving too much of themselves and being hurt.

## FOOD PREFERENCES

**Likes**
• Cold foods: raw vegetables, salads, ice cream

**Dislikes**
• Meat and cheese
• Milk (may have been reluctant to take breast milk in infancy)
• Warm foods

## FEARS

• Sharp pointed objects
• Exertion (due to lack of stamina)
• Failure in business

## GENERAL FEATURES

**Better**
• From wrapping up warmly especially the head
• In summer

**Worse**
• With cold and damp
• For the new moon
• If sweating is suppressed
• From washing or swimming
• Lying on the left side

Although *Silica* people are tenacious and stubborn, they appear fragile and passive. Despite being friendly and sensitive, they have a brittle demeanor. This is largely due to their lack of confidence and fear of responsibility, which makes them inflexible and hesitant in undertaking new tasks.

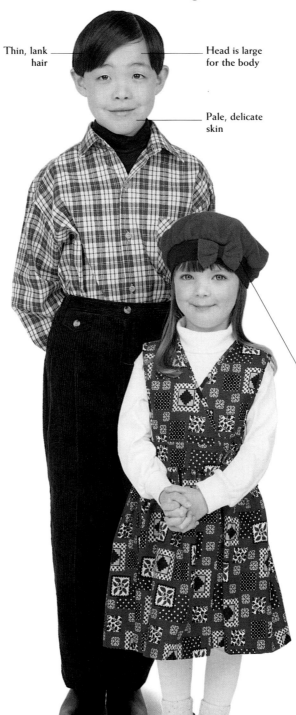

Thin, lank hair

Head is large for the body

Pale, delicate skin

Prefers to keep the head covered

### THE SILICA CHILD

• *Large, sweaty head, with pale, delicate skin, and fine hair.*

• *Small for his or her age, but well-proportioned, with small hands and feet.*

• *Feels the cold intensely and has cold, clammy extremities.*

• *Shy, delicate, and well-behaved, but self-willed and touchy, resentful of interference, and lacks stamina.*

• *Intelligent, quick-witted, and conscientious but lacks confidence.*

• *Tidy by nature and inclined to have a fixation for tiny objects, for example, small pieces of jewelry.*

• *Strong dislike and intolerance of milk.*

### Physical appearance

*Silica* types are thin and small-boned, with fine, lank hair, and a neat, tidy appearance. They are prone to cracked lips and fissures at the corners of their mouths. Their nails may be rough, brittle and yellowish. When grazed, their skin suppurates easily and is slow to heal.

### Weak areas of the body

• Nervous system
• Glands
• Bones
• Tissues
• Skin

*STRYCHNOS NUX VOMICA*

# NUX VOMICA

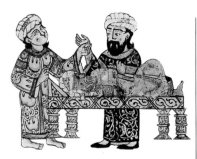

**Arabian physicians** *Strychnos nux vomica was used medicinally by 11th-century Arabian physicians.*

*Although highly poisonous, strychnine, which is extracted from the seeds of the Strychnos nux vomica tree, was used as an antidote to the plague during the Middle Ages. In small doses, it promotes the appetite, aids digestion, and increases the frequency of urination. In larger doses, it can cause severe problems in the nervous system. Digestive complaints and irritability are the key uses of the homeopathic remedy.*

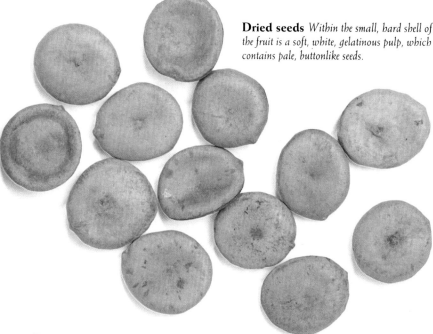

**Dried seeds** *Within the small, hard shell of the fruit is a soft, white, gelatinous pulp, which contains pale, buttonlike seeds.*

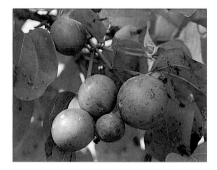

**Strychnos nux vomica** *Clusters of greenish white flowers are followed by apple-sized fruit. Strychnine is contained in the leaves, seeds, and bark of the tree.*

## REMEDY PROFILE

**Common names** Poison nut, Quaker buttons.
**Source** Grows in India, Burma, China, Thailand, and Australia.
**Parts used** Seeds.

### AILMENTS TREATED
*Nux vomica* is mainly given for extreme oversensitivity and irritability. People who need this remedy feel angry and frustrated when their expectations are not met and become ill when they bottle up their anger. This may lead them to indulge in too many stimulants, resulting in insomnia. Digestive complaints, such as indigestion, vomiting, diarrhea with painful abdominal cramps,

nausea with colicky pain, constipation, and hemorrhoids that cause rectal contractions are all helped by this remedy. These complaints may be due to the suppression of emotions, especially anger and irritability or may be brought on by overindulgence of certain foods, alcohol, and coffee.

*Nux vomica* is also good for colds with a blocked nose at night and a runny nose during the day; flu with fever and stiff, shivering, aching muscles; and coughs with retching or dry, tickly coughs with larynx pain.

Headaches and migraines, often due to a hangover, where the head feels thick or fragile on waking or as

if a nail had been driven in over the eyes, are eased by this remedy.

In women, *Nux vomica* is given for early, heavy, or irregular menstruation, and where there is faintness before menstruation. It is also used to treat cystitis; frequent urination, cramps, and morning sickness in pregnancy; and labor pain.
**Symptoms better** With warmth; from firm pressure; from washing or compresses; with sleep; when left alone; in the evening.
**Symptoms worse** In cold, dry, wintry, or windy weather; between 3 a.m. and 4 a.m.; from stimulants; from eating; from spicy foods; if touched; near noise; from mental overexertion.

# Nux vomica - the type

High-strung, energetic, competitive achievers, *Nux vomica* types work and play hard. Intolerant of criticism toward themselves, they are, however, highly critical of others, insisting on perfection.

## PERSONALITY & TEMPERAMENT

*Nux vomica* types are ambitious, thrive on challenges and decision-making, and are often found in managerial or entrepreneurial jobs. They are mentally and verbally agile and express themselves with brisk clarity and flashes of ironic wit. They are impatient and readily explode with anger. In their drive to achieve they may use alcohol or drugs to enhance their performance or to help them relax. They are likely to have a high sex drive. When ill, they are ungracious and quick to snap.

## FOOD PREFERENCES

**Likes**
- Rich, fatty foods: fatty meat cream, high-fat cheese

**Likes (and upset by)**
- Alcohol
- Coffee
- Spicy foods: chilli peppers, curries

## FEARS

- Failure in business
- Death
- Crowds and public places

## GENERAL FEATURES

**Better**
- With warmth and humidity
- Lying down for a nap or a longer sleep
- In the evening
- From applying firm pressure
- From washing or compresses

**Worse**
- In cold, dry, wintry, or windy weather
- If touched
- Near noise
- Between 3 a.m. and 4 a.m.
- From eating
- From spicy foods
- From mental overexertion

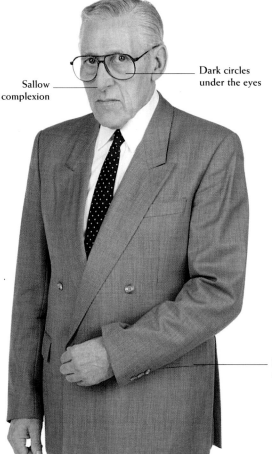

Sallow complexion

Dark circles under the eyes

Smart appearance

## THE NUX VOMICA CHILD

- *Nervous, irritable, and hyperactive.*
- *Hates to be contradicted; is inclined to throw terrible tantrums.*
- *Conscientious and competitive, but a bad loser and readily jealous.*
- *Grumpy on waking.*
- *Suffers from frequent stomachaches.*
- *As an adolescent, likely to be rebellious and defiant.*
- *Strong sense of justice and inclined to be idealistic.*

**Physical appearance**
*Nux vomica* people are lean, tense-looking, dapper individuals with an irascible air. They are inclined to have lined faces that flush in a dusky fashion when excited, sallow skin, and dark circles under the eyes.

**Weak areas of the body**
- Stomach
- Bowels
- Liver
- Lungs
- Nerves

*SULFUR*

# SULFUR

The mineral sulfur is found in every cell of the body and is especially concentrated in the hair, nails, and skin. Medicinally, it has been used for more than 2,000 years. In the past, many children were given sulfur in the form of brimstone and treacle to cleanse the bowels and skin. In orthodox medicine, sulfur is still applied externally for skin conditions such as acne. The homeopathic remedy is also used for skin and digestive complaints.

**A 16th-century hospital** *In the past, flowers of sulfur was burned to fumigate rooms occupied by those with infectious illnesses.*

### KEY USES
- Skin complaints, especially eczema where the skin is red, inflamed, itchy, and hot
- Digestive disorders
- Gynecological complaints
- Mental stress.

#### SELF-HELP
*Candidiasis* – see pp. 202–3
*Diaper rash* – see pp. 216–7
*Diarrhea* – see pp. 184–5
*Eczema* – see pp. 186–7.

**Flowers of sulfur**

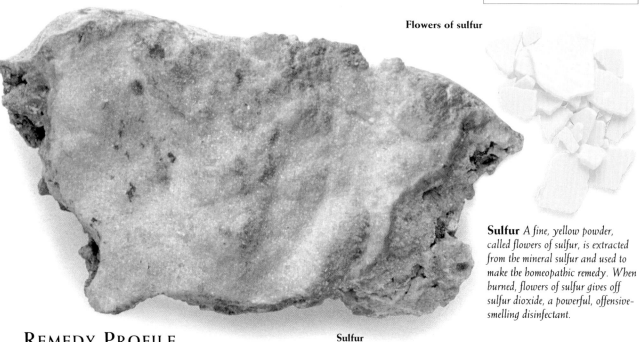

**Sulfur** *A fine, yellow powder, called flowers of sulfur, is extracted from the mineral sulfur and used to make the homeopathic remedy. When burned, flowers of sulfur gives off sulfur dioxide, a powerful, offensive-smelling disinfectant.*

**Sulfur**

## REMEDY PROFILE

**Common names** Flowers of sulfur, brimstone.
**Source** The mineral sulfur, which is found near volcanic craters and hot springs in Italy, Sicily, and the US.
**Parts used** Sulfur.

### AILMENTS TREATED
*Sulfur* is mainly used to treat skin conditions, such as eczema, candidiasis, or diaper rash where the skin looks permanently dirty and is dry, scaly, itchy, red, and worse from being scratched, and a dry scalp.

Digestive complaints that are helped by this remedy include a tendency to regurgitate food; indigestion that is worsened by drinking milk; vomiting and chronic diarrhea that occur early in the morning; hunger pain with a sinking feeling in the stomach that occurs around 11 a.m.; itchy, burning hemorrhoids; redness and itching around the anus; and anal fissures.

In women, *Sulfur* is effective for premenstrual syndrome symptoms, for example, headaches, irritability, and insomnia, and menopausal symptoms, such as flushing, dizziness, and sweating.

*Sulfur* is also given for mental stress; lack of energy and willpower; forgetfulness; irritablity; depression; disturbed sleep with nightmares; early waking; and indecision.

Other ailments helped by *Sulfur* include: fever; headaches; migraines; conjunctivitis and red eyes; chronic nasal discharge with greenish mucus; coughs with sneezing; low back pain from prolonged standing, bending, or sitting, or due to menstruation.

When ill, people who need *Sulfur* are sensitive to bad smells, and are thirsty more often than hungry.
**Symptoms better** From fresh, warm, dry air; lying on the right side.
**Symptoms worse** In the morning and at night; from alcohol; in damp and cold; in stuffy rooms; from washing; in a hot bed; wearing too many clothes; from prolonged sitting or standing; around 11 a.m.

# Sulfur-the type

Although *Sulfur* types expend a great deal of energy in imaginative and inventive thought, they are inept on a practical level. They are pedantic and egotistical with a strong need for recognition.

## PERSONALITY & TEMPERAMENT

Inclined to be belligerent and critical over minor details, *Sulfur* types can also be very open-hearted, giving generously of their time and money. They are often male executives, full of ideas and plans but surrounded by clutter. At worst, they are lazy, lacking willpower and initiative, and do not follow things through to completion.

Although easily incensed, their anger subsides quickly. They enjoy lively debate, but only on subjects of particular interest to them. Because they live life at an intellectual level, their feelings are seldom deeply affected.

## FOOD PREFERENCES

### Likes
- Sweet foods
- Fatty foods: french fries, meat fat, cream, cheese
- Spicy foods: curries
- Sour foods: pickles, lemons
- Alcohol
- Raw foods: salads
- Oysters

### Dislikes (and upset by)
- Eggs and milk
- Hot drinks

## FEARS

- Heights
- Failure in business
- Ghosts

## GENERAL FEATURES

### Better
- In fresh, dry, warm weather
- From physical exertion
- Lying on the right side

### Worse
- In stuffy rooms
- In a hot bed
- From washing
- From prolonged standing
- Around 11 a.m.

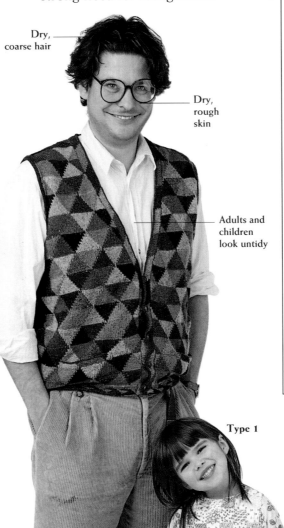

Dry, coarse hair

Dry, rough skin

Adults and children look untidy

Type 1

## THE SULFUR CHILD

### Type 1
- *Well-nourished and heavily built, with coarse, strong hair, a ruddy complexion, and red lips, ears, and eyelids.*

### Type 2
- *Thin, with spindly legs and a fairly large abdomen. Has pale, dry skin that is prone to cracking.*

### Common characteristics
- *A hearty appetite.*
- *Bright and inquisitive when stimulated, with a good memory. Adore books, but may be careless with schoolwork.*
- *Show great pride in their possessions.*
- *Tendency to show off.*
- *Lively in the evening and reluctant to go to sleep.*

### Physical appearance
*Sulfur* types have one of two appearances: they are either rotund, red-faced, and look jolly, or are lean and lanky with a slouched posture. Both types have coarse, lusterless hair, dry, scaly skin, and look unkempt, possibly in need of a bath. Even if they are smartly dressed there are generally some untidy features.

### Weak areas of the body
- Circulation
- Mucous membranes in the bowels and rectum
- Soles of the feet
- Skin
- Left side of the body

*TRIGONOCEPHALUS LACHESIS/LACHESIS MUTA*

# LACHESIS

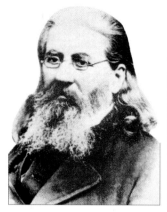

**Dr. Constantine Hering**
*(1800–80) He tested venom from the bushmaster snake on himself, thereby proving the homeopathic remedy.*

*An aggressive hunter, the bushmaster snake gets one of its common names, surukuku, from the humming noise it makes while waiting for its prey. If this snake's bite enters a vein directly, the effect can be immediately fatal because the poisons in the venom act on the nervous control of the heart. A superficial bite causes profuse bleeding and blood poisoning. The Lachesis remedy is used for circulatory problems and vascular complaints.*

## KEY USES

- Circulatory problems and vascular complaints
- Menopausal and premenstrual symptoms
- Slow-to-heal wounds
- Left-sided ailments that tend to be worse from suppressing emotions or bodily discharges.

**SELF-HELP**
*Menopause – see pp. 206–7.*

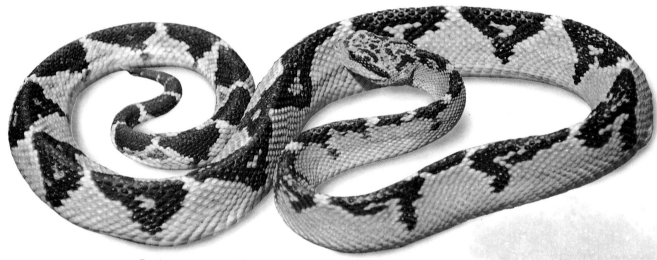

**Bushmaster snake** *The venom acts on the blood, making it more fluid and causing a tendency to hemorrhage. In turn, the homeopathic remedy made from the venom is used for wounds that bleed freely and are slow to heal.*

**Dried venom**

## REMEDY PROFILE

**Common names** Bushmaster, surukuku.
**Source** Found in South America.
**Parts used** Fresh venom.

### AILMENTS TREATED
*Lachesis* acts mainly on the blood and circulation and is used to treat engorged, throbbing veins, such as varicose veins. It is also helpful when the skin on the face, ears, fingers, and toes appears purple-blue due to circulatory problems. A weak heart; a rapid, weak, irregular pulse; palpitations; angina; and difficulty in breathing are all eased by *Lachesis*.

This is a key remedy for women during menopause and is given for menopausal hot flashes. It is also effective for premenstrual syndrome and spasmodic, congestive menstrual pain that is better for blood flow.

Throat complaints, including sore throats that are swollen and dark purple, left-sided with pain in the left ear, and worse from swallowing fluids, are helped by this remedy.

*Lachesis* is given for disorders of the nervous system, such as petit mal attacks (a type of epileptic seizure) and fainting. Other complaints it is used for include: slow-to-heal, blue-

rimmed wounds; red boils; nosebleeds; left-sided headaches; fever; hot sweats and shivering; throbbing sensations in parts of the body; ulcers and stomach pain and vomiting in appendicitis and gastrointestinal complaints; and bleeding hemorrhoids.
**Symptoms better** From having a bodily discharge; from eating; from fresh air; from cold drinks.
**Symptoms worse** From hot drinks; after hot or warm baths; with sleep; if touched; on the left side; from wearing tight clothing; from drinking alcohol; with heat or in direct sun; during menopause.

# Lachesis - the type

## PERSONALITY & TEMPERAMENT

In relationships, *Lachesis* types are inclined to be egocentric and jealous, often vacillating between love and hate for their partner. Being confined in any way is very difficult for them and they may steadfastly resist commitment. World affairs are of great concern to *Lachesis* people, who tend to embrace or reject a particular ideology. They contradict the viewpoint of others. Although they possess great creative energy, it may be sporadic and ill-sustained.

## FOOD PREFERENCES

**Likes**
- Sour foods: pickles, olives
- Starchy foods: rice, bread
- Alcohol
- Oysters

**Other factors**
- Upset by wheat and hot drinks, although *Lachesis* is one of the few types that tolerates coffee well, except during menopause

## FEARS

- Water
- Poisoning
- Burglars and strangers
- Suffocation and death

## GENERAL FEATURES

**Better**
- From having a bodily discharge, such as a bowel movement or menstruation
- From cold drinks
- From fresh air

**Worse**
- With sleep and if touched
- With heat or in direct sun
- From hot drinks
- On the left side
- From wearing tight clothing
- During menopause

*Lachesis* types are perceptive, creative, and ambitious. They live life intensely and have a sense of physical and mental congestion that can be relieved only by a form of discharge, such as a nosebleed or expressing their views.

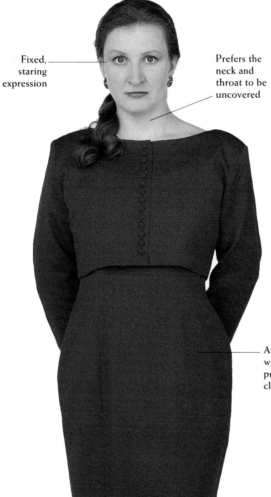

Fixed, staring expression

Prefers the neck and throat to be uncovered

Ailments are worsened by the pressure of tight clothes

## THE LACHESIS CHILD

- *Jumpy, talkative, and "hyper."*
- *Prone to behavioral and emotional problems, often due to jealousy, for example, following the birth of a sibling.*
- *Possessive of friends.*
- *May test parents and teachers to the limit, for example, inciting peers to misbehave, stealing, or tormenting pets.*
- *Can be very hurtful to peers, with a snakelike ability to pinpoint a victim's most sensitive spot.*

**Physical appearance**
*Lachesis* types are generally freckled redheads who may be overweight with a somewhat bloated appearance, or they are dark-haired, lean, and energetic. They have a pale complexion with a purplish hue. There is a tendency to flick the tip of the tongue at intervals over the top lip.

**Weak areas of the body**
- Nervous system
- Left side of the body
- Blood and circulation
- Female reproductive organs

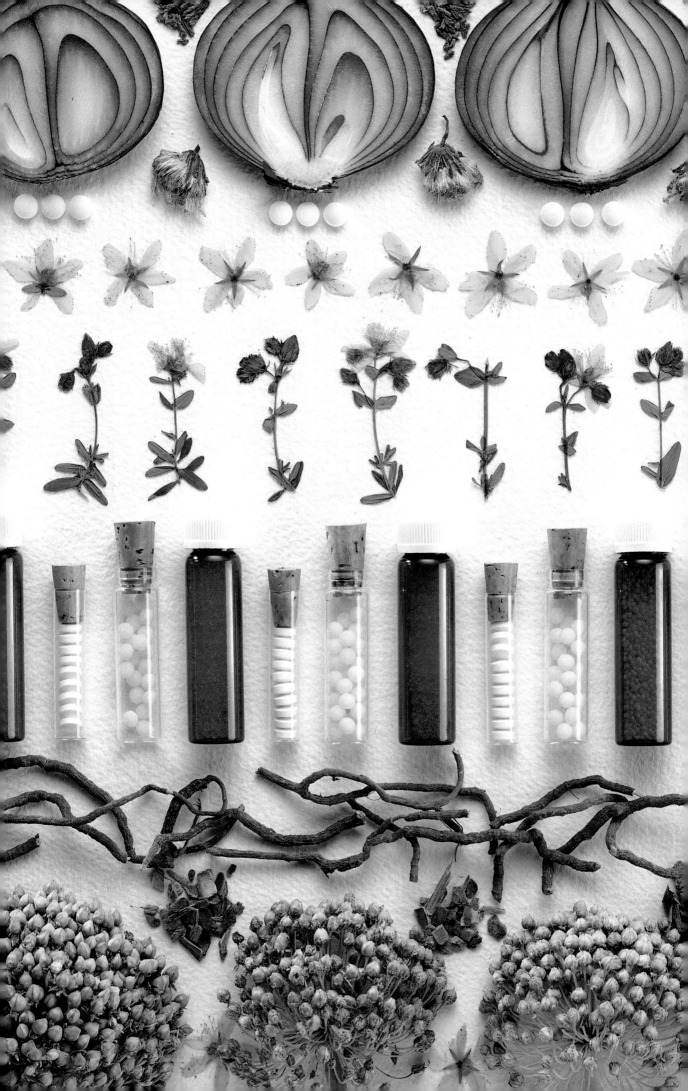

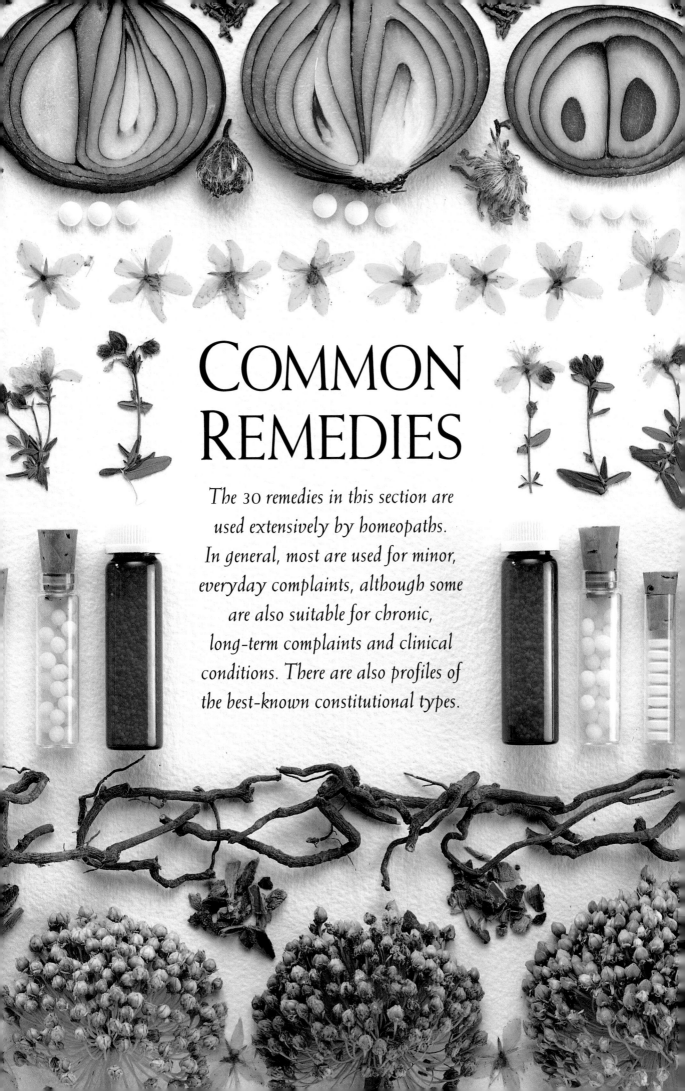

# COMMON REMEDIES

The 30 remedies in this section are
used extensively by homeopaths.
In general, most are used for minor,
everyday complaints, although some
are also suitable for chronic,
long-term complaints and clinical
conditions. There are also profiles of
the best-known constitutional types.

## ACONITUM NAPELLUS
# ACONITE

This deadly plant has been used throughout history as an arrow poison in hunting. Its name is derived from the Latin word acon for "dart." The homeopathic remedy was proved by Hahnemann in 1805 and was used extensively for fevers and sudden complaints with severe pain, which had up until then been treated by bloodletting.

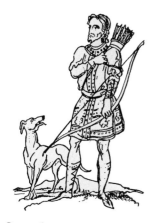

**Saxon hunter AD 730**
*Hunters dipped their arrows into the plant's juice before hunting wolves, hence the common name, wolfsbane.*

## REMEDY PROFILE

**Common names** Monkshood, friar's cap, wolfsbane.
**Source** Grows in mountainous areas of Europe.
**Parts used** Fresh root, flowers, and leaves.

### AILMENTS TREATED

*Aconite* is used to treat complaints that come on suddenly and acutely, often due to shock or a scare, exposure to dry, cold winds, and occasionally, intensely hot weather. This remedy is usually needed at the onset of symptoms of an infection, such as colds and coughs, and ear, eye, and throat complaints. It is also used for eye inflammation due to injury. Symptoms of inflammation and infection include restless, agitated sleep. The face is red, hot, flushed, and swollen, with severe burning pain, but it becomes very pale when the person gets up.

This remedy is also given for fear with associated restlessness, for example, in panic attacks with palpitations, numbness, and tingling in the body. The person looks anxious with dilated pupils; this fear often relates back to an alarming event. It is good for women who fear death during labor.
**Symptoms better** From fresh air; with warmth.
**Symptoms worse** In stuffy rooms; near music; lying on the affected area.

**Aconitum napellus**
*This highly toxic plant is the source of a remedy used for infections that come on suddenly.*

The root contains nine times more poison than the leaves

## KEY USES
- Acute infections with a sudden onset, especially in healthy people exposed to abrupt climate changes
- Fear, shock, and a fear of dying when ill
- Burning pain and numbness.

### SELF-HELP
*Absent menstruation* – see pp. 206–7
*Bereavement* – see pp. 192–3
*Coughs* – see pp. 174–5
*Fear* – see pp. 192–3
*Fear of dentists* – see pp. 164–5
*Fever in children* – see pp. 218–9
*Headaches* – see pp. 158–9
*Flu* – see pp. 174–5
*Insomnia* – see pp. 194–5
*Laryngitis* – see pp. 178–9
*Shock* – see pp. 192–3
*Sore throats* – see pp. 176–7
*Teething problems* – see pp. 216–7.

## CONSTITUTIONAL TYPE

Aconite *adults and children are strong, healthy, and full-blooded. When well, these types desire company. They tend to lack self-esteem and want to prove themselves, and may be insensitive and malicious.*
*When ill, they fear dying, even to the point of predicting the exact time of death. These people react badly to shock and have intense fears, especially of being in a crowd, and dislike going out.*

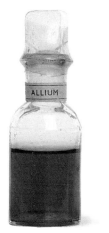

**Allium tincture** *Fresh, red onions are the source of a tincture used to make the Allium remedy.*

# ALLIUM

*The onion is among the world's oldest cultivated plants, renowned in India, China, and the Middle East for its healing properties. Onions contain a volatile oil that stimulates the tear glands and the mucous membranes of the upper respiratory tract, causing the eyes and nose to water. The homeopathic remedy is used to treat any illness in which the main symptoms include streaming eyes and a nasal discharge, such as hay fever and colds.*

## KEY USES
- Burning or neuralgic pain
- Complaints with a burning, streaming discharge, especially from the eyes and nose
- Symptoms or pains that alternate from side to side, usually from left to right.

### SELF-HELP
*Hay fever – see pp. 168–9.*

## REMEDY PROFILE

**Common name** Red onion.
**Source** Native to southwest Asia, now grown worldwide.
**Parts used** Fresh, red onion bulb.

### AILMENTS TREATED
*Allium* is used for any illness that has either burning or neuralgic pain that alternates from side to side, or a profuse, clear, watery, smarting discharge. It is especially good for colds and hay fever with watery, streaming eyes, constant sneezing, and a copious, burning nasal discharge that makes the nostrils and upper lip raw and sore. The discharge may shift from side to side, affecting only one nostril at a time. The eyelids and eyes are swollen.

This remedy is also effective for shooting neuralgic pain associated with earache in children, headaches just behind the forehead, and toothache in the molar teeth, in which the pain moves across the mouth, from one tooth to another. *Allium* is also given for the early stages of laryngitis with hoarseness; and coughs that are brought on by cold air, with a splitting, tearing sensation in the throat.
**Symptoms better** From fresh air; in cool surroundings.
**Symptoms worse** In warm, stuffy rooms; in cold, damp surroundings.

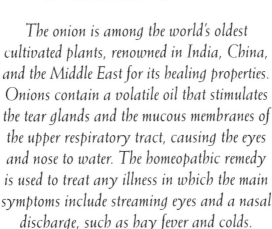

The bulb is covered in purple-red, papery skin and comprises many layers

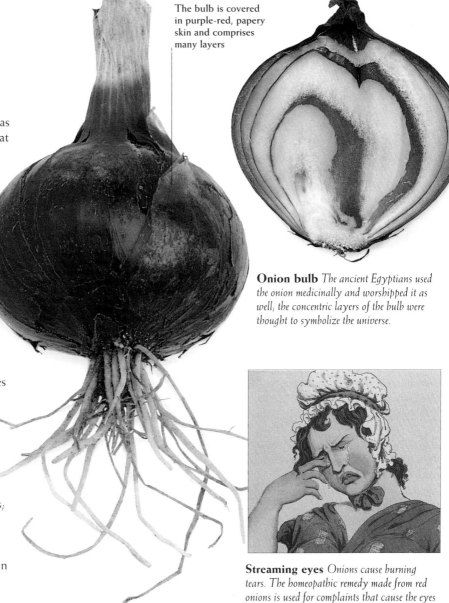

**Onion bulb** *The ancient Egyptians used the onion medicinally and worshipped it as well; the concentric layers of the bulb were thought to symbolize the universe.*

**Streaming eyes** *Onions cause burning tears. The homeopathic remedy made from red onions is used for complaints that cause the eyes to sting or water, such as hay fever.*

*APIS MELLIFICA/A.MELLIFERA*

# APIS

*Honeybees are remarkable insects and provide a range of medicinal substances. The whole bee, honey, beeswax, propolis (a sticky resin used to seal holes in the hive), royal jelly (a gel secreted to feed young queen bees), and pollen are all used. In homeopathy, the Apis remedy is used for inflammation with burning, stinging pain, especially in skin complaints where the skin is itchy, swollen and extremely sensitive to touch.*

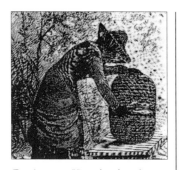

**Beekeeper** *Honeybees have been kept for honey, beeswax, and propolis, which is a natural antibiotic. In the past, propolis was given for wounds.*

x

## KEY USES

- Burning, stinging pain that is worse with heat and better with cold
- Tight, blisterlike swellings that are sensitive to touch and pressure
- Fever with a lack of thirst and dry skin
- Symptoms that start on the right side and then move to the left side.

### SELF-HELP
*Insect stings – see p. 221*
*Sore throats – see pp. 176–7*
*Hives (urticaria) – see pp. 188–9.*

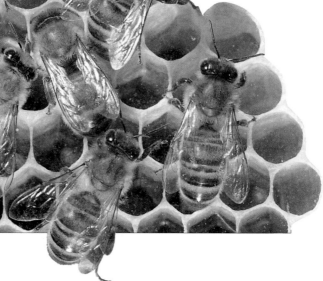

**Honeybees** *The* Apis *remedy is made from the whole bee, including the stinger. One of its main uses is to treat insect stings.*

**Actual size**

## REMEDY PROFILE

**Common name** Honeybee.
**Source** Found in Europe, Canada, the US and many other countries.
**Parts used** Whole, live bee.

### AILMENTS TREATED
*Apis* is used for skin complaints, such as hives (urticaria), bites, and stings, in which the skin becomes swollen, itchy, or burning, and sensitive to touch. It is given for urinary tract infections, such as cystitis, where there is burning, stinging pain on passing urine, and for urine retention.

Edema (fluid retention in the body tissues) and allergic conditions in the eyes, mouth, and throat (such as watery swellings on the eyelids or in the mouth that spread to the throat and obstruct breathing) are helped by *Apis*. It is also good for fever with a lack of thirst and dry, sensitive skin, a sore throat, and headaches where the head feels hot with stabbing pain.

*Apis* is given for conditions that affect the lining of the joints, chest, and abdomen, for example, arthritis, pleurisy, and peritonitis.
**Symptoms better** From bathing; from cold compresses; in cool surroundings.
**Symptoms worse** From touch; from pressure; with sleep; with heat; in hot, stuffy rooms.

**Caution** Avoid the *Apis* remedy below 30c potency during pregnancy.

### CONSTITUTIONAL TYPE

Apis *types are fiercely overprotective of their environment and jealous of any newcomer. They spend hours frantically sorting things out, but tend not to accomplish much. They are irritable, nervous, restless, and hard to please, and are often described as "queen bees" who love to organize everybody, but have a stinger in their tail for those who upset them.*

### ARNICA MONTANA
# ARNICA

*The importance of Arnica montana as a healing herb was first recognized in the 16th century. It was well-known to country people as a remedy for muscular aches and bruises. In orthodox medicine it has been used for dysentery, gout, malaria, and rheumatism. Today, it is used internally only in homeopathic doses for shock, for example, after an injury, and arnica cream is used externally for bruises and sprains.*

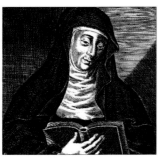

**St. Hildegard of Bingen**
*(1099–1179) A nun well-versed in medicine, St. Hildegard wrote extensively about Arnica montana.*

## KEY USES
• Shock, pain, bruising, and other injuries, and bleeding caused by injuries
• Emotional shock, for example, from bereavement.

### SELF-HELP
*Bereavement* – see pp. 192–3
*Burns & scalds* – see p. 220
*Cramps* – see pp. 156–7
*Cuts & grazes* – see p. 220
*Discomfort after dental treatment* – see pp. 164–5
*Eye injuries* – see p. 223
*Nosebleeds* – see p. 221
*Osteoarthritis* – see pp. 154–5
*Sprains & strains* – see p. 223.

## REMEDY PROFILE

**Common names** Leopard's bane, mountain tobacco, sneezewort.
**Source** Grows in the mountains of Europe, and in Siberia.
**Parts used** Whole, fresh plant in flower.

### AILMENTS TREATED
*Arnica* is an excellent first-aid remedy and is used for physical and emotional shock and injury, for example, following bereavement, an accident, surgery, dental treatment, or childbirth. Given internally, it promotes healing of damaged tissues and helps control bleeding.

It is an effective remedy, internally and externally, for joint and muscle problems, such as osteoarthritis, sore muscles due to unaccustomed exercise, cramps, bruises, and sprains.

It is also given internally for skin complaints, such as eczema and boils, concussion and black eyes, eyestrain, and fever when the head feels hot but the body feels cold.

In children, *Arnica* is given for a whooping cough, and bedwetting due to nightmares.
**Symptoms better** On starting to move; lying down with the head lower than the feet.
**Symptoms worse** With continued movement; from light pressure; with prolonged rest; with heat.
**Caution** Do not use arnica cream on broken skin as it may cause a rash.

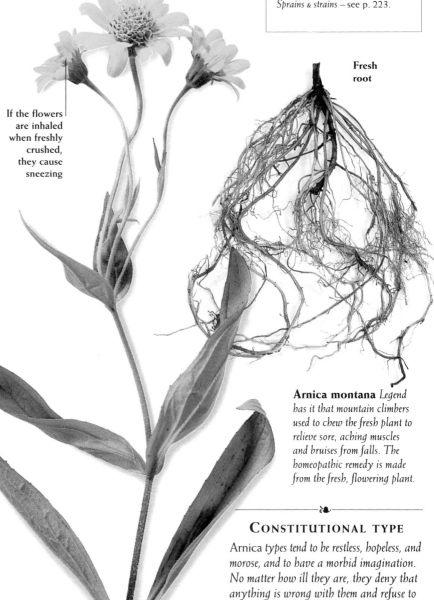

If the flowers are inhaled when freshly crushed, they cause sneezing

**Fresh root**

**Arnica montana** *Legend has it that mountain climbers used to chew the fresh plant to relieve sore, aching muscles and bruises from falls. The homeopathic remedy is made from the fresh, flowering plant.*

### CONSTITUTIONAL TYPE
*Arnica types tend to be restless, hopeless, and morose, and to have a morbid imagination. No matter how ill they are, they deny that anything is wrong with them and refuse to see a doctor. They prefer to be left alone.*

*ATROPA BELLADONNA*

# BELLADONNA

*Deadly nightshade was allegedly used in witchcraft and magic during the Middle Ages. It was also used by Italian women in eyedrops to dilate their pupils and make their eyes more attractive; bella donna means "beautiful woman." The plant contains the alkaloids atropine and hyoscine, which are used in orthodox medicine for spasms, nausea, and vertigo. Hahnemann proved the remedy in 1799 and used it to treat scarlet fever.*

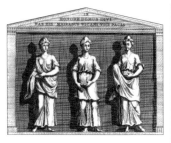

**The Greek Fates** *The generic name, Atropa, comes from the name of the Greek fate Atropus, who cuts the thread of life – a reference to the plant's poisonous nature.*

## KEY USES

- Acute complaints of sudden and violent onset with flushing and throbbing due to increased blood circulation, particularly in the head
- High fever with dilated pupils and staring eyes
- Ailments accompanied by extreme sensitivity to light, noise, touch, pressure, pain, and jarring.

### SELF-HELP

*Boils – see pp. 188–9*
*Breastfeeding problems – see pp. 212–3*
*Earache – see pp. 166–7*
*Fever in children – see pp. 218–19*
*Flu – see pp. 174–5*
*Headaches – see pp. 158–9*
*Teething problems – see pp. 216–7*
*Tonsillitis – see pp. 178–9*
*Toothache – see pp. 162–3.*

## REMEDY PROFILE

**Common name** Deadly nightshade.
**Source** Grows throughout Europe.
**Parts used** Fresh leaves and flowers.

### AILMENTS TREATED

*Belladonna* is used to treat complaints of sudden onset and infections with inflammation, such as acute fever with staring eyes, flu, tonsillitis, a sore throat, a dry, tickly cough that is made worse by talking, and earache (especially right-sided), which is worse from getting the head wet or cold. Symptoms include: throbbing pain; a pale mouth and lips; a bright red tongue; a red, hot face; and dry, flushed skin but with cold hands and feet.

Other conditions helped by *Belladonna* include: pounding headaches in which the slightest eye movement intensifies the pain; boils; seizures; labor pain; swollen, red breasts from breastfeeding; cystitis; nephritis (inflammation of the kidneys); and restless sleep. It is also given to children for teething pain and to reduce a high fever.
**Symptoms better** With warmth; standing or sitting upright; from applying warm compresses to the affected part.
**Symptoms worse** On the right side; at night; with movement, noise, and jarring; in light and sun; lying down; from pressure; in cool surroundings.

*The leaves and flowers are chopped and pounded to a pulp to make the homeopathic remedy*

**Atropa belladonna** *Although every part of this plant is poisonous, it has been used throughout history for infections and inflammations.*

## CONSTITUTIONAL TYPE

*Belladonna types are fit and very healthy, with a strong, energetic mind and body. They are lively, entertaining people. When they fall ill, they become violent and obstinate, and may hit, bite, or kick those around them. Their illnesses are always characterized by restless, agitated behavior with extreme sensitivity to light, noise, movement, or being touched.*

*AURUM METALLICUM*

# AURUM MET.

*AURUM METALLICUM*

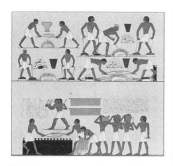

**Gold processing** *Ancient Egypt was once the richest country in gold, with over 100 mines in Nubia. Gold ornaments were symbols of rank.*

*Gold was esteemed by Arabian physicians in the 12th century for heart conditions. Medicinally, it was not used again until the early 20th century for treating tuberculosis and in a blood test for syphilis. Today, it is used in orthodox medicine for rheumatoid arthritis and in the treatment of cancer. The homeopathic remedy Aurum met. is given for specific clinical complaints ranging from depression to heart disease.*

## KEY USES

• Depression and suicidal thoughts
• Congestion of blood in various organs associated with vascular complaints, including heart disease
• Ailments characterized by general oversensitivity to noise, smell, touch, taste, and music.

**Gold** *This dense, precious, lustrous metal is still used today in orthodox medicine and dentistry.*

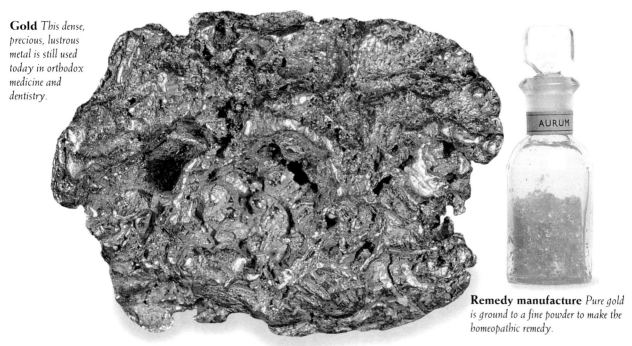

**Remedy manufacture** *Pure gold is ground to a fine powder to make the homeopathic remedy.*

## REMEDY PROFILE

**Common name** Gold.
**Source** Found in Australia, South Africa, the US, and Canada.
**Parts used** Gold.

### AILMENTS TREATED
Aurum met. is given for mental illnesses, such as depression with suicidal thoughts. People who need this remedy are very sensitive to being contradicted and may explode in anger, flushing easily, and trembling.

It is also used for increased blood circulation that causes congestion of blood in the head or other organs, for example, a headache, with obvious pulsation in the temples.

Heart disease is also helped by *Aurum met.* Cardiac symptoms include breathlessness, intermittent chest pain behind the breastbone, a feeling that the blood vessels are hot, and a feeling that the heart is going to stop. *Aurum met.* is given for liver problems, such as jaundice; sinus congestion; and bone pain associated with bone loss, where the bones are very sensitive to touch.

The remedy is also used for un-descended testicles in young boys, particularly on the right side, and for chronic inflammation of the testes.
**Symptoms better** From fresh air; after a cold bath; walking; with rest.

**Symptoms worse** From emotional stress; from mental concentration or exertion, particularly at night.

### CONSTITUTIONAL TYPE
Aurum met. *types set high goals for themselves and their driving ambition makes them workaholics. They have an excessive sense of duty and always feel that they have not done as well as they should; this makes them sensitive to others' opinions and vulnerable to being hurt. If they believe that they have failed they may become despairing. In extreme cases, this leads to severe clinical depression and suicide.*

*BRYONIA ALBA*

# BRYONIA

*Bryony was used medicinally by the ancient Greeks and Romans for the treatment of epilepsy, vertigo, paralysis, gout, hysteria, wounds, and coughs. Bryony root smells and tastes bitter, and is very poisonous, causing death within hours, usually from inflammation of the digestive tract. The homeopathic remedy, which was proved in 1834, is used primarily for slow-starting ailments with pain on the slightest movement.*

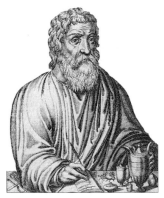

**Hippocrates** *(460–370 BC) This ancient Greek physician used bryony in his repetoire of remedies.*

## KEY USES

• Acute conditions that develop slowly with pain on the slightest movement and great thirst
• Ailments characterized by dryness, for example, of the mouth, lips, chest, and eyes.

### SELF-HELP

*Breast pain* – see pp. 210–11
*Colic in babies* – see pp. 214–5
*Coughs* – see pp. 174–5
*Flu* – see pp. 174–5
*Headaches* – see pp. 158–9
*Osteoarthritis* – see pp. 154–5
*Rheumatism* – see pp. 156–7.

## REMEDY PROFILE

**Common names** White bryony, common bryony, wild hops.
**Source** Grows in central and southern Europe.
**Parts used** Fresh root.

### AILMENTS TREATED
*Bryonia* is used to treat coughs, flu, violent headaches, and other acute conditions that develop slowly, with pain on the slightest movement, dryness, and great thirst. This remedy is also effective for inflammation in the lining of the joints, chest, and abdomen, and is given for osteoarthritis, and rheumatism with joints that are painfully hot and swollen.

Other ailments helped by this remedy include: pneumonia and pleurisy with severe chest pain near the rib cage; constipation; and colic. Symptoms include stabbing pain, a heavy feeling in the eyelids, excessive sweating, and a constricted throat.

Women who are pregnant or breastfeeding and have swollen, hard, painful breasts also benefit from this remedy.

When ill, people who need *Bryonia* are reluctant to move or speak and feel irritable and weary.
**Symptoms better** With rest; from pressure applied to the affected part.
**Symptoms worse** With movement; bending forward; with exercise.

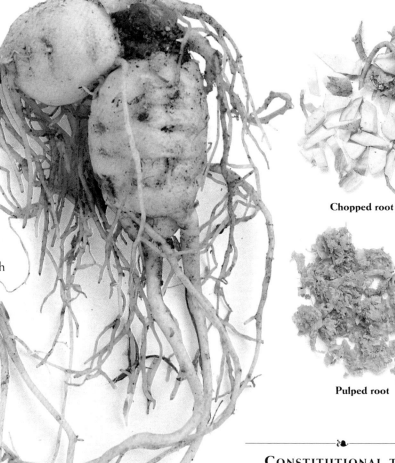

**Chopped root**

**Pulped root**

**Bryonia alba** *The fresh root is chopped and then pounded to a pulp to make the homeopathic remedy.*

### CONSTITUTIONAL TYPE

*Bryonia types tend to be very materialistic; they see life as a struggle for financial security and often have a great fear of poverty, even if they are financially successful. They are clean-living, critical, meticulous, reliable individuals. If their material security is threatened, they become irritable, anxious, and depressed.*

*CALCAREA PHOSPHORICA*

# CALC. PHOS.

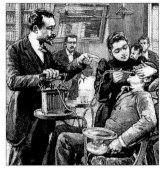

**Tooth polishing** *The mineral calcium phosphate has long been used as a polishing powder in dentistry.*

*The mineral salt calcium phosphate is the main constituent of bones and teeth. It is also found in nature in the mineral apatite. Mixed with calcium sulfate, calcium phosphate is used as a plant food. It is also used in the manufacturing of glass and porcelain. The homeopathic remedy Calc. phos. is a Schussler tissue salt (see p. 227) and is good for bone and teeth problems, including teething pain and slow growth.*

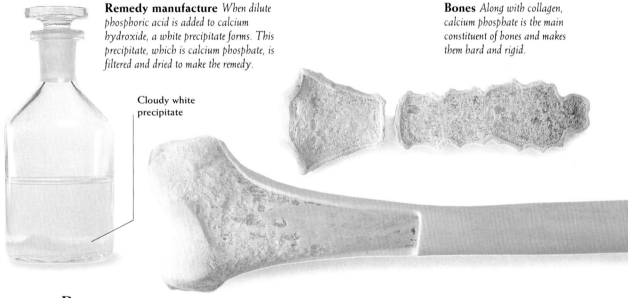

**Remedy manufacture** *When dilute phosphoric acid is added to calcium hydroxide, a white precipitate forms. This precipitate, which is calcium phosphate, is filtered and dried to make the remedy.*

Cloudy white precipitate

**Bones** *Along with collagen, calcium phosphate is the main constituent of bones and makes them hard and rigid.*

## REMEDY PROFILE

**Common name** Calcium phosphate.
**Source** Prepared chemically from dilute phosphoric acid and calcium hydroxide.
**Parts used** Calcium phosphate.

### AILMENTS TREATED
Calcium phosphate is an important mineral salt that is essential for the healthy growth of bones, teeth, and soft tissues. The *Calc. phos.* remedy is mainly used to treat bone complaints, for example, painful bones and joints, or slow-to-heal fractures and rapid tooth decay. This remedy is also good for problems such as slow growth, and growing pain in children and adolescents, with numbness or crawling sensations in the hands and feet. In children,

*Calc. phos.* is effective for problems associated with growth, such as a fontanel that is slow to close and delayed or difficult teething.

Weakness, exhaustion, and fatigue after illness can be helped by *Calc. phos.* It is also a key remedy for digestive tract disorders, such as indigestion or diarrhea with pain after eating, and is used for swollen glands due to tonsillitis or recurrent throat infections.

People who need *Calc. phos.* are unhappy and discontented. When ill, they may crave bacon rind.
**Symptoms better** In the summer; in warm, dry weather.
**Symptoms worse** In cold, damp weather; from worry or grief; lifting and overexertion; from sexual excess.

### CONSTITUTIONAL TYPE
Calc. phos. *babies are irritable, require constant attention, and they may be late walkers. As they grow older they become more sensitive and often cannot cope with school. They may become phobic or develop headaches or stomach pain. Often they appear to be bored and unhappy and are angry without any real cause.*

Calc. phos. *adults continue to feel the discontentment and unhappiness that was present as a child. They cannot understand what is wrong with them, which makes them irritable and dissatisfied. Although they appear friendly and open, they complain constantly that nothing is right. They are restless, dislike routine, need stimulation, and have trouble getting up in the morning.*

*CARBO VEGITABILIS*

# CARBO VEG.

Charcoal is made by heating wood in the absence of air. The partly-burned wood is very hard and in the past it was used to stake out property boundaries. Medicinally, charcoal is thought to be a deodorant and disinfectant and is used for gas, poorly digested food in the stomach, septic diseases, and ulceration. In orthodox medicine, it is still used in the form of charcoal tablets for gas in the lower intestine.

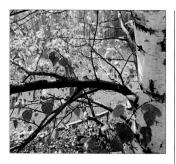

**Silver birch** *Woods from different trees make charcoals with different properties. Silver birch, beech, or poplar trees are used in homeopathy.*

## KEY USES
- Low vitality and exhaustion
- Cold, clammy skin, and a hot feeling inside the body associated with shock
- Conditions affecting the venous circulation and digestion.

### SELF-HELP
*Bloating & flatulence – see pp. 184–5*
*Cold hands & feet – see pp. 198–9*
*Indigestion – see pp. 180–1.*

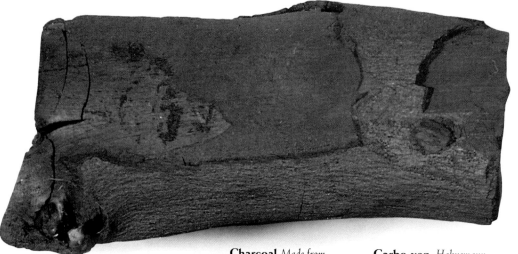

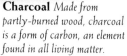

**Charcoal** *Made from partly-burned wood, charcoal is a form of carbon, an element found in all living matter.*

**Carbo veg.** *Hahnemann proved the remedy after he learned that doctors were using charcoal as a mouthwash for ulcers.*

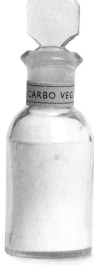

## REMEDY PROFILE

**Common name** Charcoal.
**Source** Charcoal made from beech, silver birch, or poplar trees, which grow in the Northern Hemisphere.
**Parts used** Charcoal.

### AILMENTS TREATED
*Carbo veg.* is mainly given for exhaustion, weakness, and low vitality that follows an operation or illness. Shock, paticularly after an operation, where the skin feels cold and the person looks pale but feels hot inside, is eased by this remedy.

It is also given for lack of oxygenation in the tissues due to poor venous circulation. Symptoms include cold, bluish skin on the hands, feet, and face, bleeding varicose veins, or puffy, cold legs. There may be a cold tongue and breath, hoarseness, lack of coordination, and reduced energy.

Digestive problems, regardless of diet, such as gas, indigestion, and heartburn are all helped by this remedy. Symptoms include a salty taste in the mouth, sour burping, and regurgitation of food. *Carbo veg.* is also used to alleviate headaches that occur in the morning, especially after overeating, and when the head feels heavy and hot, with nausea, dizziness, and a tendency to faint.

This remedy is helpful for asthma and spasmodic coughing, as in whooping cough, with choking, gagging, and vomiting of mucus, and in bronchitis in the elderly.

**Symptoms better** After burping; from cold, fresh air.
**Symptoms worse** In warm, wet weather; from fatty foods, milk, coffee, and wine; in the evening; lying down despite exhaustion.

### CONSTITUTIONAL TYPE

Carbo veg. *types lack interest in current affairs, fear the supernatural, prefer daylight to darkness, and tend to have very fixed ideas. They complain of never having felt really well since they had a particular illness or accident. Often, they are very tired and in a state of physical and mental collapse; they lack energy, have slow thought processes, and a patchy memory.*

*CEPHAELIS IPECACUANHA*

# IPECAC.

The medicinal use of Cephaelis ipecacuanha, *which induces vomiting, was first recorded by a Portuguese friar who lived in Brazil around 1600. It was brought to Europe about 70 years later. Today, the homeopathic remedy made from the root is mainly used for nausea and vomiting. In orthodox medicine, a drug made from the plant is used to induce vomiting in those who have taken poison or an overdose of drugs.*

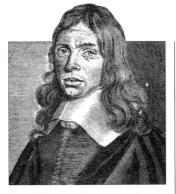

**Dr. Helvetius** (1625–1709)
*In 1670, he was selling a herbal treatment made from ipecacuanha for nausea and vomiting.*

| KEY USES |

## KEY USES
• Constant nausea, with or without vomiting
• Difficulty in breathing and a feeling of suffocation.

### SELF-HELP
*Migraines* – see pp. 160–1
*Morning sickness* – see pp. 208–9
*Nausea & vomiting* – see pp. 182–3.

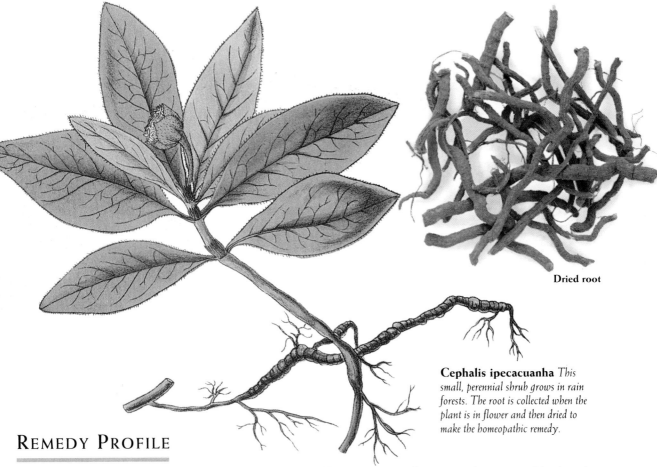

**Dried root**

**Cephalis ipecacuanha** *This small, perennial shrub grows in rain forests. The root is collected when the plant is in flower and then dried to make the homeopathic remedy.*

## REMEDY PROFILE

**Common name** Ipecacuanha.
**Source** Grows in the tropical rain forests of South and Central America.
**Parts used** Dried root.

### AILMENTS TREATED

*Ipecac.* is an excellent remedy for nausea and vomiting. Physical symptoms helped include: persistent nausea with a pale face and lips; cold or hot sweats and clamminess; nausea associated with migraines; nausea

that is not relieved by vomiting; and vomiting that is worse when bending over. Stomach ailments accompanied by a weak pulse, lack of thirst, fainting, and constant saliva production are also helped by *Ipecac.* It is effective for breathing difficulties, such as asthma, spasmodic coughing that leads to choking, and a need to cough and vomit at the same time.

Profuse bleeding with loss of bright red blood that is slow to clot, for

example, in a nosebleed, is also helped by this remedy.

A key feature of all ailments is that the tongue feels clean, not thickly coated. The person may feel continually cold on the outside and hot on the inside. Those who need this remedy are anxious, and fear death.
**Symptoms better** From fresh air.
**Symptoms worse** In winter; with movement; lying down; from stress or embarrassment; with warmth and heat.

### CHINA OFFICINALIS/CINCHONA SUCCIRUBRA

# CHINA

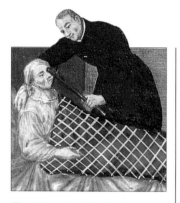

**Tending the sick** *The Jesuits introduced quinine, extracted from Peruvian bark, as a cure for malaria during the 17th century.*

*Made from Peruvian bark, the China remedy is of particular historical importance to homeopaths. The bark was the first substance that Hahnemann tested on himself, thus recording the first proving of a medicine in homeopathy (see pp. 12–15). He noted that in large doses, quinine, which is extracted from the bark, causes similar symptoms to malaria, which it cures. Today, China is an important remedy for exhaustion.*

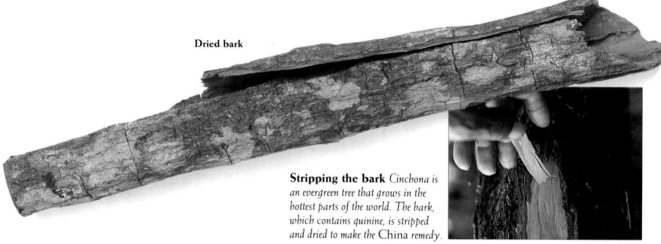

**KEY USES**
• Nervous exhaustion that results from debilitating conditions
• Weakness that results from severe loss of bodily fluids, such as from sweating, diarrhea, or vomiting.

**Dried bark**

**Stripping the bark** *Cinchona is an evergreen tree that grows in the hottest parts of the world. The bark, which contains quinine, is stripped and dried to make the China remedy.*

## REMEDY PROFILE

**Common names** Peruvian bark, cinchona bark, Jesuits' bark.
**Source** Native to the tropical forests of South America, now grown in India, Sri Lanka, and southeast Asia.
**Parts used** Dried bark.

### AILMENTS TREATED

*China* is used mainly for nervous exhaustion that results from a debilitating illness, weakness from breastfeeding, or an extreme loss of bodily fluids, for example, from sweating, vomiting, or diarrhea.

This remedy is also good for the following: headaches that are better from applying firm pressure to the painful area but are worse with light touch, such as combing the hair; neuralgia; convulsions; dizziness; tinnitus (ringing in the ears); twitchy muscles associated with fatigue; and hemorrhages and nosebleeds.

It is also given for profuse sweating, shivering, and flushing with or without fever. During sweats the person refuses to drink, but during chills wants to. The complexion appears yellowish and sallow, and the skin is very sensitive to the slightest touch.

*China* also acts on the digestive system and is good for stomach flu, gallbladder problems, and gas exacerbated by movement.

*China* is helpful for mental symptoms including lack of concentration, apathy and indifference, edginess, and uncharacteristic, angry outbursts. Sleep may be restless and difficult.

People who need this remedy may have swollen ankles, indigestion that is not relieved by burping, and a sensation of food being stuck behind the breastbone. They dislike butter and fatty foods and crave alcohol.

**Symptoms better** With sleep; with warmth; from applying firm pressure to affected parts.
**Symptoms worse** From being cold or in a draft; at night; in the autumn.

### CONSTITUTIONAL TYPE

*China types tend to be hypersensitive, idealistic, and are easily offended. Their intense, artistic personality makes it difficult for them to share their feelings with others. Instead, they express themselves creatively and are very sensitive to nature. They dislike social chat and prefer to talk about more meaningful issues. This intensity is in itself very tiring and may make them lazy, depressed, irritable, edgy, or even violent. China types are extremely imaginative, especially at night when they dream up great plans for the future or fantasize about performing heroic deeds. Such thoughts later embarrass them.*

*CIMICIFUGA RACEMOSA/ACTAEA RACEMOSA*

# CIMIC.

The rhizome of this plant was used by Native Americans as a cure for rattlesnake bites (hence its common name, rattle root) and for menstrual and labor pain. The root was also chewed as a sedative and to alleviate depression. A tea made with the herb was sprinkled in rooms to prevent evil spirits from entering. In herbalism, the root is still used as a diuretic, a cough suppressant, and to reduce inflammation and rheumatic pain.

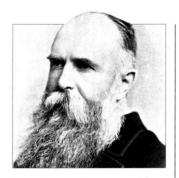

**Dr. Hughes** (1836–1902) *This English homeopath extensively proved* Cimic. *as a treatment for neck stiffness that causes headaches.*

### KEY USES
- Complaints associated with menstruation, pregnancy and birth, and menopause
- Headaches and problems in the nape of the neck
- Sighing and sadness
- Ailments characterized by marked chilliness.

**SELF-HELP**
*Headaches – see pp. 160–1.*

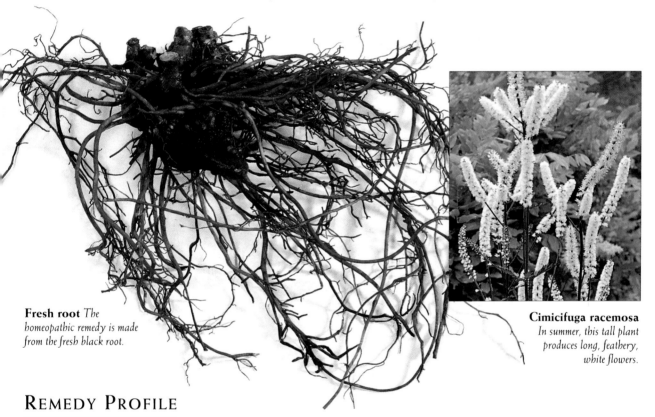

**Fresh root** *The homeopathic remedy is made from the fresh black root.*

**Cimicifuga racemosa**
*In summer, this tall plant produces long, feathery, white flowers.*

## REMEDY PROFILE

**Common names** Bugbane, black snakeroot, black cohosh, rattle root.
**Source** Grows in the US and Canada.
**Parts used** Fresh root and rhizome.

### AILMENTS TREATED
*Cimic.* is largely a women's remedy that acts on the nerves and muscles of the uterus. It is used for menstrual symptoms, such as congestion in the head before menstruation and heaviness and cramps in the small of the back during menstruation. This remedy is good for early miscarriage

and it is also helpful for common complaints in pregnancy, such as nausea and vomiting, sleeplessness and shooting pain in the uterus. Post-partum depression and menopausal symptoms, such as fainting spells and hot flashes are also helped by *Cimic.*

Neck stiffness that causes headaches is helped by *Cimic.*, as well as emotional symptoms due to a hormonal imbalance, such as sighing, sadness, anxiety, and irritability.
**Symptoms better** From wrapping up warmly; from fresh air; from pressure; with gentle, continued movement.

**Symptoms worse** With cold and damp; in a draft; from a change in weather; from alcohol; excitement.

### CONSTITUTIONAL TYPE
*These types are usually women who can be excitable, extroverted, forceful, and talkative, jumping from subject to subject, or sad, depressed, and repeatedly sighing. They have an intense emotional life and strong fears, such as death and insanity (especially during menopause).*

*CITRULLUS COLOCYNTHIS*

# COLOCYNTHIS

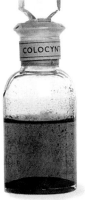

**Colocynthis tincture** *Since 1834 a remedy for digestive upsets has been made from Colocynthis tincture.*

*Ancient Greek physicians used this fruit as a drastic purgative and for dropsy, lethargy, mania, and to induce abortion. The seeds are thought to be highly nutritious, but if the bulk of the fruit is eaten, a resinous substance called colocynthin is released, which acts on the bowels, causing inflammation and cramps. The homeopathic remedy is used for these same symptoms as well as colicky pain and other digestive complaints.*

### KEY USES
- Extreme anger and indignation that causes colicky or neuralgic pain
- Digestive upsets
- Headaches associated with anger or embarrassment.

### SELF-HELP
*Colic in babies – see pp. 214–5*
*Stomach flu – see pp. 182–3.*

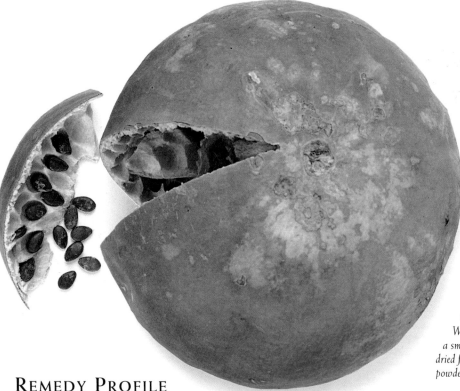

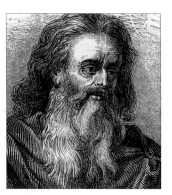

**Prophet Elisha** *It is said that the prophet Elisha turned bitter apple, a poisonous gourd, into an edible fruit during a famine in Gilgal.*

**Citrullus colocynthis**
*When dried, the fruit resembles a small, orange pumpkin. The dried fruit, without the seeds, is powdered to make the remedy.*

## REMEDY PROFILE

**Common names** Bitter apple, bitter cucumber.
**Source** Grows in hot, dry regions worldwide.
**Parts used** Dried fruit, without the seeds.

### AILMENTS TREATED
The main conditions treated with *Colocynthis* are characterized by colicky or neuralgic pain caused by suppressed anger. It is very effective for headaches, facial neuralgia, stomach pain accompanied by nausea or vomiting, severe abdominal pain

that is eased by lying down with the knees drawn up, and abdominal pain with diarrhea. Nerve pain around the kidneys or ovaries, gout, sciatica (pain that spreads along the sciatic nerve), rheumatism, and dizziness caused by holding the head to one side due to rheumatism in the neck, are all helped by this remedy.

People who need *Colocynthis* suffer from pent-up anger. Often this anger or irritability is made worse by questioning or indignation.
**Symptoms better** With warmth; from pressure; from passing gas.

**Symptoms worse** From eating and drinking; in damp, cold weather; from being angry or indignant.

### CONSTITUTIONAL TYPE
*These types are reserved, with a strong sense of justice and of what is right and wrong. If their opinion is contradicted they become very upset, especially if they feel slighted or humiliated. After becoming angry or indignant they may suffer physical complaints, such as cramps, digestive complaints, and neuralgia.*

*CUPRUM METALLICUM*

# CUPRUM MET.

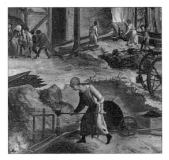

**Mining** *Copper was the first metal used to make tools and weapons. It is often mixed with other metals, for example with tin, to make bronze.*

*Medicinally, copper was once used as an ointment to heal wounds. Copper poisoning was first recognized in coppersmiths, some of whom suffered from colic, coughs, and malnutrition. In large doses, copper is toxic and can lead to convulsions, paralysis, and even death. Today, nervous system problems and respiratory complaints are among the conditions treated with this homeopathic remedy, which was proved in 1834.*

### KEY USES
• Cramps and muscular spasms
• Tiredness or exhaustion from mental exertion
• Respiratory problems.

**SELF-HELP**
*Cramps – see pp. 156–7.*

**Copper** *This reddish gold metal is powdered to make the homeopathic remedy. Copper, which is found in many foods, is essential for bone growth.*

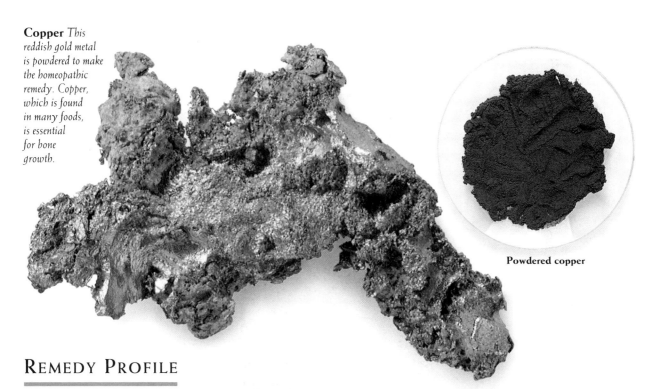

**Powdered copper**

## REMEDY PROFILE

**Common name** Copper.
**Source** Found in rocks worldwide.
**Parts used** Copper.

### AILMENTS TREATED
*Cuprum met.* mainly affects the nervous system and is used to treat cramps that start with twitching and jerking in the toes and then spread deep into the feet, ankles, and calves. This remedy is effective in the treatment of epilepsy, with muscular spasms and convulsions that start in the fingers and toes and spread to the center of the body. It is also an important remedy for exhaustion caused by mental exertion.

*Cuprum met.* is good for respiratory problems, such as asthma and whooping cough, in which there may be short periods when breathing seems to stop. The person looks pale and they may turn blue; when drinking they may make a gurgling noise.

People who need this remedy are changeable and alternate from being yielding to headstrong. They may cry before lapsing into sullenness. Suppression of any emotions, such as anger, or bodily discharges, such as perspiration by using antiperspirants, aggravates their symptoms.
**Symptoms better** From cold drinks; from perspiring.

**Symptoms worse** In hot weather; from vomiting; if touched.

### CONSTITUTIONAL TYPE
Cuprum met. *types are serious, self-critical, and have intense emotions that are strongly suppressed. Because they do not express their feelings, they seem extremely unforthcoming. Problems often start in adolescence, when they suppress their sexual urges. Cuprum met. children may be destructive. They cannot bear others to be near them and will hold their breath from anger until they turn blue in the face.*

## *DROSERA ROTUNDIFOLIA*
# DROSERA

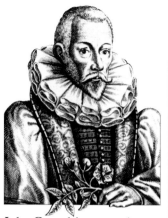

**John Gerard** (1545–1612)
*According to Gerard, the sundew plant was used by 16th-century physicians to treat tuberculosis.*

*This small, carnivorous plant traps insects inside its leaves and digests them with a fluid secreted from glands on the upper surface. The plant was used by Asian physicians for skin eruptions and during the Middle Ages it was used to treat the plague. When eaten by sheep, the fresh plant causes a severe, spasmodic cough similar to that of whooping cough. This led to the homeopathic proving and its use as a cough remedy.*

### KEY USES
- Violent, hollow-sounding coughs, such as in whooping cough, that are worse after midnight
- Growing pains and bone pain
  - Restlessness and obstinacy.

## REMEDY PROFILE

**Common names** Sundew, red rot, youthwort, moorgrass.
**Source** Grows in Europe, India, China, South America, and the US.
**Parts used** Whole, fresh plant in flower.

**Drosera rotundifolia**
*Found in bogs and heaths, this tiny plant grows low to the ground. The juice of the fresh plant is caustic, acting on the respiratory system.*

The flowers open in the early morning and close up in full sun

### AILMENTS TREATED
*Drosera* is mainly a cough remedy, and it is used to treat violent coughs that are spasmodic, deep, barking, and hollow, such as in whooping cough. The sensation of a feather or crumb in the larynx sets off the cough. The cough is worse after midnight and, in the acute stages, ends in gagging, vomiting, nosebleeds, and cold sweating followed by talkativeness.

This remedy is also good for growing pains, with a tingling sensation in the leg bones, and bone pain that is better for stretching. Other symptoms helped by *Drosera* include: a hoarse, deep, and toneless voice; stiffness; and inflexible ankles.

When ill, people who need this remedy are restless, obstinate, anxious when alone, have difficulty concentrating, fear ghosts, have a sense of persecution, and suspect they will be told bad news.
**Symptoms better** From pressure; from fresh air; from walking; with movement; sitting up in bed; in quiet.
**Symptoms worse** After midnight; lying down; from talking, singing, eating cold food and drinking; from weeping; in a warm bed.

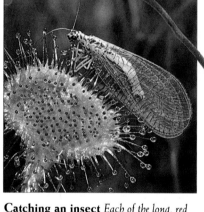

**Catching an insect** *Each of the long, red hairs on the leaves of the sundew plant contains a gland that secretes a fluid that traps and digests insects. This secretion is most prolific in full sun.*

*EUPHRASIA OFFICINALIS/E. STRICTA*

# EUPHRASIA

*This small wildflower was first mentioned in 1305 as a medicine for the eyes. In the 14th and 15th centuries, Scottish highlanders used an infusion of* Euphrasia officinalis *for affected eyes. In the 19th century it was also given for coughs, hoarseness, earache, and headaches. Today, it is used by herbalists as an antiseptic and to reduce inflammation.*

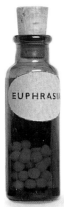

**Euphrasia remedy** *Homeopaths use* Euphrasia *primarily as a first aid remedy for the eyes, ranging from sore, tired, swollen eyes to eye injuries.*

### KEY USES
• Eye complaints characterized by watery, burning, stinging eyes
• Eye injuries or inflammation
• Hay fever with an irritating discharge from the eyes but a bland nasal discharge.

**SELF-HELP**
Conjunctivitis – see pp. 168–9
Eye injuries – see p. 223
Hay fever – see pp. 168–9

## REMEDY PROFILE

**Common name** Eyebright.
**Source** Grows in Europe and the US.
**Parts used** Whole, fresh plant in flower.

### AILMENTS TREATED
*Euphrasia* is mainly used for eye complaints such as conjunctivitis, blepharitis (inflammation of the eyelids), iritis (inflammation of the iris), dimmed vision, intolerance of bright light, sticky mucus, or small blisters on the cornea (surface of the eye), and dry eyes that accompany menopause. It is also effective for eye injuries or whenever the eyes are watery or stinging, with a copious, burning, sticky discharge.

Colds and hay fever accompanied by hot, red cheeks and watery mucus benefit from this remedy. Hay fever sufferers, for whom the eyes are mainly affected, are helped by *Euphrasia*. The eyes become swollen and irritated, but there is a bland nasal discharge.

It is also used to treat splitting headaches, constipation, and the early stages of measles. In women, it is given for short, painful menstruation in which the flow lasts only one hour a day, and in men for inflammation of the prostate gland.
**Symptoms better** From coffee; lying down in a darkened room.
**Symptoms worse** In warm, windy weather; in bright light; from being indoors; in the evening.

**Euphrasia officinalis** *This plant's delicate flowers are white, lilac, or purple and variegated with yellow. It has long been used as a cure for eye complaints.*

**The Three Graces** Euphrasia, *which preserves eyesight, is derived from euphrosyne, the Greek word for "gladness." Euphrosyne, one of the three Graces, was well known for her joy. It is thought that the plant was named for her because of its ability to help eyesight, which brings happiness to the life of the sufferer.*

*FERRUM PHOSPHORICUM*

# FERRUM PHOS.

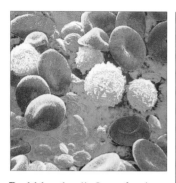

**Red blood cells** *Iron is found in red blood cells as part of hemoglobin, which carries oxygen around the body.*

*Made from iron phosphate, Ferrum phos. is a Schussler tissue salt (see p. 227). Schussler believed Ferrum phos. was most beneficial in the first stages of inflammation, when extra blood flows into the affected tissues and can cause congestion. In such cases it strengthens the blood vessel walls, thereby reducing the likelihood of congestion. The homeopathic remedy is also used for the early stages of inflammatory conditions.*

## KEY USES

• The early stages of inflammation, fever, and infection before any other definite symptoms have appeared
• Coughs and colds with a slow onset.

### SELF-HELP
*Colds – see pp. 172–3*
*Fever in children – see pp. 218–9.*

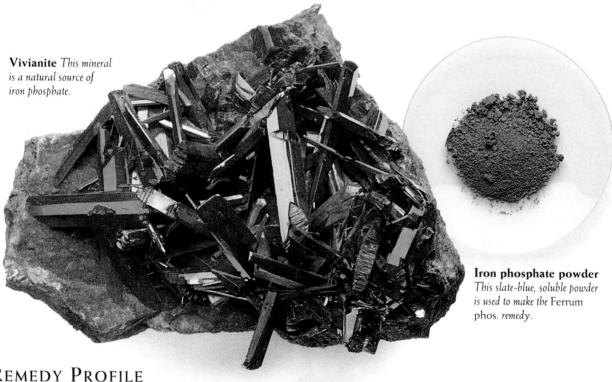

**Vivianite** *This mineral is a natural source of iron phosphate.*

**Iron phosphate powder** *This slate-blue, soluble powder is used to make the Ferrum phos. remedy.*

## REMEDY PROFILE

**Common name** Iron phosphate.
**Source** Prepared chemically from iron sulfate, sodium phosphate, and sodium acetate.
**Parts used** Iron phosphate.

### AILMENTS TREATED
*Ferrum phos.* is used for the onset of infections and inflammations. The following are helped by it: colds that start slowly and may be accompanied by a nosebleed; slow-starting fevers and dry, hacking coughs with chest pain; laryngitis; headaches that are eased by cool compresses; earache; rheumatism accompanied by a

temperature and shooting pain that recedes with gentle exercise; indigestion with sour burping; gastritis with vomiting of undigested food; and the early stages of dysentery with blood in the stools.

Other symptoms helped by *Ferrum phos.* include a pale face that flushes easily, a weak and rapid pulse, and chills starting in the early afternoon.

In women, *Ferrum phos.* is given for a short menstrual cycle, dragging pain in the uterus; vaginal dryness, and stress incontinence at night. People who need this remedy dislike meat and milk and crave caffeine.

**Symptoms better** From gentle exercise; from cold compresses.
**Symptoms worse** With heat; in the sun; from jarring and movement; if touched; lying on the right side; suppressing perspiration; at night; between 4 a.m. and 6 a.m.

### CONSTITUTIONAL TYPE

Ferrum phos. *types are thin, often with a slight flush to their skin. Open-natured and alert, they have an abundance of ideas. They tend to suffer from gastrointestinal and respiratory problems.*

*GELSEMIUM SEMPERVIRENS*

# GELSEMIUM

*This beautiful climbing plant with fragrant yellow flowers is poisonous. In large doses it interferes with breathing and movement, causing paralysis. Medicinally, it has been used since the 1840s, when it is said a Mississippi farmer who ate the root in error was cured of the fever he had. This fortuitous recovery eventually led to the plant's use as a fever cure in herbalism and, subsequently, the homeopathic proving.*

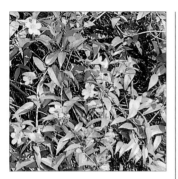

**Carolina jasmine** *This striking plant grows beside streams and along the sea coast from Virginia to Florida.*

## KEY USES

- Conditions of the nervous system
- Headaches and eye problems
- Colds and flu
- Fears and phobias.

### SELF-HELP
*Fear of dentists – see pp.164–5*
*Flu – see pp. 174–5*
*Shock – see pp. 194–5*
*Sore throats – see pp. 176–7.*

## REMEDY PROFILE

**Common names** Carolina jasmine, yellow jasmine, false jasmine.
**Source** Native to the southern US.
**Parts used** Fresh root.

### AILMENTS TREATED
*Gelsemium* mainly affects the brain and spinal cord, the motor nerves, muscles, eyelids, and mucous membranes. It alleviates the following: headaches that intensify with movement or bright light and feel as if there is a tight band around the head; a sore scalp due to nerve inflammation; muscle pain associated with fever; nervous disorders, such as multiple sclerosis; uterine pain and painful menstruation; drooping, heavy eyelids; achy right-eye pain; a sore throat with red tonsils, difficulty swallowing and earache; and summer colds.

It is given for feverish symptoms, such as a sweaty, flushed face, an unpleasant taste in the mouth, a furred, trembling tongue, twitching muscles that feel cold and tingly, chills with waves of heat along the spine, and a lack of thirst.

It is also used for fears and phobias, such as surgery or going to the dentist, and fear after a shock. All are accompanied by trembling. Over-excitement that causes the heart to miss a beat, drowsiness, and insomnia are also helped by *Gelsemium*.

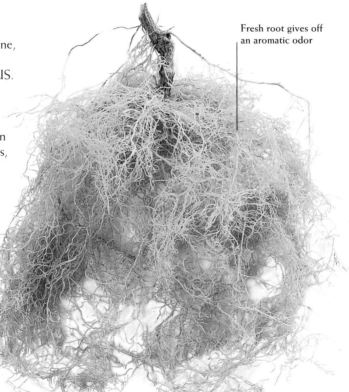

Fresh root gives off an aromatic odor

**Gelsemium sempervirens root**
*Bitter and extremely toxic, the fresh root acts on the spinal cord, and affects the respiratory system, slowing breathing.*

**Symptoms better** After urinating; from stimulants or alcohol; from perspiring; bending forward.
**Symptoms worse** In the sun; in heat and humidity; in damp and fog; near tobacco smoke; from excitement, stress, or worry about symptoms of an illness or a public performance.

**Gelsemium remedy** *This remedy is used for ailments ranging from fears and phobias to infections with feverish symptoms.*

### CONSTITUTIONAL TYPE

Gelsemium *types look dull and heavy with a blue tinge to their skin and are often heavy smokers. Their main complaint is weakness. They tend to be cowardly and the remedy has often been used to counteract cowardice on the battlefield. It is also one of the main remedies for performers who suffer from stage fright. Due to mental weakness, fears, and phobias, this type may be unable to lead an active life.*

*HAMAMELIS VIRGINIANA*

# HAMAMELIS

*The bark of the twigs and outer layer of the root of witch hazel, which draws body tissues together, is used in herbalism to treat inflamed veins, such as hemorrhoids. In orthodox medicine, it was once used as a lotion for skin rashes, burns, and insect bites. The homeopathic remedy was proved by Dr. Hering in 1850 (see p. 17) and is used for varicose veins and chilblains.*

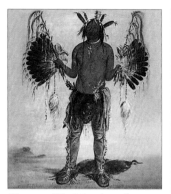

**Shaman** *Witch hazel was first used by Native Americans.*

### KEY USES

- Weak, inflamed veins and bleeding
- Bruising and soreness
- Nosebleeds
- Weakness from blood loss caused by a burst inflamed vein
- Depression.

**SELF-HELP**
*Hemorrhoids – see pp. 184–5*
*Varicose veins – see pp. 198–9.*

## REMEDY PROFILE

**Common names** Witch hazel, spotted alder, snapping hazelnut.
**Source** Native to the eastern and central US and Canada, now grown in Europe.
**Parts used** Fresh bark of twigs and outer layer of the root.

### AILMENTS TREATED

The chief use of *Hamamelis* is to treat hemorrhoids and varicose veins where the veins are weak and inflamed, and venous bleeding that is slow to stop, such as in nosebleeds. It is good for chilblains associated with inflamed veins.

This remedy also alleviates: headaches that are better after nosebleeds; sore, bruising pain due to injury; painful, bloodshot, or black eyes; and coughs with blood-flecked phlegm.

Pain during ovulation or from heavy menstrual bleeding, with a bruised feeling in the abdomen and inflammation of the uterus or ovaries, is also eased by this remedy.

*Hamamelis* is useful in the treatment of depression, when the person wishes to be left alone, wants others to show respect, and feels restless and irritable, with grandiose ideas.
**Symptoms better** From fresh air; from reading, thinking, or talking.
**Symptoms worse** From warm, damp air; from pressure; with movement.

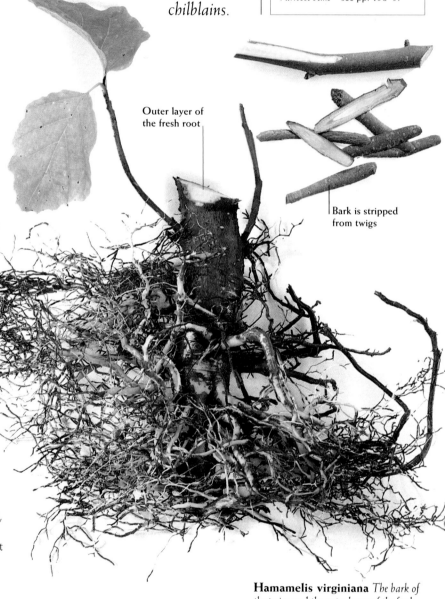

Outer layer of the fresh root

Bark is stripped from twigs

**Hamamelis virginiana** *The bark of the twigs and the outer layer of the fresh root are chopped and pounded to a pulp to make the remedy. The binding and contracting properties of the bark make Hamamelis an excellent remedy for internal and external bleeding.*

*HEPAR SULFURIS CALCAREUM*

# HEPAR SULF.

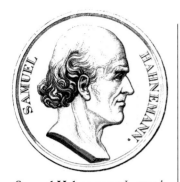

**Samuel Hahnemann** *In 1794 he prepared calcium sulfide by using calcium carbonate from oyster shells and heating it with flowers of sulfur.*

*Before Hahnemann's time, calcium sulfide was used externally to treat itching, rheumatism, gout, goiter, and tubercular swellings. In the 18th century, Hahnemann used the homeopathic remedy made from calcium sulfide as an antidote for the side effects of mercury, which was used extensively in the treatment of many illnesses. In orthodox medicine, calcium sulfide has been used for acne and boils.*

## KEY USES
- Infection, especially with the formation of pus
- Ailments characterized by sharp pain, sour smelling secretions, and sensitivity to touch, pain, and noise
- Sore throat with ear pain on swallowing.

### SELF-HELP
*Acne* – see pp. 188–9
*Boils* – see pp. 188–9
*Earache* – see pp. 166–7
*Sinus congestion* – see pp. 170–1
*Tonsillitis* – see pp. 178–9.

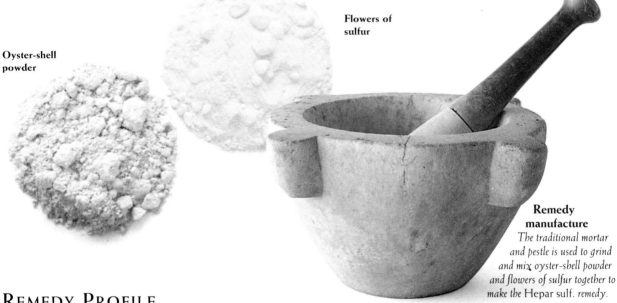

**Oyster-shell powder**

**Flowers of sulfur**

**Remedy manufacture**
*The traditional mortar and pestle is used to grind and mix oyster-shell powder and flowers of sulfur together to make the Hepar sulf. remedy.*

## REMEDY PROFILE

**Common names** Crude calcium sulfide.
**Source** Prepared chemically by heating together oyster-shell powder and flowers of sulfur.
**Parts used** Impure calcium sulfide.

### AILMENTS TREATED
*Hepar sulf.* is mainly used when there is an infection, for example, in tonsillitis, earache, and skin complaints where the skin is sensitive to touch, moist, and suppurates easily. This remedy helps expel pus, such as in infected pimples in acne, or boils that are very sensitive to touch and ready to burst. It is also given for the following: sore throat with ear pain on swallowing and loss of voice or

hoarseness; sinus congestion; ulceration or inflammation of the eyes; cold sores and mouth ulcers; colds that start with an itchy, tickly throat; a dry, hoarse cough or a crowing cough with loose, rattling phlegm in the chest; a chesty cough brought on by exposure to cold air; and flu with a fever, sneezing, sweating, and a need for warmth.

When ill, people helped by this remedy are very sensitive to cold air, touch, pain, and any kind of disturbance. All of their bodily secretions, such as urine, persipiration, and stools smell sour. They are anxious and irritable, with unreasonable likes and dislikes, and tend to be hasty and to take offense easily.

**Symptoms better** From eating; from applying warm compresses to the affected parts; from being warm; from wrapping up the head.
**Symptoms worse** From cold air; from getting cold on undressing; from touching affected parts.

### CONSTITUTIONAL TYPE
*These types are overweight, flabby, pale, sluggish, and rather depressed. They look as though they have been through a lot. They are vulnerable and sensitive to pain, and often complain in a way that is out of proportion to their disease. They are restless, but this is concealed by outward calm and by looking hard done by.*

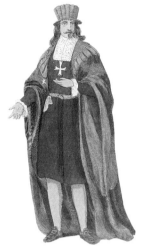

**Knight of St. John** *It is said that St.-John's-wort takes its name from the Knights of St. John of Jerusalem.*

## HYPERICUM PERFORATUM
# HYPERICUM

*The 16th-century herbalist John Gerard described this brightly flowering herb as "a most precious remedy for deep wounds." Because the juice from the crushed flowers is blood red, it was thought to be a good wound herb. Today, it is still used in herbalism to treat jaundice and fevers, and as a tonic for the kidneys and nervous system. In homeopathy its main use has always been, and still is, to treat nerve pain after injury.*

### KEY USES
- Injuries to the nerves with nerve pain
- Severe shooting pain that travels upward
- The effects of head injuries
- Asthma that is worse in foggy weather.

### SELF-HELP
*Cuts & grazes* – see p. 220
*Discomfort after dental treatment* – see pp. 164–5.

## REMEDY PROFILE

**Common name** St.-John's-wort.
**Source** Native to Europe and Asia, now grown worldwide.
**Parts used** Whole, fresh plant in flower.

### AILMENTS TREATED
*Hypericum* is used to treat shooting nerve pain that usually travels upward and nerve injuries, for example, after an operation or accident. It is the most important remedy to use whenever there is an injury to any part of the body with a high concentration of nerve endings, for example, the fingers, toes, spine, eyes, lips, nailbeds, and head. *Hypericum* is effective for concussion with sensations in the head, such as an ice-cold feeling, and eye injuries. It acts on the spinal nerves, and is given for severe back pain that travels up or down the spine.

This is an excellent first-aid remedy for any kind of puncture wound, for example, from nails, splinters, or bites, and crushed fingers or toes.

Other ailments for which the remedy is used include: asthma that is worse in foggy weather; toothache with pulling or tearing pain; and discomfort after dental treatment.

*Hypericum* is also used for nausea; indigestion, when a person has a coated tongue with a clear tip; diarrhea; bleeding, painful hemorrhoids; nerve pain in the rectum; and late menstruation accompanied by a headache. It is useful in the treatment of depression and drowsiness.

**Symptoms better** Tilting the head backward.
**Symptoms worse** In cold, damp, or foggy weather; in hot, stuffy rooms; if touched; getting cold on undressing.

When bruised, the flowers produce a red juice

**Hypericum perforatum** *The dark green leaves are full of tiny holes, which are glands that secrete the blood-red essential oil. The tincture (see p. 221) is good for cuts, scrapes, and grazes.*

*KALI BICHROMICUM*

# KALI BICH.

*The source of Kali bich., potassium dichromate is a caustic and corrosive compound. It is widely used in industry in dyestuff manufacture, calico printing, photography, and for electric batteries. The homeopathic remedy was first proved in 1844. Like many of the "Kali" remedies, it is excellent for the treatment of mucus and other types of discharge, for example, from the vagina, urethra, and stomach.*

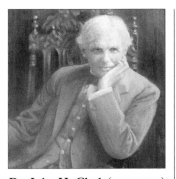

**Dr. John H. Clark** (*1853–1931*)
*This famous homeopath proved Kali bich. to be a good remedy for vomiting.*

## KEY USES
• Thick, stringy, yellow or white mucus and other forms of discharge
• Pain that shifts rapidly from one part of the body to another and appears and disappears regularly.

### SELF-HELP
*Glue ear* – see pp. 218–9
*Sinus congestion*– see pp. 170–1.

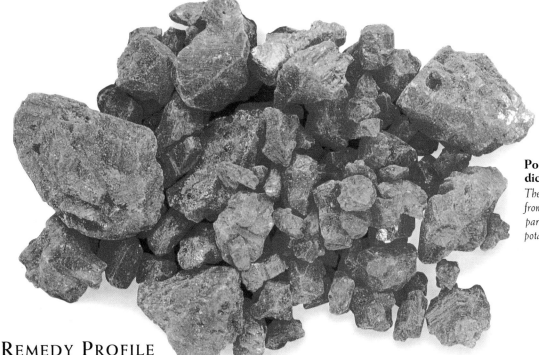

**Potassium dichromate**
*The remedy is made from the bright orange particles of pure potassium dichromate.*

## REMEDY PROFILE

**Common names** Potassium dichromate; potassium bichromate.
**Source** Prepared chemically by adding yellow potassium chromate in solution to a stronger acid.
**Parts used** Potassium dichromate.

### AILMENTS TREATED
*Kali bich.* is usually given for complaints affecting the mucous membranes, especially in the nose, throat, vagina, urethra, and stomach. It is an important remedy for conditions with excessive mucus, colds that turn into sinus congestion with pressure and fullness in the nose, and glue ear (fluid in the middle ear), with a sensation of fullness in the ear.

It is also used to treat joint problems with rheumatic pain that appears and disappears suddenly, moves around the affected part rapidly, and is aggravated by a sudden change to hot weather. Digestive disorders, such as nausea and vomiting of yellow mucus, also benefit from *Kali bich.*

Migraines, which start at night, or are better from firm pressure at the root of the nose but worse bending over, are eased by this remedy.

When ill, people who need *Kali bich.* are chilly and extremely sensitive to the cold. However, they feel worse in hot summer weather.
**Symptoms better** With heat; with movement; from eating; vomiting.

**Symptoms worse** Between 3 a.m. and 5 a.m.; in cold, wet weather; in the summer; from waking; from getting cold on undressing; alcohol.

### CONSTITUTIONAL TYPE
Kali bich. *types are conservative, proper, down-to-earth, and very moral. They are sticklers for detail and want everything to be done on a regular basis. As a result their life has to be lived according to a strict routine. They eat, sleep, and work following a rigid timetable. Strong conformists, they tend to be rather narrow-minded and self-interested.*

*KALI PHOSPHORICUM*

# KALI PHOS.

*Potassium phosphate is an essential nutrient. The body uses potassium, found in the brain and nerve cells, in many ways, for example, to help store energy in cells and to ensure healthy nerve function. In orthodox medicine potassium phosphate is given to patients who are fed intravenously. Kali phos. is a Schussler tissue salt (see p. 227) and is a key homeopathic remedy for disorders of the nervous system and exhaustion.*

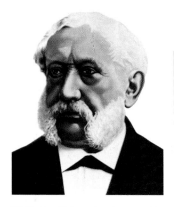

**Wilhelm Schussler** (1821–98)
*An eminent German homeopath, Schussler founded the system of tissue salt medicine in 1873.*

## KEY USES

• Physical and mental exhaustion with an associated aversion to company and marked chilliness
• Pus-filled discharges.

### SELF-HELP
*Chronic fatigue syndrome –* see pp. 196–7.

## REMEDY PROFILE

**Common names** Potassium phosphate, phosphate of potash.
**Source** Prepared chemically by adding dilute phosphoric acid to a solution of potassium carbonate.
**Parts used** Potassium phosphate.

### AILMENTS TREATED
*Kali phos.* is given for mental and physical exhaustion, with nervousness and oversensitivity caused by extreme stress or over-exertion. It is often needed by students who have studied too hard and suffer a breakdown. Those in a state of exhaustion may flinch at the slightest sound and they become shy, preferring to be alone. They may even develop an aversion to their own family. Their weakness is frustrating and makes them irritable and angry.

Physical symptoms of exhaustion include: sensitivity to cold; a yellow-coated tongue; a yellow or pus-filled discharge from the vagina, bladder, lungs, or with stools; extreme muscular weakness; and waking at 5 a.m. with hunger and a gnawing pain in the stomach.

People with exhaustion or chronic fatigue syndrome who need this remedy tend to sweat on the face or head from excitement or after meals, but otherwise do not perspire easily. When hungry, they develop a headache and an empty, nervous feeling in their stomach. They tend to dislike bread and eat sweet foods.

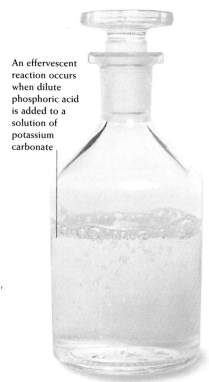

An effervescent reaction occurs when dilute phosphoric acid is added to a solution of potassium carbonate

**Potassium phosphate** *To make the Kali phos. remedy, dilute phosphoric acid is added to a solution of potassium carbonate. Potassium carbonate is derived from wood that is burned until there is no charcoal left, only a white powder, called potash.*

**Symptoms better** From eating; in cloudy weather; with heat; with gentle movement.
**Symptoms worse** From the slightest mental excitement; from worry; if touched; with pain; from cold, dry air; from cold drinks; from physical exertion; during and from sleep; in winter; near noise; from talking.

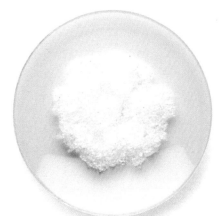

**Potassium carbonate**

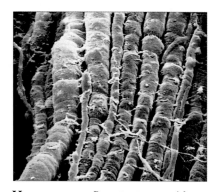

**Human nerves** *Potassium is essential for the proper functioning of the nervous system. It is responsible for the passage of impulses along the nerves.*

### CONSTITUTIONAL TYPE
Kali phos. *types have a conservative outlook, are often extroverted, and see things clearly. Bad news, or news of famine or violence in distant parts of the world, upsets them easily. They are easily exhausted by stress and overworking.*

# LEDUM PALUSTRE
# LEDUM

Wild rosemary gets its generic name from the Greek word ledos, which means "woolly robe," and refers to the woolly hairs on the underside of the plant's leaves. The fresh herb has an antiseptic smell and since the 13th century it has been used by the Finns to get rid of pests and vermin. In 1773, after the infamous tea tax was introduced to the American colonies, Ledum palustre became for a time a tea substitute.

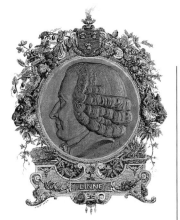

**Karl Linnaeus** (1707–78) *This Swedish botanist was the first to use Ledum palustre medicinally for throat infections and coughs.*

## KEY USES
• To prevent infection in wounds
• Stings, cuts, and grazes
• Eye injuries
• Rheumatic pain that moves upward, with marked chilliness of the affected part.

### SELF-HELP
*Cuts & grazes* – see p. 220
*Eye injuries* – see p. 223.
*Insect stings*– see p. 221.

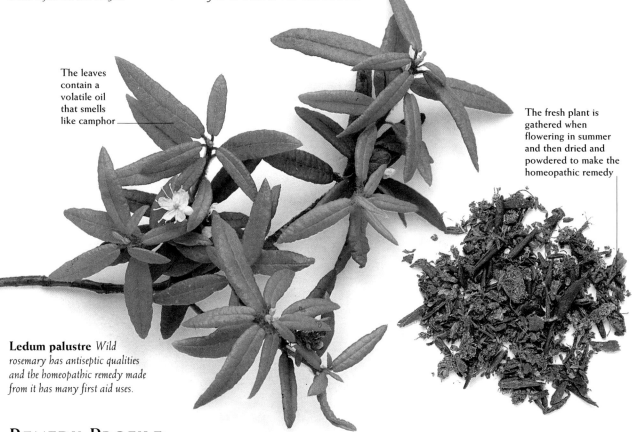

The leaves contain a volatile oil that smells like camphor

The fresh plant is gathered when flowering in summer and then dried and powdered to make the homeopathic remedy

**Ledum palustre** *Wild rosemary has antiseptic qualities and the homeopathic remedy made from it has many first aid uses.*

## REMEDY PROFILE

**Common names** Wild rosemary, marsh tea.
**Source** Grows in the Northern Hemisphere, especially in Canada, the US, Scandinavia, and Ireland.
**Parts used** Fresh plant in flower, dried and powdered.

### AILMENTS TREATED
*Ledum* helps to prevent infection and is an important first-aid remedy, which is taken internally. It is especially useful for acute complaints

such as insect stings, black eyes, and other eye injuries, cuts and grazes and puncture wounds. *Ledum* is effective for injuries or stings where there is severe bruising, with puffy, purplish skin and stinging pain.

*Ledum* is also given for the following: rheumatic pain that starts in the feet and moves upward; stiff, painful joints where the person feels hot inside but the affected limb is cold to the touch and is relieved by cold compresses; pain in the balls of

the big toes due to gout; and painful swollen, and stiff tendons.

When ill, people who need this remedy suffer night sweats and throw off the bedclothes. Their feet and ankles may feel intensely itchy. They are prone to sprained ankles and may feel very angry, impatient, timid, and anxious, and prefer to be left alone.
**Symptoms better** From applying cold compresses to the affected part.
**Symptoms worse** At night; with warmth; if touched.

**The effects of tarantism** *It was said that people afflicted with this disease would exhibit maniacal behavior and leap, dance, and shriek.*

*LYCOSA TARENTULA/TARENTULA HISPANICA*

# TARENTULA

*The wolf spider gets the species name Tarentula from Tarentum, a town in Italy where the spider is widely found. Unlike the South American tarentula, which if it bites can cause mania, twitching, and a sensation of choking, the wolf spider is not dangerous to humans. However, it was once believed that if anyone was bitten by the spider "tarantism" would result, a disease that could cause either melancholy or mania.*

## KEY USES
- Extreme restlessness, both physical and mental
- Heart disorders
- Ovarian disease
- Sensitive genitalia in women
- Complaints that are characterized by a tendency to roll from side to side to relieve symptoms, and which become better for music.

## REMEDY PROFILE

**Common names** Wolf spider, Spanish spider.
**Source** Found in Europe.
**Parts used** Whole, live spider.

### AILMENTS TREATED
Disorders of the nervous system, for example, mental and physical restlessness, and mania with extreme impatience and restlessness, are the ailments most commonly treated with *Tarentula*. It is also used to treat heart disorders, such as angina and heart disease.

In women, this remedy is given for ovarian disease where the sufferer feels worse on the left side, and for sensitive genitalia with itching of the vulva and vagina, which become dry, hot, and raw and are worse from scratching and heavy menstruation. *Tarentula* is also used for headaches with a sensation of needles pricking the brain, and respiratory problems, such as coughing.

All complaints treated with *Tarentula* are characterized by physical symptoms that include: edginess and an inability to keep still, with restless legs that are worse from walking; jerking and twitching; and a tendency to roll from side to side in an attempt to ease symptoms.

People who need this remedy may have sudden mood changes when they are ill, for example, one minute they can be laughing and the next become spiteful and destructive.

**Symptoms better** From seeing bright colors; near music; from fresh air; from rolling from side to side; and curiously, from smoking.
**Symptoms worse** At the same time each year; with movement; touch; near noise; seeing others in trouble.

**Tarentula remedy** *The remedy is made from a tincture of the whole, live spider and is used for restless behavior.*

**Lycosa tarentula** *It is commonly called a wolf spider because it chases its prey rather than catches it in a web.*

### CONSTITUTIONAL TYPE
*Tarentula types suffer from overstimulation of the nervous system. At first this appears as hyperactive behavior and an inability to stop working, but as the sense of hurry and impatience grows, mental symptoms develop, such as extreme restlessness and mood swings, ranging from maniacal laughter to violence and destructivenss. These types also tend to be manipulative.*

*LYTTA VESICATORIA/CANTHARIS VESICATORIA*

# CANTHARIS

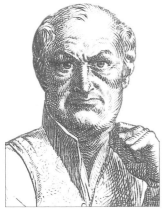

**Marquis de Sade** (*1740–1814*)
*Tried for murdering women, the Marquis gave Lytta vesicatoria to his victims; it was said to be an aphrodisiac.*

*This bright green beetle secretes an irritant substance called cantharidin, which has been used since ancient times to remove warts. It has also been used for rheumatic problems and as an aphrodisiac in love potions. Cantharidin is a powerful poison if taken in large doses, attacking mainly the urinary tract and causing violent vomiting and burning pains. The homeopathic remedy is given for complaints with burning symptoms.*

### KEY USES
- Ailments characterized by burning, stinging pain and a great thirst but no desire to drink
- Burns and stings
- Conditions that worsen rapidly.

#### SELF-HELP
*Blisters* – see p. 222
*Burns & scalds* – see p. 220
*Cystitis* – see pp. 200–1.

## REMEDY PROFILE

**Common name** Spanish fly.
**Source** Found mainly in southern France and Spain.
**Parts used** Whole, live beetle.

### AILMENTS TREATED
*Cantharis* is mainly used to treat severe cystitis with a burning, scalding pain that gets worse as urine is passed. It is also given for other urinary tract infections and for scalds and burns that are helped by cold compresses.

This remedy is also effective for: irritation of the digestive tract that leads to a distended abdomen; burning pain and scalding diarrhea; a burning sensation on the soles of the feet at night; icy hands with red, hot fingernails; pus-filled rashes on the hands; and black-centered stings. Conditions treated with *Cantharis* worsen quickly.

Other physical symptoms eased by this remedy include loss of appetite, burning sensations in the throat, and a great thirst but no desire to drink.

Mental problems alleviated by *Cantharis* include an excessive desire for sexual intercourse, fits of rage, irritability leading to violence, severe anxiety, screaming, and insolence.
**Symptoms better** With warmth; with gentle massage; after burping and passing gas; at night.
**Symptoms worse** With movement; from coffee and cold water.

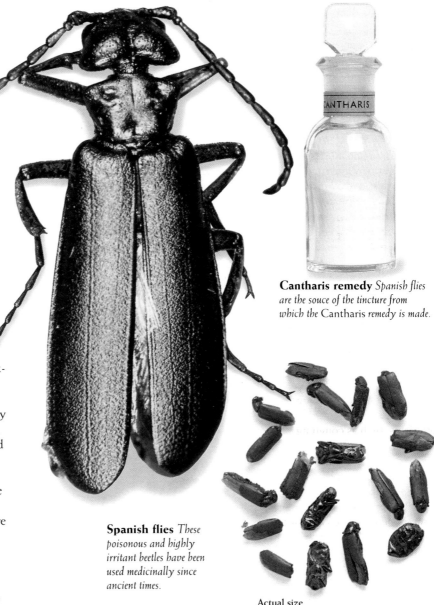

**Cantharis remedy** *Spanish flies are the souce of the tincture from which the Cantharis remedy is made.*

**Spanish flies** *These poisonous and highly irritant beetles have been used medicinally since ancient times.*

Actual size

*RHUS TOXICODENDRON/R. RADICANS*

# RHUS TOX.

*If touched, poison ivy causes a violent skin eruption, often with fever, loss of appetite, a headache, and swollen glands. Poison ivy was first used medicinally in the 18th century when a doctor observed that a patient was cured of herpes of the wrist after being poisoned by it. The plant has been used in orthodox medicine for rheumatism. The homeopathic remedy is mainly given for rheumatic pain and skin complaints.*

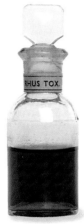

**Rhus tox. tinture** *Fresh poison ivy leaves are used to make the tincture for the Rhus tox. remedy.*

## KEY USES
• Skin complaints where the skin is itchy, red, swollen, and burning
• Joint and muscle ailments where stiffness and pain are better with continued movement but worse on first starting to move.

### SELF-HELP
Blisters – see p. 222
Diaper rash – see pp. 216–7
Osteoarthritis – see pp. 154–5
Restless legs – see pp. 156–7
Rheumatism – see pp. 156–7
Sprains & strains – see p. 223.

## REMEDY PROFILE

**Common names** Poison ivy, poison oak.
**Source** Grows throughout Canada and the US.
**Parts used** Fresh leaves.

### AILMENTS TREATED
*Rhus tox.* is mainly used to treat skin complaints with burning, itchy, red, swollen skin, and a tendency to scaling, such as herpes, diaper rash, blisters, and eczema, and musculo-skeletal problems, such as osteo-arthritis, rheumatism, restless legs, cramps, sprains, and strains.

Other physical symptoms treated, for example of rheumatic fever, flu, and other viral infections include: high temperature with confusion and delirium; dizziness made worse by standing up or walking; swollen eyes with painful stinging tears; sensitive scalp; blocked nose in the evening; dry, cracked, brownish, red-tipped tongue; bitter taste in the mouth; irritating coughs that clear up when talking or singing; stiffness in the lower back; numb arms and legs; nausea and vomiting; and stitchlike pain made worse by cold and damp.

Women's problems helped by the remedy include heavy, prolonged, early menstruation, burning pain in the vagina, and abdominal pain alleviated by lying down. People who need this remedy may be irritable; depressed, with a suicidal inclination; and may cry with no cause. They lack sensual enjoyment, are anxious and fear being poisoned by drugs, and are extremely sensitive to cold and damp.

**Symptoms better** With continued movement and frequent changes of position; with dry warmth.
**Symptoms worse** With rest; from starting to move after resting; from getting cold on undressing; in windy, stormy weather; at night.

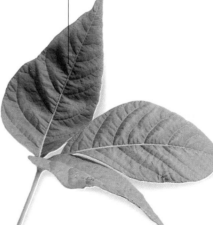

The slightest contact with the fresh leaves can cause a violent rash

The leaves contain a milky white sap that is extremely poisonous

**Poison ivy** *The leaves are collected before the plant flowers, when the poison is considered most active, and pounded to a pulp to make the homeopathic remedy.*

### CONSTITUTIONAL TYPE
Rhus tox. *types tend to be cheerful, lively, humorous, quick-witted, and are good company, although a bit timid at first. They are often serious, hard-working, and rather driven people. They may feel an inner restlessness and agitation and become irritable, frustrated, depressed, and gloomy if suffering from a long-standing illness, as pain wears them down. They may suffer from compulsive and ritualistic behavior.*

*RUTA GRAVEOLENS*

# RUTA GRAV.

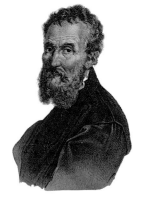

*Rue was used for indigestion by the ancient Greeks and has since been used in folk medicine to cure coughs, croup, colic, headaches, and as an antidote to poisoning by mushrooms, snake bites, and insect stings. In large doses, it causes gastric upset with vomiting, swelling of the tongue, confusion, and convulsive twitchings. The homeopathic remedy made from rue has been used since the 1820s.*

**Michelangelo** (1475–1564) *This great Renaissance painter believed, along with other painters, that rue would improve the eyesight.*

## KEY USES
• Bruised, aching bones and muscles
• Eyestrain from fine, detailed work.

### SELF-HELP
*Eyestrain* – see pp. 166–7
*Rheumatism* – see pp. 156–7
*Sprains & strains* – see p. 223.

## REMEDY PROFILE

**Common names** Rue, bitter herb, herb-of-grace.
**Source** Native to southern Europe, now grown worldwide.
**Parts used** Juice extracted from the whole, fresh plant before flowering.

### AILMENTS TREATED
*Ruta grav.* is an important remedy for bruising of the periosteum (the lining of the bones) with deep aching pain, rheumatism, tendon injuries, painful bruises, and sciatica (pain along the sciatic nerve) that is worse at night and when lying down. It is also given for eyestrain, with hot, red-looking eyes, and eyestrain-induced headaches, often caused by reading small print.

The remedy is also used to treat chest weakness and breathing difficulty with pain over the breastbone, as in coughs and croup; infection of the tooth socket after a tooth extraction; prolapse of the rectum that is worse for stooping and crouching; constipation alternating with loose, blood- and mucus-filled stools; and tearing or stitchlike pain in the rectum, as with rectal prolapse.

When ill, people who need *Ruta grav.* may be depressed and lack personal satisfaction. They may also be critical of others and anxious.
**Symptoms better** With movement.
**Symptoms worse** Lying down; with rest; in cold and damp.

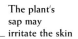
The plant's sap may irritate the skin

The leaves contain a pungent oil that has a wide range of uses

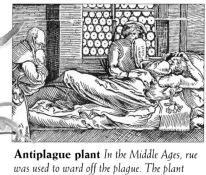

**Antiplague plant** *In the Middle Ages, rue was used to ward off the plague. The plant has an extremely potent, noxious smell.*

**Ruta graveolens**
*This plant has been used medicinally throughout history. The homeopathic remedy made from it is a key treatment for deep, aching pain.*

*THUJA OCCIDENTALIS*

# THUJA

*The generic name of this conifer tree, Thuja, is derived from the Greek word* thero, *which means "to fumigate or sacrifice." Although Native Americans used the leaves and twigs to treat malaria, coughs, gout, and rheumatism, extracts of the tree have never been used in orthodox medicine. In aromatherapy, the essential oil of Thuja occidentalis is used to treat hair loss and acne.*

**Sacrifice to the gods** *The arbor vitae tree was burned at pagan sacrifices.*

## KEY USES

• Warts and other skin complaints
• Nail problems
• Genitourinary tract conditions
• Ailments characterized by yellowish green or green phlegm.

**SELF-HELP**
*Warts – see pp. 188–9.*

**Fresh plant**
*The aromatic leaves and twigs of Thuja occidentalis are pounded to a pulp to make the homeopathic remedy and are also made into a cream, which helps rheumatism.*

*Fresh leafy twigs have a pungent scent that resembles camphor*

**Thuja occidentalis** *The leaves and young twigs of this slow-growing evergreen have been used in herbal remedies for centuries.*

## REMEDY PROFILE

**Common names** Arbor vitae, tree of life, white cedar.
**Source** Native to the US and Canada.
**Parts used** Fresh leaves and twigs.

### AILMENTS TREATED
As well as being a key remedy for warts, *Thuja* is used for other skin complaints, such as oily skin and to treat weak nails. It also acts on the genitourinary tract and is given for urethral and vaginal infections.

Physical symptoms it is given for include: offensive smelling perspiration; headaches brought on by stress, too much excitement or exhaustion; tooth decay and swollen gums; chronic greenish yellow or green phlegm; and loss of appetite in the morning. *Thuja* is also effective for menstrual problems, such as early and scanty bleeding and cramps.

People who need this remedy are very sensitive, paranoid about others trying to manipulate them, sleep badly, and talk in their sleep.
**Symptoms better** With movement.
**Symptoms worse** In cold and damp; on the left side; at night.

### CONSTITUTIONAL TYPE
Thuja *types have a marked lack of self-esteem. At first they spend a lot of energy trying to present a pleasing and wholesome image to the world, but are badly upset by negative reactions, which make them secretive and depressed, and lack interest in their appearance. However, they have fixed ideas about the way they look. They have pale, greasy, waxlike skin.*

Thuja *children tend to be small, fine-boned, and find self-expression difficult. They have a manipulative character.*

*URTICA URENS*

# URTICA

*Stinging nettles have been used medicinally thoughout history. The 16th-century herbalist John Gerard used the plant as an antidote to poisoning and curiously, the juice of the nettle provides an excellent antidote for its own sting. This common weed is used in herbalism, to treat hemorrhoids, stomach problems, diabetes, and nosebleeds. Hives (urticaria), which looks very similar to nettle rash, is treated with the homeopathic remedy.*

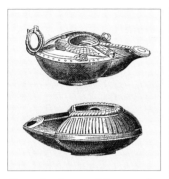

**Egyptian lamps** *Oil expressed from the seeds of stinging nettle was burned in lamps in ancient Egypt.*

## KEY USES

- Burning and stinging skin complaints
- Rheumatic pain
- Burns with itching and swelling
- Insect stings.

### SELF-HELP
*Burns & scalds* – see p. 220
*Hives (urticaria)* – see pp. 188–9.

## REMEDY PROFILE

**Common name** Dwarf stinging nettle.
**Source** A common weed that grows worldwide.
**Parts used** Whole, fresh plant.

### AILMENTS TREATED
This remedy, taken either internally or applied as an ointment externally, is mainly used for skin problems, especially if the skin is burning and stinging due to an allergic reaction. *Urtica* is an excellent remedy for skin rashes, for example, hives (urticaria) caused in particular by insect stings, and by eating shellfish, such as shrimp. Burns, where the skin is hot and blistered, and eczema, especially when the skin is itchy or blotchy, are both helped by this remedy. Skin eruptions that are suppressed by steroid ointments, for example, can lead to diarrhea, which is eased by this remedy.

    *Urtica* is also an effective remedy for rheumatism and is given for acute gout, neuritis (nerve inflammation), and neuralgia.

    In women, *Urtica* is a remedy for vulval itching and scanty breast milk in lactating mothers.

    It is also good for burning urine that causes itching and may be associated with cystitis.
**Symptoms better** From rubbing the affected area; lying down.
**Symptoms worse** From cold, damp air; from being in water and snow; if touched; from eating shellfish.

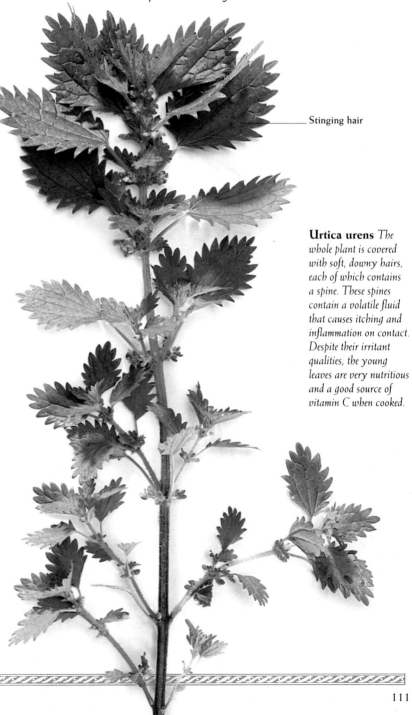

Stinging hair

**Urtica urens** *The whole plant is covered with soft, downy hairs, each of which contains a spine. These spines contain a volatile fluid that causes itching and inflammation on contact. Despite their irritant qualities, the young leaves are very nutritious and a good source of vitamin C when cooked.*

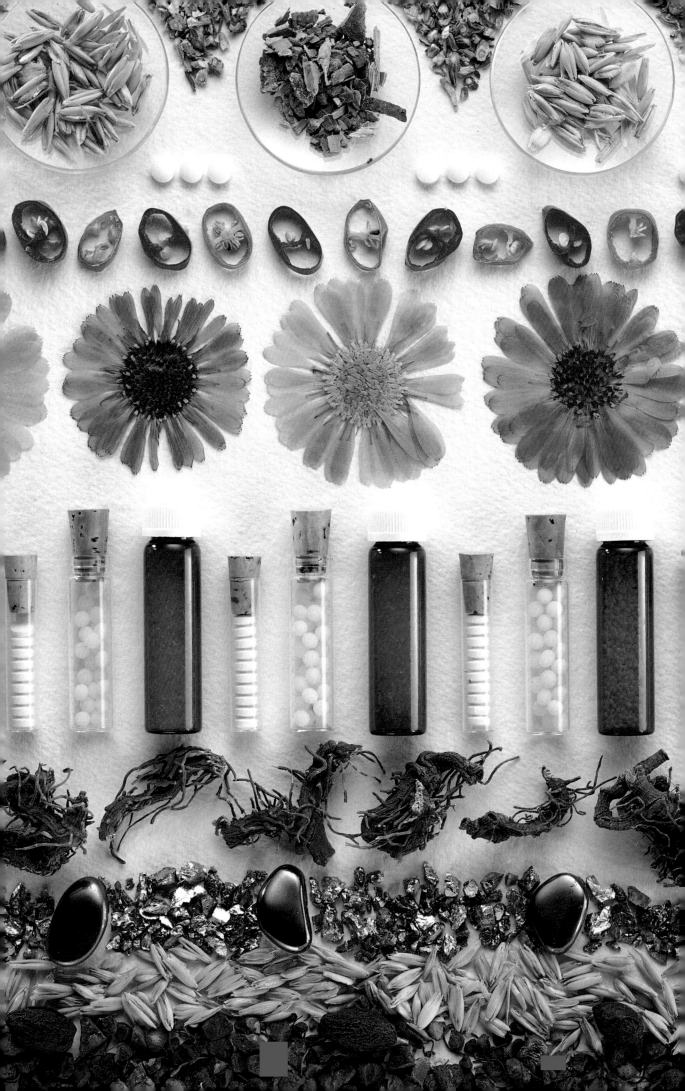

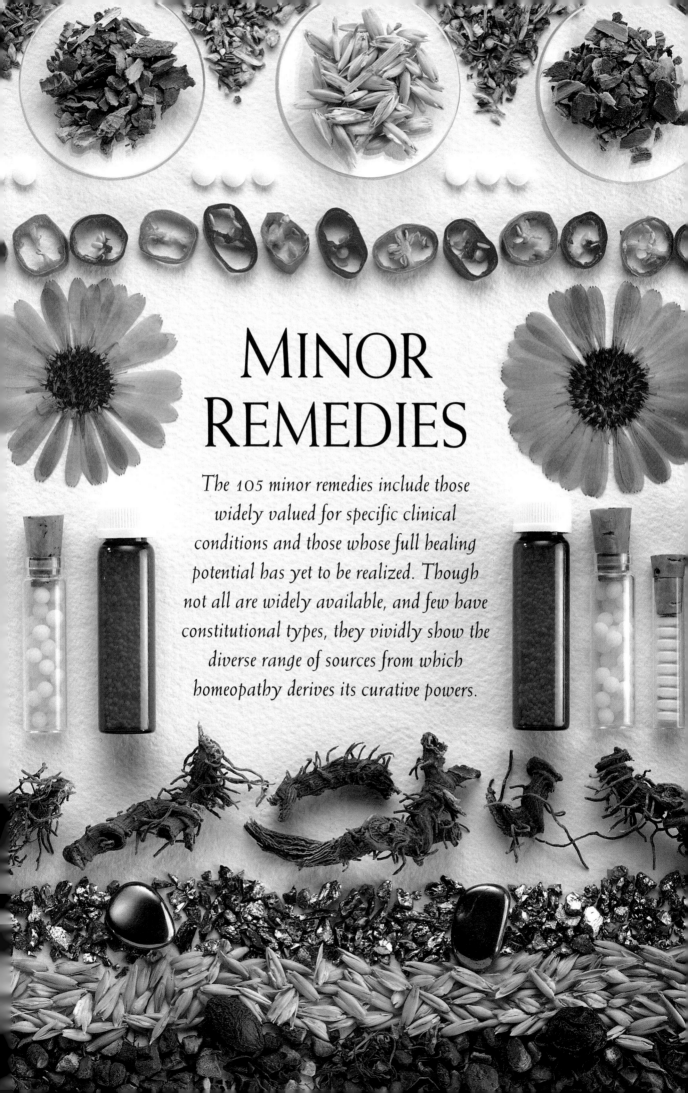

# MINOR REMEDIES

The 105 minor remedies include those widely valued for specific clinical conditions and those whose full healing potential has yet to be realized. Though not all are widely available, and few have constitutional types, they vividly show the diverse range of sources from which homeopathy derives its curative powers.

## AETHUSA CYNAPIUM

# AETHUSA

The plant's name is derived from ai, an Arabic word meaning "to burn," which reflects its tendency to cause burning and rawness. Its common name, fool's parsley, corresponds to its homeopathic use for inability to think clearly or concentrate.

**Common name** Fool's parsley.
**Source** A common weed native to Europe, now grown in the US and Canada.
**Parts used** Fresh plant in flower.

### AILMENTS TREATED
*Aethusa* chiefly affects the nervous system and gastrointestinal system. It is used to treat violent vomiting, pains, convulsions, and even delirium, which all lead to exhaustion and sleepiness. Babies suffering from an inability to digest milk and from diarrhea, especially when they are teething or in hot weather, are often helped by *Aethusa*. The remedy is also used to strengthen the mind when it is weak and when concentration is difficult.
**Symptoms better** From fresh air; with company.
**Symptoms worse** With warmth; in the evening; between 3 a.m. and 4 a.m.; in the summer.

*AETHUSA CYNAPIUM Known as fool's parsley, this herb is distinguished from garden parsley by the peculiar, disagreeable smell of its leaves.*

## AGARICUS MUSCARIUS/ AMANITA MUSCARIA

# AGARICUS

This toxic, common toadstool is called fly agaric because it is used to kill flies. It is highly poisonous and hallucinogenic and was used by Siberian medicine men to encourage visionary states.

**Common name** Fly agaric.
**Source** Grows in parts of Scotland, Scandinavia, and other parts of Europe, as well as Asia, the US, and Canada.
**Parts used** Whole fresh fungus.

### AILMENTS TREATED
This is an important homeopathic remedy for chilblains and nervous disorders in which jerking, twitching, trembling, and itching are predominant, for example in epilepsy and chorea. It is also given for delirium tremens associated with alcoholism and for the effects of senile dementia, or when there is marked dizziness, an impulse to fall backward, redness and puffiness of the face without heat, and an increase in appetite. Those who need *Agaricus* are sensitive to the cold, particularly when ill.
**Symptoms better** With slow movement.
**Symptoms worse** From being cold; in cool surroundings; before a thunderstorm; from eating.

**MAIN SELF-HELP USE**
Chilblains – see pp. 198–9.

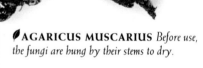

*AGARICUS MUSCARIUS Before use, the fungi are hung by their stems to dry.*

## AILANTHUS GLANDULOSA/A. ALTISSIMA

# AILANTHUS

This deciduous tree is popular in urban centers. Observations about its homeopathic use were first recorded in 1953 by an American homeopath, who described the range of digestive illnesses that occurred in those who inhaled the sickening smell of its flowers.

**Common names** Chinese sumac, tree of heaven, shade tree, copal tree.
**Source** Native to China, now grows worldwide.
**Parts used** Fresh flowers.

### AILMENTS TREATED
*Ailanthus* is used to treat glandular fever with a characteristic swelling and redness of the tonsils, white mucus, and a very sore throat that makes swallowing difficult and

painful. The glandular fever may be accompanied by a headache, chronic fatigue, and muscular pains.
**Symptoms better** From pressure.
**Symptoms worse** In the morning; from fresh air; lying down; in light; bending forward; swallowing.

---

*ALOE SOCOTRINA/A. FEROX*

# ALOE

The aloe has been used in medicine from early times both as a purgative and tonic. The Greeks and Romans thought aloe was good for stimulating bile flow in order to cure abdominal afflictions. In the early part of the 20th century, aloe was frequently used as a purgative. The homeopathic remedy was first proved by Dr. Constantine Hering in 1864 (see p. 17).

**Common name** Aloe.
**Source** Grows in southern Africa.
**Parts used** Powdered resin. The resin is made from drained juice.

## CONSTITUTIONAL TYPE
People who benefit from *Aloe* tend to be irritable, particularly in cloudy weather. They are dissatisfied and angry with themselves, especially when they are constipated. They feel weary and are unwilling to work. Curiously, these types crave beer, even though it makes them sick.

## AILMENTS TREATED
This remedy is used to treat congestion, especially in the pelvic organs, abdomen, and head; for example minor prolapse of the uterus, prostate problems, constipation, and headaches. It is also useful for diarrhea with painful urination brought on by food intolerance. This is a common remedy for people who have a very sedentary lifestyle, especially the elderly and those who suffer fatigue. *Aloe* is also useful for those who have drunk too much alcohol, especially beer.
**Symptoms better** In cold weather; from cold compresses; passing gas.
**Symptoms worse** In summer; in hot, dry weather; in the early morning; from eating or drinking.

### 🐚 MAIN SELF-HELP USE
Diarrhea – see pp. 182–3.

---

*ALUMINUM OXIDE*

# ALUMINA

Aluminum is widely used in indigestion remedies for its antacid effects. It is also used to make cooking utensils. There is concern that as aluminum is found in greater amounts in the brains of people suffering from Alzheimer's disease, it may be partly to blame for this condition. Interestingly, the homeopathic remedy is used to treat senile dementia.

**Common name** Alumina.
**Source** Bauxite, which is found in France, Italy, Hungary, Ghana, the US, Jamaica, Indonesia, and Russia.
**Parts used** Aluminum oxide.

## CONSTITUTIONAL TYPE
This remedy is used for elderly people who are confused or senile with a poor memory. They tend to be thin, with dried-up gray skin. They have a peculiar sensitivity to seeing sharp objects and knives and fear insanity because of this. They feel that something awful is about to happen, which leads to deep despair. *Alumina* types crave inedible things including pencils, chalk, coffee grounds, and tea leaves, but dislike meat and beer.

## AILMENTS TREATED
Sluggishness is the keynote running through *Alumina*. This is an excellent remedy for severe constipation in which the bowels are sluggish and even small, soft stools are difficult to pass. This is common in pregnant women and children.

*Alumina* is also used for dizziness on closing the eyes, a sensation of cobwebs over the face, heaviness, a lack of coordination, and paralysis of the limbs, as in multiple sclerosis, and difficulty urinating due to sluggishness.

### 🐚 ALUMINUM
**OXIDE** *The* Alumina *remedy is made from bauxite, a rock composed of hydrated aluminum oxides.*

---

**Symptoms better** In the evening; from cold compresses; from fresh air.
**Symptoms worse** From cold air; in the morning; from salty, starchy food.

### 🐚 MAIN SELF-HELP USE
Constipation – see pp. 184–5.

---

*AMMONIUM CARBONICUM*

# AMMON. CARB.

Ammonium carbonate was once used as smelling salts to revive those who had fainted. It was also used for centuries to treat blood-poisoning from scarlet fever. Hahnemann found it to have a much wider range of actions when potentized.

**Common names** Ammonium carbonate, sal volatile.
**Source** Prepared chemically from sodium carbonate and ammonium chloride.
**Parts used** Ammonium carbonate.

## CONSTITUTIONAL TYPE
*Ammon. carb.* types tend to be forgetful, bad-tempered, gloomy, and weepy, especially during cloudy weather. They are often stout and suffer marked fatigue.

## AILMENTS TREATED
This remedy is used when there is a lack of oxygenation to the tissues, for example in respiratory problems and mild heart failure. It has also been given for chronic fatigue syndrome.
**Symptoms better** From pressure; in warm, dry rooms; raising the feet.
**Symptoms worse** In cloudy weather; with continued movement.

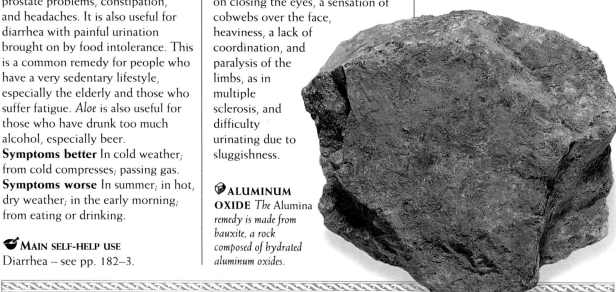

## AMMONIUM MURIATICUM

# AMMON. MUR.

*When it was introduced to the West in the 2nd century, ammonium chloride was of great importance to alchemists. Today, it is used as an electrolyte in batteries and in galvanizing, tinning, and soldering. It is also used in orthodox cough and cold medicines. Up until the 9th century ammonium chloride came from a single source, the Fire Mountain in central Asia; now it is manufactured.*

**Common names** Ammonium chloride, sal-ammoniac.
**Source** Prepared chemically.
**Parts used** Ammonium chloride.

### CONSTITUTIONAL TYPE
*Ammon. mur.* types tend to be fat and puffy, but with thin legs and arms. They are gloomy, weepy, fear darkness, and tend to take a strange dislike to certain people. Physically, their circulation is irregular and this causes burning and throbbing pain. There is a characteristic pain or ulcer on the heel of the foot.

### AILMENTS TREATED
*Ammon. mur.* is given for lung conditions, such as bronchitis, coughs, and pneumonia in which thick, tenacious mucus is produced. Symptoms include a slimy feeling in the mouth and throat, swollen glands

**AMMONIUM MURIATICUM** *This mineral is ammonium chloride, or sal-ammoniac. The remedy is made from chemically prepared ammonium chloride.*

and neck, a low backache, and tendons that feel tight, as if they are too short. This remedy is also given for lumbago and sciatica that is worse on the left side.
**Symptoms better** From fresh air; with rapid movement.
**Symptoms worse** In the morning and afternoon; between 2 a.m. and 4 a.m.

## ANACARDIUM ORIENTALE/ SEMECARPUS ANACARDIUM

# ANACARD. OR.

*The nuts from this tree have been used by Hindus for all kinds of skin complaints. The acrid black juice, found between the external rind and the nut, was used to burn off warts and to clean leg ulcers. The Hindus also mixed it with chalk to make an ink for marking linen. The Arabians used the juice chiefly for mental illness, loss of memory, paralysis, and spasms.*

**Common name** Marking nut tree.
**Source** Grows mainly in the East Indies and other parts of Asia.
**Parts used** Oily black juice from around the nut.

### CONSTITUTIONAL TYPE
*Anacard. or.* is used for people who have an inferiority complex and work hard to prove themselves. They have often been belittled from an early age and lack self-confidence. This makes them feel detached from themselves, as if they are split into two wills. The remedy is often needed by students who give up their studies due to memory loss. These

types may display cruel behavior and confuse reality and fantasy.

### AILMENTS TREATED
This remedy is used when there is a sensation of constricted pain, as if the gut or anus is plugged, and the body feels as if there are bands around it. These symptoms may be associated with hemorrhoids and indigestion. *Anacard. or.* is also given for constipation, rheumatism, and duodenal ulcers that feel better after eating but cause acute discomfort once food has been digested.
**Symptoms better** From fasting.
**Symptoms worse** From eating, after a hot bath; from compresses; at midnight.

## ANTIMONIUM TARTARICUM

# ANTIM. TART.

*Antimony potassium tartrate is used in the textile industry to bind dyes to fabrics. It was once used in orthodox medicine as an expectorant, to induce vomiting, and in the treatment of fungal infections and worms.*

**Common names** Antimony potassium tartrate, tartar emetic.
**Source** Prepared chemically from oxide of antimony and potassium tartrate.
**Parts used** Antimony potassium tartrate.

### AILMENTS TREATED
This remedy is used in the very old and very young who are wheezing but too weak to cough up phlegm, drowsy, and irritable. It is also given for headaches with a sensation of a tight band around the head, which is made worse by coughing.
Generally these ailments are characterized by the face feeling cold to the touch and the tongue being thickly coated and red in the center and around the edges. Usually there is a lack of thirst. Legs may be puffy from fluid retention. Nausea is relieved by vomiting.
**Symptoms better** From cold air; sitting up.
**Symptoms worse** In warm rooms; in damp and cold; with movement; lying down.

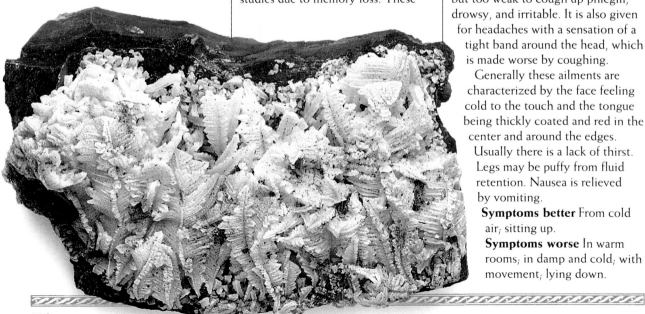

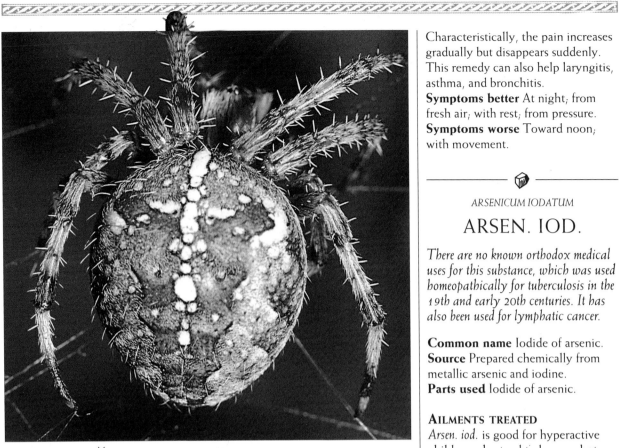

Characteristically, the pain increases gradually but disappears suddenly. This remedy can also help laryngitis, asthma, and bronchitis.

**Symptoms better** At night; from fresh air; with rest; from pressure.
**Symptoms worse** Toward noon; with movement.

### *ARSENICUM IODATUM*
# ARSEN. IOD.

*There are no known orthodox medical uses for this substance, which was used homeopathically for tuberculosis in the 19th and early 20th centuries. It has also been used for lymphatic cancer.*

**Common name** Iodide of arsenic.
**Source** Prepared chemically from metallic arsenic and iodine.
**Parts used** Iodide of arsenic.

**AILMENTS TREATED**
*Arsen. iod.* is good for hyperactive children who tend to be very hot (although some are cold). It is also used to treat psoriasis and chest complaints such as bronchitis. Any nasal discharges are burning; this is very evident in hay fever or allergic rhinitis in which the upper lip becomes raw. Asthma may accompany the hay fever. This remedy is also given for hard lymph glands due to psoriasis and eczema.
**Symptoms better** From fresh air.
**Symptoms worse** At night, especially after midnight.

**MAIN SELF-HELP USE**
Hay fever – see pp. 168–9.

---

ARANEA DIADEMA/A. DIADEMATUS
# ARANEA DIAD.

*This spider uses venom, passed through small holes in its jaw, to numb its victim. The homeopathic remedy was first proved by the German homeopath von Grauvogl in the mid-19th century. He promoted Aranea diad. as a key remedy for people with an abnormal sensitivity to cold and damp.*

**Common name** Papal cross spider.
**Source** Commonly found in the Northern Hemisphere.
**Parts used** Whole live spider.

**AILMENTS TREATED**
*Aranea diad.* is used mainly for disorders of the nervous system characterized by neuralgia with sudden, violent pain that causes wincing and occurs at regular intervals. Facial neuralgia is an example. Severe burning nerve pain affects the cheek, lips, gums, or chin on one side of the face. Other symptoms of neuralgia include numbness and a sensation of heaviness.
**Symptoms better** In summer; and, curiously, from smoking.
**Symptoms worse** In cold and damp; from cold compresses.

**ARANEA DIADEMA** *The remedy made from this spider is primarily used for disorders of the nervous system.*

### *ARGENTUM METALLICUM*
# ARGENT. MET.

*Pure silver rarely occurs on its own in nature but is usually found in ore deposits with other minerals such as copper, iron, and zinc. It is used in heat and electrical conduction, photographic film, and to make mirrors. In orthodox medicine, it was given as a diuretic and for palpitations and bad breath.*

**Common name** Silver.
**Source** Ore deposits, which are mainly found in the US and South America.
**Parts used** Silver.

**AILMENTS TREATED**
*Argent. met.* is used for arthritis and rheumatism where the joints of the hands, fingers, feet, and toes are sore. It is given for raw pain in the internal organs.

**ARGENTUM METALLICUM** *Silver has been mined since ancient times. The remedy made from it is used for arthritis.*

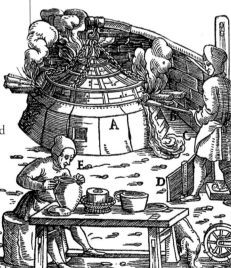

---

### ARUM TRIPHYLLUM

# ARUM TRIPH.

*This native perennial plant of North America is noted for the unusual shape of its leaves and is a well-known wildflower, appearing in late spring. Arum comes from* ar, *an Arabic word meaning "fire."*

**Common names** Jack-in-the-Pulpit, wild turnip, Indian turnip.
**Source** Grows in Canada and the US.
**Parts used** Fresh root.

#### AILMENTS TREATED
*Arum triph.* is used mainly to treat hay fever, especially when the left nostril is the worst affected, and colds. Symptoms include redness around the mouth and lower face with cracked, painful, and bleeding lips. The nose and inside of the mouth are also cracked and bleeding and there are cracks at the corners of the mouth. There is a hot nasal discharge and the saliva is hot. In addition, this remedy is given for chronic hoarseness and loss of voice caused by exposure to cold, windy weather and too much singing.
**Symptoms better** From coffee; in the morning.
**Symptoms worse** In cold, windy weather; lying down.

---

### AVENA SATIVA

# AVENA

*Wild oats were first found growing in western Europe as a weed among barley and have been cultivated ever since. Most oats are used for feeding livestock, but some are processed for breakfast foods. Oats are a nutritive food and are used as a nerve tonic in both herbalism and homeopathy.*

**Common name** Wild oats.
**Source** Grows in the temperate regions of the world.
**Parts used** Fresh green plant in flower.

#### AILMENTS TREATED
*Avena* is used mainly as a tincture to strengthen the nerves, in nervous exhaustion, or for worry

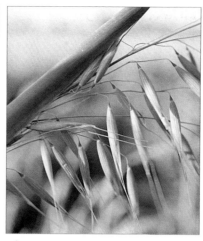

 **AVENA SATIVA** *Wild oats are used to make the remedy, which is given for nervous exhaustion, insomnia, and anxiety.*

and anxiety. It is also said to help impotence and is very useful in treating nervousness and insomnia in alcoholics and heavy drinkers.
**Symptoms better** With sleep.
**Symptoms worse** From alcohol.

---

### BAPTISIA TINCTORIA

# BAPTISIA

*In high doses, this perennial plant is poisonous, mainly affecting the gastro-intestinal tract. Native to the US and Canada, its medicinal properties were first discovered by Native Americans, who also used it as a dye. The root is still used today in herbalism as an antibacterial, antiseptic, and as a cooling agent, for example, to treat throat infections.*

**Common name** Wild indigo.
**Source** Grows throughout Canada and the US.
**Parts used** Fresh root, including its bark.

#### AILMENTS TREATED
The main use of *Baptisia* is to treat acute complaints, especially feverish illnesses. It is used extensively for severe influenza and typhoid fever. Symptoms of the acute complaints treated include falling asleep in the middle of answering a question and being unable to return to sleep because the mind feels scattered and delirious. The tongue is coated brown and is dry in the center, there are sores on the gums, the breath smells extremely offensive, and diarrhea with foul-smelling, painless stools may come on suddenly.
**Symptoms better** From walking in fresh air.
**Symptoms worse** In humid heat.

---

### BARYTA CARBONICA

# BARYTA CARB.

*Barium carbonate (also called witherite) is used to make the Baryta carb. remedy. Witherite was first discovered by William Withering in 1783. Medicinally, it was given for tuberculosis and glandular swellings. Barium is an element found in the earth's crust in minerals such as barite and witherite. It glows in the dark after heating and its compounds are used in radiology. It is also used to make fine glassware and optical glass.*

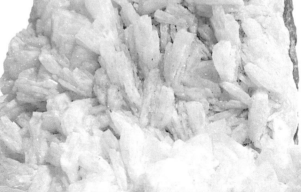

**BARYTA CARBONICA** *White crystals of barite and witherite are found together; the latter is the source of barium carbonate.*

**Common name** Barium carbonate, witherite.
**Source** Witherite, which is found in Scotland, England, Italy, and the US.
**Parts used** Barium carbonate.

## CONSTITUTIONAL TYPE

Emotionally, *Baryta carb.* types tend to lack self-confidence and are childish, timid, insecure, and unable to make decisions. They have an offensive smelling foot sweat and bite their nails. Occasionally, they have an odd sensation, as if they are inhaling smoke.

## AILMENTS TREATED

*Baryta carb.* is used mainly for children and the elderly. A keynote for the remedy is slow physical, intellectual, or emotional development. Both children and elderly people requiring *Baryta carb.* may be intellectually challenged.

Children who need this remedy tend to be late walkers and talkers, with large heads. The genitals and other parts of the body may not have grown properly. They may suffer from short stature or Down's syndrome. Because they are susceptible to infection, they have acute, recurrent tonsillitis.

Elderly people who require this remedy may have senile dementia or may have suffered a stroke with a possible handicap.
**Symptoms better** From wrapping up warmly; from walking in fresh air.
**Symptoms worse** With the least exposure to cold and damp.

*BELLIS PERENNIS*

# BELLIS

*The roots and leaves of the garden daisy were used during the Middle Ages to treat wounds. The plant was considered good for removing blood from bruises and was commonly known as bruisewort. Today, it is still used to ease painful bruising.*

**Common names** European daisy, garden daisy, bruisewort.
**Source** Grows throughout Europe and in eastern parts of the US.
**Parts used** Fresh plant in flower.

## AILMENTS TREATED

This remedy is taken for bruising and soreness, to ease pain, and to speed recovery, for example, after an injury or operation. It can also help prevent infection and is used to treat abscesses. *Bellis* is very useful after accidents that cause the lymph glands to swell up or the limbs to become swollen and cold. Complaints are generally worse for becoming suddenly chilled when overheated.

In women, *Bellis* is excellent for uterine pain during pregnancy.
**Symptoms better** With movement; from rubbing the affected area.
**Symptoms worse** From getting wet; from cold drinks when overheated; sweating; being too warm in bed.

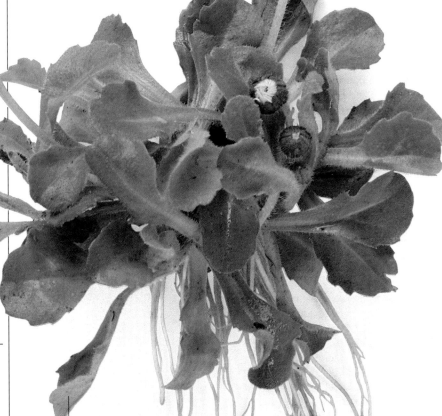

**BELLIS PERENNIS** *Despite its delicate appearance, the common daisy is a very potent plant. It is the source of a remedy that is particularly effective for bruises and injuries.*

The leaves contain an acrid juice

## BENZ. AC.

*BENZOICUM ACIDUM*

*Benzoic acid is found in gum benzoin, a vegetable resin. When benzoic acid is mixed with sodium salts it forms sodium benzoate, which is widely used as a food preservative. Homeopathic provings have shown that people who are sensitive to benzoic acid may develop medical problems if they consume too much sodium benzoate.*

**Common name** Benzoic acid.
**Source** Gum benzoin, which occurs naturally in some plants and is also prepared chemically.
**Parts used** Benzoic acid.

### AILMENTS TREATED
*Benz. ac.* is used mainly to treat arthritis and gout, where the joints crack on moving. It is also used for kidney stones. These ailments are characterized by a combination of tearing pain, urine that smells very offensive, and chilliness.
**Symptoms better** With heat.
**Symptoms worse** From fresh air; from getting cold on undressing.

## BERBERIS

*BERBERIS VULGARIS*

*This plant was used by Greek and Arabian physicians, as well as the 16th-century herbalist Gerard. It was believed to cool the blood in fevers and was used for bleeding, jaundice, diarrhea, and dysentery. Today, it is still used to treat jaundice as well as gallstones and other liver problems.*

**Common names** Barberry, pipperidge bush.
**Source** Grows throughout Europe.
**Parts used** Fresh root.

### AILMENTS TREATED
The main use of *Berberis* is to treat kidney infections, especially when there is tenderness in the region of the kidneys. Urine may be dark or abnormal in some other way. Sudden movement, stepping too hard down stairs, or getting up after sitting may aggravate weakness and soreness in the lower back. This remedy is also given for gallstones that lead to biliary colic and jaundice with pale stools. People who need *Berberis* look pale with sunken cheeks and hollow eyes. The mucous membranes are dry and their symptoms may change rapidly.
**Symptoms better** From stretching or exerting the muscles.
**Symptoms worse** From standing.

## BOTHROPS

*BOTHROPS LANCEOLATUS/LACHESIS LANCEOLATUS*

*This is an extremely poisonous snake. It is gray or brown and marked by a series of black-edged diamonds, often bordered in a lighter color. Its bite can be fatal to humans. If a limb is bitten it swells rapidly to an enormous size and becomes infected and gangrenous.*

Raised area behind the eye

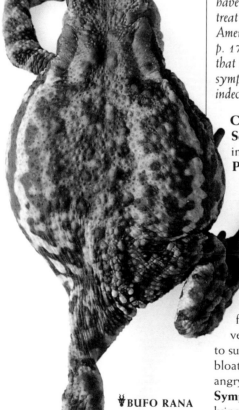

**Common names** Yellow pit viper, fer de lance.
**Source** Found on the island of Martinique in the Caribbean.
**Parts used** Fresh venom.

### AILMENTS TREATED
*Bothrops* is used mainly for thrombosis or hemorrhaging. It can also be used for left-sided strokes with right-sided paralysis and an inability to articulate or to remember correct words. Generally, people who require this remedy are sluggish or weary and experience nervous trembling.
**Symptoms better** No specific factors.
**Symptoms worse** On the right side.

## BUFO

*BUFO RANA*

*When molested, the common toad ejects a poison that irritates the eyes and mucous membranes. The poison can affect animals as large as dogs, causing paralysis and even death. The Chinese have long used dried toad poison to treat various ailments. When the American homeopath Kent (see p. 17) first proved this remedy he noted that it produced "a disgusting set of symptoms," from imbecility and indecency to apathy.*

**Common name** Common toad.
**Source** Found worldwide except in Australia and Madagascar.
**Parts used** Poison.

### AILMENTS TREATED
The main use of *Bufo* is for epilepsy followed by a violent headache. Symptoms include lapping of the tongue and intolerance of music or brilliant objects before an epileptic fit; the pain follows the line of the lymph vessels. *Bufo* types generally tend to suffer fluid retention and look bloated and besotted. They become angry if misunderstood.
**Symptoms better** In the morning; lying down.
**Symptoms worse** At night; when asleep; during menstruation.

**⍦BUFO RANA**
*The poison-secreting glands are found in the warts, mostly in the raised areas behind the eyes.*

*CACTUS GRANDIFLORUS/SELINECEREUS GRANDIFLORUS*

# CACTUS GRAND.

*This cactus has large, fleshy stems. The Cactus grand. remedy was first proved by Dr. Rubins in 1862. The symptoms he noted included severe constricting sensations in the heart with chest pain, and Cactus grand. is therefore an important heart remedy. Some varieties of cactus have been used in folk medicine.*

**Common name** Night-blooming cactus.
**Source** Grows in dry, desert regions in the US and South America.
**Parts used** Young, tender stems and flowers.

### AILMENTS TREATED
*Cactus grand.* is used for angina with violent, constricting pain. The chest feels very tight, as if gripped by an iron hand, especially when the heart is working hard, for example during exercise or when stressed. The pain is violent, worse when lying on the left side, and there may be associated palpitations. There may also be associated swelling or a tingling sensation in the left hand. Sufferers feel that they will die and that there is no cure.
**Symptoms better** Lying on the right side with the head raised.
**Symptoms worse** At 11 a.m. and 11 p.m.

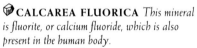
**CALCAREA FLUORICA** *This mineral is fluorite, or calcium fluoride, which is also present in the human body.*

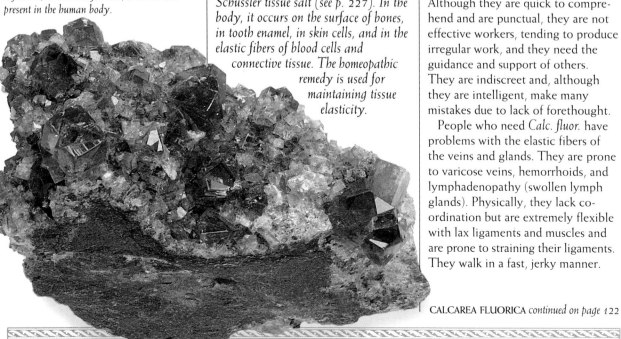

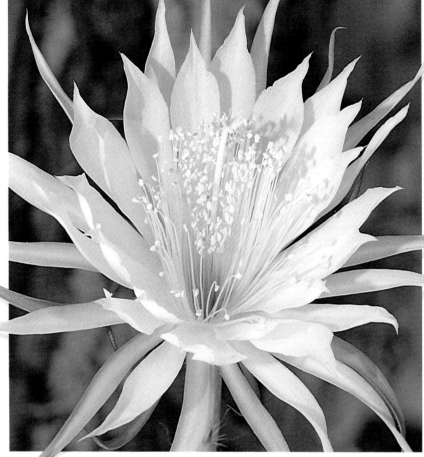

**CACTUS GRANDIFLORUS**
*The remedy made from the young, tender stems and flowers is good for angina.*

*CALCAREA FLUORICA*

# CALC. FLUOR.

*Calcium fluoride, or fluorite, is a Schussler tissue salt (see p. 227). In the body, it occurs on the surface of bones, in tooth enamel, in skin cells, and in the elastic fibers of blood cells and connective tissue. The homeopathic remedy is used for maintaining tissue elasticity.*

**Common name** Calcium fluoride, fluorite.
**Source** Fluorite, which is found in Italy, Mexico, England, Brazil, Norway, Canada, and the US.
**Parts used** Calcium fluoride.

### CONSTITUTIONAL TYPE
Mentally, these types tend to worry about their health and fear poverty. Although they are quick to comprehend and are punctual, they are not effective workers, tending to produce irregular work, and they need the guidance and support of others. They are indiscreet and, although they are intelligent, make many mistakes due to lack of forethought.

People who need *Calc. fluor.* have problems with the elastic fibers of the veins and glands. They are prone to varicose veins, hemorrhoids, and lymphadenopathy (swollen lymph glands). Physically, they lack coordination but are extremely flexible with lax ligaments and muscles and are prone to straining their ligaments. They walk in a fast, jerky manner.

CALCAREA FLUORICA *continued on page 122*

### CALCAREA FLUORICA *continued*

#### AILMENTS TREATED

*Calc. fluor.* is primarily used for maintaining tissue elasticity and dispersing outgrowths of hard bone. It is also good for overstretched muscles, ligaments, and joints, deficient tooth enamel, lumbago and other back pain, and enlarged adenoids. In children, it is given for the slow development of bones and associated difficulty in learning to walk, and enlarged adenoids that become stony and hard after recurrent ear, nose, and throat infections.
**Symptoms better** With continued movement; with heat; from warm compresses.
**Symptoms worse** On starting to move; from cold and damp; in a draft.

### CALCAREA SULFURICA

# CALC. SULF.

*Calc. sulf., commonly known as calcium sulfate, is used to make plaster casts, cement, and white pigment. Schussler, who identified it as a tissue salt (see p. 227), believed that a deficiency of calcium sulfate prevented worn-out red blood cells from breaking down correctly, causing tissues to become infected and filled with pus.*

**Common names** Calcium sulfate, gypsum, plaster of Paris.
**Source** Gypsum, which is found in Canada, the US, Italy, and France.
**Parts used** Calcium sulfate.

#### CONSTITUTIONAL TYPE

A key characteristic of *Calc. sulf.* types is jealousy. This can lead to a state of melancholy and irritability. Curiously, these types crave unripe fruit. They are intolerant of heat and prefer to be uncovered even when it is cold.

#### AILMENTS TREATED

This remedy is used whenever there is a discharge of pus, or for wounds that are slow to heal, for example, abscesses, boils, carbuncles, cysts, or infected eczema. Associated symptoms include a yellow coating at the base of the tongue, swollen glands, and a burning sensation on the soles of the feet.

**Symptoms better** From fresh air; from eating; from drinking tea.
**Symptoms worse** In cold, wet weather.

### CALENDULA OFFICINALIS

# CALENDULA

*Calendula officinalis is a common garden plant. Its antiseptic and anti-inflammatory properties have been employed since ancient times to treat a variety of complaints, ranging from skin problems to cancer. Today, it is one of the most commonly used medicinal herbs, especially for skin problems. In addition to the remedy, the tincture is used externally for cuts.*

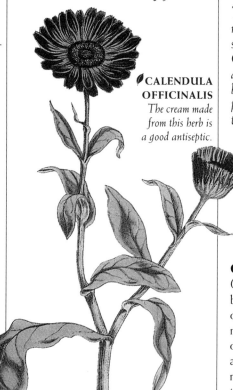

**CALENDULA OFFICINALIS**
The cream made from this herb is a good antiseptic.

**Common names** Calendula, pot marigold.
**Source** Native to France, now grown worldwide.
**Parts used** Fresh leaves and flowers.

#### AILMENTS TREATED

*Calendula*, which is mainly used externally in the form of a cream or tincture, is a popular homeopathic antiseptic and can be used to promote healing, even if the skin is broken. It helps control bleeding, for example from minor cuts, and abrasions. It is widely used in midwifery to treat perineal tears after childbirth.

The antiseptic properties of the tincture make it an effective gargle for mouth ulcers and sore throats and it helps control bleeding after tooth extractions. *Calendula* has been given internally for jaundice and fever where there is associated irritability and nervousness and acute hearing.
**Symptoms better** Lying completely still; from walking.
**Symptoms worse** In damp, cloudy weather; in a draft; from eating.

### CAPSICUM FRUTESCENS

# CAPSICUM

*The homeopathic remedy Capsicum is made from the chilli pepper, which is still known in homeopathy by the name C. annuum. Medicinally, chillies are a powerful stimulant for the whole body, increasing blood flow and promoting perspiration. In the past they were used to treat infections.*

**Common names** Chilli pepper, red cayenne pepper.
**Source** Native to the East and West Indies and South America, now grown worldwide.
**Parts used** Dried capsules and seeds from the mature fruit.

#### CONSTITUTIONAL TYPE

*Capsicum* types have light hair and blue eyes. They tend to be unfit or overweight, with lax muscles. Too much stimulation, either from work or overindulgence of caffeine, alcohol, spicy foods, or tobacco makes them sluggish. Children tend to be clumsy, adults are awkward and both tend to be lazy, unclean, sad, nostalgic and prone to homesickness.

#### AILMENTS TREATED

Complaints helped by this remedy are characterized by stinging pain in the bladder, thighs, back, ears, neck, and, when coughing, the chest. The pain resembles the burning sensation caused by eating or touching hot peppers. *Capsicum* is given for mouth ulcers, diarrhea, hemorrhoids, heartburn, rheumatism, and sore throats. People who need *Capsicum* crave stimulants such as coffee, although these aggravate the burning pain.

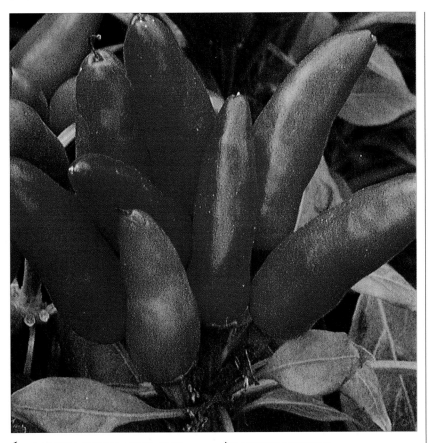

*CAUSTICUM HAHNEMANNI*

# CAUSTICUM

Causticum *is a potassium compound that is unique to homeopathy. It was manufactured and proved by Hahnemann in the early 19th century; he noted that it caused an astringent sensation and burning taste on the back of the tongue.*

**Common name** Potassium hydrate.
**Source** Prepared chemically by distilling freshly burned lime, potassium bisulfate, and water.
**Parts used** Clear distillate.

### CONSTITUTIONAL TYPE
*Causticum* types are dark-haired, dark-eyed, and sallow-skinned. They are weak, rigid-thinking people who suffer prolonged effects from grief and are sympathetic to the suffering of others. They tend to feel chilly and have warts around the nails, and on the eyelids, face, and nose.

### AILMENTS TREATED
This remedy is mainly used for weakness or paralysis of the nerves and muscles in the bladder, larynx, vocal cords, upper eyelids, or the right side of the face. In the bladder, this can lead to bedwetting, especially if the person is very cold, and leakage of urine when sneezing, coughing, walking, or blowing the nose. Hoarseness and laryngitis are often associated with a dry, deep cough where it is difficult to bring up mucus. Raw, burning pain is characteristic, especially in rheumatism, and in heartburn in pregnancy.
**Symptoms better** From cold drinks; with warmth; from washing.
**Symptoms worse** In dry, cold winds; in the evening; from exertion.

**MAIN SELF-HELP USES**
Bedwetting – see pp. 218–9
Heartburn in pregnancy – see pp. 210–11
Laryngitis – see pp. 178–9
Rheumatism – see pp. 156–7
Stress incontinence – see pp. 200–1.

---

*CAPSICUM FRUTESCENS Chillies, or red cayenne peppers, are used medicinally for their stimulant properties.*

**Symptoms better** With continued movement; from eating; with heat.
**Symptoms worse** In cool surroundings; starting to move; in a draft.

**MAIN SELF-HELP USE** Heartburn in pregnancy – see pp. 210–11.

---

*CAULOPHYLLUM THALICTROIDES*

# CAULOPHYLLUM

*The root of this plant was used as an herbal remedy by Native Americans to prevent long and painful labors and to quicken childbirth. The plant is still used in herbal medicine as a tonic and uterine stimulant. Caulophyllum was first introduced to homeopathy in 1875 by Dr. Hale, a well-known American homeopath.*

**Common names**
Blue cohosh, squaw root, papoose root.
**Source** Grows in Canada and the US.
**Parts used** Fresh root.

### AILMENTS TREATED
*Caulophyllum* has two main uses in homeopathy: the first is for rheumatism that affects the small joints of the hands and feet with erratic, shooting cramping pain; the second is to help labor that does not progress properly, for example, when there is weak, irregular labor pain, or very painful but ineffectual contractions. It is also given for false labor pain.

This remedy can help prevent habitual miscarriages and to ease severe pain following childbirth and menstrual pain. Because it is a uterine stimulant it may stimulate menstruation in women suffering absent menstruation.
**Symptoms better** With warmth.
**Symptoms worse** In pregnancy; from suppressed menstruation.

*CAULOPHYLLUM THALICTROIDES The root is used to make a remedy.*

123

### CEANOTHUS AMERICANUS

# CEANOTHUS

*The leaves of this tall, deciduous plant were used as a tea substitute during the American Revolution. Its homeopathic use was first discovered in the mid-19th century, but it was not until 1900, after further study, that it became known as a remedy for pain and enlargement of the spleen.*

**Common names** Jersey tea root, red root.
**Source** Native to the US and Canada.
**Parts used** Fresh leaves from the flowering plant.

#### AILMENTS TREATED
*Ceanothus* is used mainly for pain, inflammation, enlargement or a sensation of fullness in the left side of the abdomen, and cutting pain that is worse when lying on the left side. People who need this remedy are very chilly and need to sit close to a source of heat to keep warm.
**Symptoms better** With rest.
**Symptoms worse** Lying on the left side; with movement.

### CEANOTHUS AMERICANUS
*The leaves of this ornamental shrub are used to make a remedy that is mainly given for abdominal pain.*

### CHELIDONIUM MAJUS

# CHELIDONIUM

*According to the Doctrine of Signatures (see p. 11), the yellow juice of this plant meant that it was good for liver disorders, such as jaundice. In fact, the juice is poisonous. Commonly known as wartweed for its power to remove warts, it belongs to the same plant family as the poppy.*

**Common names** Greater celandine, wartweed.
**Source** Native to Europe, now grown in many countries.
**Parts used** Fresh plant in flower.

#### CONSTITUTIONAL TYPE
*Chelidonium* types are usually thin, fair, lethargic people who tend to be depressed, anxious, pessimistic, and despondent. They are sluggish mentally and unwilling to make any effort. They tend to have headaches accompanied by great lethargy and heaviness and crave cheese and hot drinks.

#### AILMENTS TREATED
This remedy is used for liver and bile disorders, for example gallstones, indigestion, jaundice, and hepatitis. Characteristically there is often a bruised, aching pain on the lower part of the right shoulder blade, with an upset stomach, nausea, vomiting, and possibly distension of the upper abdomen. Abdominal symptoms are relieved by passing stools. Symptoms are usually right-sided. Externally, the remedy is used to treat warts.

When ill, people who need this remedy feel generally "liverish" or nauseous, and depressed with a dull headache. They have a sallow, yellowish complexion. One foot may feel hot and the other cold.
**Symptoms better** From drinking milk and hot drinks; from eating; from firm pressure.
**Symptoms worse** With heat; from changes in the weather; early in the morning; around 4 a.m. and 4 p.m.

### CICUTA VIROSA

# CICUTA

*Orthodox medicine still uses this plant occasionally to treat gout. The fresh root is extremely toxic and causes symptoms of poisoning similar to those of strychnine poisoning with spasms, excessive salivation, sweating, and hyperventilation.*

**Common name** Water hemlock.
**Source** Grows in Europe, Siberia, the US, and Canada.
**Parts used** Fresh root.

#### AILMENTS TREATED
*Cicuta* is used for twitching and spasmodic jerks, especially where the head is bent backward, for example, in epilepsy, meningitis, eclampsia, and paralysis, and for the after-effects of head injuries. People who need this remedy may have a desire to eat inedible things such as chalk.
**Symptoms better** With heat; from passing gas.
**Symptoms worse** From jarring or touch; in cool surroundings.

## COFFEA

*COFFEA ARABICA/C. CRUDA*

*Coffee was reportedly first drunk in Persia and introduced to Aden in the 15th century. Caffeine, its main ingredient, has been used medicinally as a stimulant, painkiller, diuretic, and digestive tonic. Today, it is still used in combination with aspirin and other common analgesics.*

**Common name** Coffee.
**Source** Native to Arabia and Ethiopia, now grown in the West Indies and Central America.
**Parts used** Unroasted coffee beans.

### AILMENTS TREATED

*Coffea* is used to treat excessive mental activity that leads to insomnia and extreme sensitivity to pain, such as a bad toothache or labor pain. All five senses are acute and any noise is intolerable. *Coffea* is also given for menopause and overexcitement.
**Symptoms better** From ice-cold water in the mouth; with rest.
**Symptoms worse** In cold, windy weather; near noise or odors; if touched.

### ⚕ MAIN SELF-HELP USES

Insomnia – see pp. 194–5
Labor pain – see pp. 212–13
Sleeplessness in children – see pp. 216–17
Toothache – see pp. 162–3.

---

## COLCHICUM

*COLCHICUM AUTUMNALE*

*The ancient Greeks found this plant to be invaluable in the treatment of gout and rheumatism, and it was called "the soul of the joints." It has also been used for bronchitis, dropsy, fevers, venereal disease, neuroses, and convulsions.*

⚕**COLCHICUM AUTUMNALE**
*A remedy is made from the fresh bulb.*

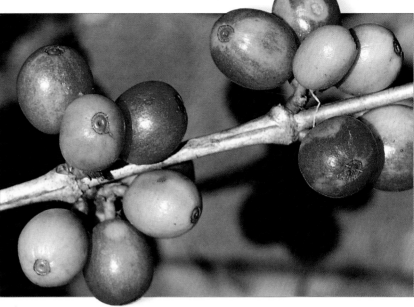

⚕**COFFEA ARABICA** *The ripe, red berries contain coffee beans. These are used to make the Coffea remedy, which is given for insomnia.*

**Common names** Meadow saffron, naked ladies.
**Source** Grows in Europe, Asia Minor, the US, and Canada.
**Parts used** Fresh bulb.

### AILMENTS TREATED

The key use of *Colchicum* is for gout where the pain is severe and touch or the slightest motion is unbearable. Characteristically, the big toe is the most affected and the pain causes extreme sensitivity.
  *Colchicum* is also used to treat digestive disorders such as heartburn, nausea, vomiting, and diarrhea, which are better for bending forward. It also helps heart disorders and muscle and joint complaints.
**Symptoms better** With warmth; with rest and quiet.
**Symptoms worse** With movement; if touched; in cold, damp conditions, especially in autumn.

---

## CONIUM

*CONIUM MACULATUM*

*Also known as hemlock, this toxic herb was used by the ancient Greeks as a "state poison" to kill criminals; Socrates was forced to drink its juice. The Romans, Dioscorides, and Pliny used the plant medicinally for skin disorders, complaints of the nervous system and liver, breast tumors, and cancer, to calm sexual urges, and as a painkiller.*

**Common names** Common hemlock, spotted hemlock.
**Source** Grows in Europe, eastern Asia, the US, Canada, and Chile.
**Parts used** Juice expressed from the leaves and flowering stems.

### CONSTITUTIONAL TYPE

Emotionally, people who need this remedy have a limited outlook that leads to a sensation of dullness, indifference to external impressions, and depression with fixed ideas and superstitions. This emotional paralysis may be caused by either sexual excess or sexual frustration. They become depressed when they lose their sexual partners.

### AILMENTS TREATED

*Conium* is used for glandular enlargements such as cancerous tumors, especially in the breast, and nervous disorders with gradual paralysis in the muscles from the feet upward. This paralysis may be accompanied by sensitivity to light.
  The remedy is also given for dizziness that is worse when lying down or turning the head; sore breasts before and during menstruation and in pregnancy; premature ejaculation; and prostate enlargement.
**Symptoms better** From pressure; from passing gas; with continued movement.
**Symptoms worse** Looking at moving objects; from alcohol; from sexual excess or celibacy.

### ⚕ MAIN SELF-HELP USE

Breast pain – see pp. 210–11.

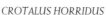

## CROCUS SATIVUS
# CROCUS

*The long red stigmas of Crocus sativus, which are the source of saffron, were first used medicinally by Hippocrates as a purgative and emollient and for their aphrodisiac properties. The ancient Arabians used saffron to treat a difficult labor and liver disease. Since then, saffron has been used in orthodox medicine for a wide range of conditions, including mental illness, arthritis, and asthma.*

**Common name** Saffron crocus.
**Source** Native to western Asia, now grown throughout Europe.
**Parts used** Stigma and part of the style.

### AILMENTS TREATED
*Crocus* is used to treat emotional symptoms, such as the sudden onset of sadness, even while reading something absorbing and interesting. Moods alternate from angry to calm and from humorous to sad. There is a curious sensation as if everything in the body is twitching, which can be a symptom of a mental illness, such as schizophrenia.

Other symptoms treated include menstrual bleeding or nasal bleeding that is black, clotted, and stringy.
**Symptoms better** From fresh air; from eating breakfast.
**Symptoms worse** Near music; in warm rooms.

## CROTALUS HORRIDUS
# CROTALUS HOR.

*The rattlesnake is distinctive because of its tail, which makes a rattling sound when it is about to strike. The homeopathic remedy was first proved by Dr. Hering in 1837 (see p. 17) and is used today for a range of serious illnesses.*

**Common names** Rattlesnake, pit viper.
**Source** Found in arid regions of Canada, the US, and South America.
**Parts used** Fresh venom.

### AILMENTS TREATED
*Crotalus hor.* helps stop bleeding from any orifice, especially when it is slow and the blood is dark, thin, and does not clot. The remedy is used for jaundice, sepsis, and total collapse. It is also given for right-sided strokes, cancer, and heart problems where the person is worse lying on the left side and the pain extends to the left hand. Sometimes it is given for swelling in the whole body; for example in liver failure and blood poisoning. It can also be helpful for alcoholism.
**Symptoms better** From fresh air.
**Symptoms worse** In warm, wet weather; complaints tend to be right-sided but are aggravated by lying on the left side; wearing tight clothes.

**CROTALUS HORRIDUS** *The venom of this snake is the source of a remedy used to treat serious ailments, such as strokes.*

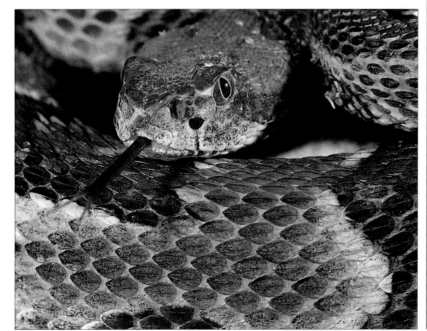

## CYCLAMEN EUROPAEUM
# CYCLAMEN

*This flowering plant was used extensively in ancient times by Greek, Roman, and Arabian physicians for phlegm, an enlarged spleen, liver diseases, such as jaundice and hepatitis, and to promote menstruation.*

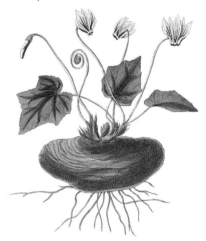

**CYCLAMEN EUROPAEUM** *The large, tuberous root was used as a purgative in herbalism because it is extremely acrid.*

**Common name** Sowbread.
**Source** Grows in southern Europe and North Africa.
**Parts used** Juice from the fresh root.

### AILMENTS TREATED
*Cyclamen* is used to regulate the menstrual cycle and to treat violent headaches with flickering before the eyes. It is also good for burning pain in the skin and muscles. People who require this remedy may have an aversion to fatty foods and desire inedible things like chalk, earth, and worms. They are often depressed and full of remorse.
**Symptoms better** With movement; from crying.
**Symptoms worse** From fresh air.

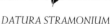

## DATURA STRAMONIUM
# STRAMONIUM

*This plant is strongly narcotic and its main use in medicine has been as a pain reliever for rheumatism, neuralgia, and sciatica. In 16th-century Europe it was eaten by soldiers to dull their emotions before a battle. It is poisonous and causes sedation and hallucinations.*

**Common names** Thornapple, devil's apple, Jamestown-weed.
**Source** Grows in Europe, Asia, and the US.
**Parts used** Juice expressed from the fresh plant before it flowers, or seeds.

## AILMENTS TREATED

The main use of *Stramonium* is for disorders of the nervous system with associated fears and violent muscle spasms, cramps, and even convulsions. The main fears are of darkness, water, and violence. It is used as a remedy for night terrors or for conditions that occur after a scare, especially in children. Children and adults needing the remedy often stammer due to nervousness. Other symptoms may include diminished urine or perspiration, and recurrent twitching and jerking as in restless legs, epilepsy, meningitis, and strokes, and great thirst, especially for acidic drinks. It is also an important remedy for high fever in children.
**Symptoms better** In light; around company; with warmth.
**Symptoms worse** With sleep, especially a long sleep; in cloudy weather; when alone; when attempting to swallow, particularly liquids.

---

*DELPHINIUM STAPHYSAGRIA*

# STAPHYSAGRIA

*This remedy was known to the ancient Greeks and Romans. It was taken internally to cause vomiting and to purge the bowels, and used externally in the form of an ointment as an antidote to stings and bites.*

**Common names** Stavesacre, palmated larkspur.
**Source** Grows in southern Europe and Asia.
**Parts used** Seeds.

## CONSTITUTIONAL TYPE

These types have deeply suppressed emotions, especially rage. They seem mild and yielding, but are very sensitive to rudeness and insults. They fear losing self-control and tend to have a high sex drive. Their sweat, stools, and gas may smell of rotten eggs. They are addicted to work and crave alcohol and sweet foods.

## AILMENTS TREATED

The remedy is most often used for complaints involving the nerves, such as neuralgia, teething problems, cystitis, sties, blepharitis (inflammation of the eyelid), and headaches that feel as if a weight is pressing out from the forehead. It is also useful for women with new sexual partners, who have pain during sexual intercourse.
**Symptoms better** With warmth.
**Symptoms worse** After an afternoon nap; from eating breakfast; when emotions are suppressed.

 **MAIN SELF-HELP USES**
Cystitis – see pp. 200–1
Sties – see pp. 168–9.

---

*DIGITALIS PURPUREA*

# DIGITALIS

*Foxglove was used by the ancient Britons to cure wounds. Many hundreds of years later, in 1785, Dr. William Withering discovered its properties for treating dropsy. It is still used in orthodox medicine to treat heart failure and heartbeat irregularities, and in homeopathy it is a key heart remedy.*

**Common name** Foxglove.
**Source** Native to Europe.
**Parts used** Juice expressed from young, fresh leaves.

## AILMENTS TREATED

*Digitalis* is used to treat a very slow pulse or an irregular, intermittent pulse associated with the following: heart failure; weakness with a faint, sinking feeling in the stomach; and nausea at the sight or smell of food. The heart feels as if it will stop beating with the slightest movement. There may be associated liver problems, such as hepatitis.
**Symptoms better** From fresh air; from having an empty stomach.
**Symptoms worse** Sitting up; from eating; near music.
**Caution** Available only by prescription in the US and Canada.

This biennial has large, pendulous, purple flowers

**DIGITALIS PURPUREA**
*Foxglove leaves gathered in spring before the plant flowers are the source of an effective heart remedy.*

## ELAPS

*The coral snake rarely bites when handled, but the venom can kill humans. The poison acts as an anticoagulant (stops blood from clotting), which leads to hemorrhaging. The homeopathic remedy, which is made from the venom, was first proved by an American homeopath in the 19th century. It is used to treat bleeding and strokes.*

**Common name** Coral snake.
**Source** True coral snakes are found only in Canada, the US, and South America, especially in Brazil, but similar forms are found in Asia and Africa.
**Parts used** Fresh venom.

### AILMENTS TREATED
*Elaps* is used for heavy bleeding and black discharges, such as in nosebleeds and menorrhagia (excessive loss of blood during menstruation) and to treat right-sided strokes, especially when there are spasms followed by paralysis. Symptoms of these disorders are associated with a sensation of internal coldness and a craving for oranges, and ice. Curiously, cold food and drink, fruit, the approach of a thunderstorm, humidity, and bed warmth aggravate the symptoms. People who need this remedy are fearful of rain, being alone, snakes, strokes, and death.
**Symptoms better** At night.
**Symptoms worse** From walking; lying on the abdomen; from cold drinks.

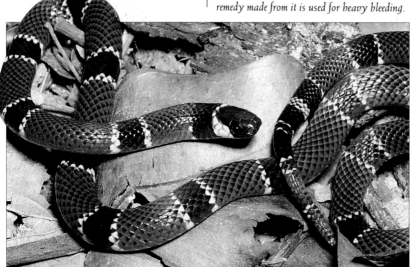

## EQUISETUM

*This prehistoric plant is related to trees that grew on earth during the Carboniferous period. Although poisonous to livestock, it has been used to heal wounds since ancient times. Chinese doctors use the herb to treat eye disorders, dysentery, flu, and hemorrhoids.*

**Common names** Horsetail, scouring rush.
**Source** E. hiemale grows in the East, particularly China. E. arvense grows in many places except in Australasia.
**Parts used** Whole, fresh plant.

### AILMENTS TREATED
*Equisetum* is used for symptoms associated with an irritable bladder, for example, pain that is worse at the end of urination; a sensation of pressure with an aching, full, tender bladder; a constant desire to pass urine; and dribbling of urine or mucus in the urine. Although the symptoms are similar to cystitis, there is no infection present. The remedy is also good for treating bedwetting in children that occurs during dreams or nightmares.
**Symptoms better** Lying on the back.
**Symptoms worse** With movement; from pressure; if touched.

### MAIN SELF-HELP USE
Bedwetting – see pp. 218–9.

**ELAPS CORALLINUS** *The coral snake is very poisonous and marked with tricolored bands. Its venom causes hemorrhaging and the remedy made from it is used for heavy bleeding.*

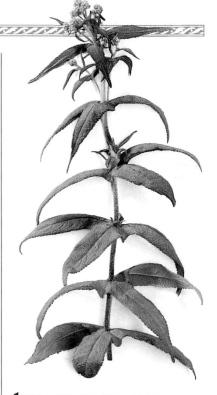

**EUPATORIUM PERFOLIATUM**
*This aromatic plant is the source of an excellent fever remedy, which is used for fever with muscle and bone pain.*

## EUPATOR.

*Boneset was traditionally used for fevers and is said to be a principal Native American remedy for malaria. It became known to the European settlers and was used in New York in 1830 to treat malaria. It is also said to have been recommended in ancient times by Dioscorides for ulcers, dysentery, reptile bites, chronic fevers, and liver disease. The plant is used in herbal medicine for flu with aches and pains.*

**Common names** Boneset, agueweed, thoroughwort.
**Source** Native to Canada and the US, now grown in Europe.
**Parts used** Whole, fresh plant in flower.

### AILMENTS TREATED
*Eupator.* is used mainly to treat flu and other feverish illnesses where characteristically there is tremendous bone pain and fever with scanty perspiration and restlessness because of the pain. The bones often feel as if they have been broken. The head, eyeballs, and chest are sore and there is a desire for ice-cold water and cold food. There may be a cough that

exacerbates symptoms and can be relieved by going on all fours.
**Symptoms better** From being indoors; from conversation; after vomiting bile.
**Symptoms worse** From fresh air; movement; between 7 a.m. and 9 a.m.

*FERRUM METALLICUM*

# FERRUM MET.

*Iron is widely used in orthodox medicine in the form of dietary supplements. A deficiency of iron in the diet or in its absorption leads to anemia with resultant fatigue and breathlessness. Although there is no direct link between a dietary lack of iron and the homeopathic remedy, some homeopaths believe that the remedy helps the body to absorb and utilize iron in the diet more efficiently.*

**Common name** Iron.
**Source** Iron, from iron ores such as hematite, which is found in Canada, the US, and Venezuela.
**Parts used** Iron.

### AILMENTS TREATED
*Ferrum met.* is often needed by well-built people who look healthy but who tend to be weak, feel the cold, and suffer from circulatory problems or anemia. This weakness affects them mentally, making them very sensitive to noise, intolerant of contradiction, and changeable in mood. They dislike moving around because of fatigue and prefer to sit down, but curiously, because of pain or restlessness, they are forced to keep moving. *Ferrum met.* types dislike eggs and fatty foods, which may upset their digestion, but like tomatoes and sour foods.
**Symptoms better** With gentle movement.
**Symptoms worse** At night.

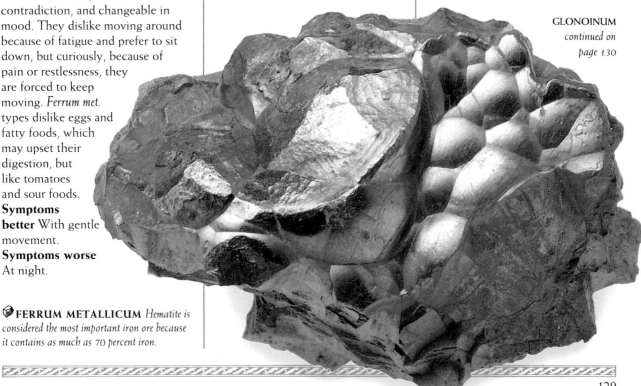

⚘ **FERRUM METALLICUM** *Hematite is considered the most important iron ore because it contains as much as 70 percent iron.*

*FLUORICUM ACIDUM*

# FLUOR. AC.

Fluoricum acidum, *also known as hydrofluoric acid, is used in large quantities in industry to clean metals and for polishing, frosting, and etching glass. Hydrofluoric acid contains fluorine, which is stored in teeth and bones. A deficiency of fluorine can lead to tooth decay. Fluoride, a compound of fluorine, is often added to the water supply to prevent tooth decay.*

**Common name** Hydrofluoric acid.
**Source** Prepared chemically by distilling calcium fluoride (the calcium salt of fluorine) with sulfuric acid to produce hydrogen fluoride gas, which is then dissolved in water to give hydrofluoric acid.
**Parts used** Hydrofluoric acid.

### CONSTITUTIONAL TYPE
*Fluor. ac.* types are materialistic with few spiritual values, domineering, and obsessed with sex. They tend to be selfish, giving no attention to their loved ones or family. This may mean they cut themselves off from others, or alternatively, it may be because they are self-satisfied and egotistical and do not wish to commit themselves to others or to be held responsible. These types are very energetic, do not feel the cold, and do not suffer from muscle fatigue. A short sleep revives them.

### AILMENTS TREATED
Conditions that affect fibrous tissues, such as veins and bones, are treated with *Fluor. ac.* These include varicose veins, pain in the coccyx, and more serious conditions such as bone tumors. The remedy is also used for tooth decay.
**Symptoms better** From cold compresses; from fresh air.
**Symptoms worse** With heat.

*GLONOINUM*

# GLONOIN.

*Glonoinum, or glyceryl trinitrate, is a colorless, oily, toxic liquid. It was discovered by an Italian chemist, A. Sobrero, in 1846. In 1867 the Swedish scientist, Alfred Nobel, added kiesel-guhr to it to produce dynamite, which is one of the most powerful explosives known. Glyceryl trinitrate has a potent effect on the circulation and is used in orthodox medicine to treat angina.*

**Common names** Glyceryl trinitrate, nitroglycerine.
**Source** Prepared chemically by adding glycerine to a mixture of nitric and sulfuric acids.
**Parts used** Glyceryl trinitrate.

### AILMENTS TREATED
This remedy is mainly used for complaints, such as heatstroke, that involve the nervous control of the

**GLONOINUM**
*continued on page 130*

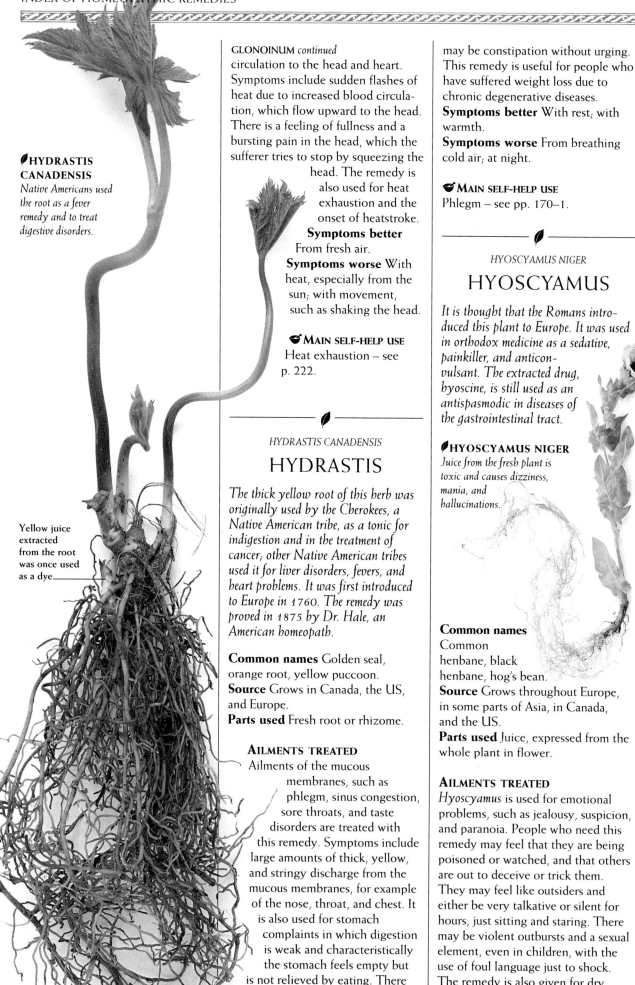

**HYDRASTIS CANADENSIS**
*Native Americans used the root as a fever remedy and to treat digestive disorders.*

Yellow juice extracted from the root was once used as a dye

**GLONOINUM** *continued*
circulation to the head and heart. Symptoms include sudden flashes of heat due to increased blood circulation, which flow upward to the head. There is a feeling of fullness and a bursting pain in the head, which the sufferer tries to stop by squeezing the head. The remedy is also used for heat exhaustion and the onset of heatstroke.
**Symptoms better** From fresh air.
**Symptoms worse** With heat, especially from the sun; with movement, such as shaking the head.

**MAIN SELF-HELP USE**
Heat exhaustion – see p. 222.

---

*HYDRASTIS CANADENSIS*

# HYDRASTIS

The thick yellow root of this herb was originally used by the Cherokees, a Native American tribe, as a tonic for indigestion and in the treatment of cancer; other Native American tribes used it for liver disorders, fevers, and heart problems. It was first introduced to Europe in 1760. The remedy was proved in 1875 by Dr. Hale, an American homeopath.

**Common names** Golden seal, orange root, yellow puccoon.
**Source** Grows in Canada, the US, and Europe.
**Parts used** Fresh root or rhizome.

**AILMENTS TREATED**
Ailments of the mucous membranes, such as phlegm, sinus congestion, sore throats, and taste disorders are treated with this remedy. Symptoms include large amounts of thick, yellow, and stringy discharge from the mucous membranes, for example of the nose, throat, and chest. It is also used for stomach complaints in which digestion is weak and characteristically the stomach feels empty but is not relieved by eating. There

may be constipation without urging. This remedy is useful for people who have suffered weight loss due to chronic degenerative diseases.
**Symptoms better** With rest; with warmth.
**Symptoms worse** From breathing cold air; at night.

**MAIN SELF-HELP USE**
Phlegm – see pp. 170–1.

---

*HYOSCYAMUS NIGER*

# HYOSCYAMUS

It is thought that the Romans introduced this plant to Europe. It was used in orthodox medicine as a sedative, painkiller, and anticonvulsant. The extracted drug, hyoscine, is still used as an antispasmodic in diseases of the gastrointestinal tract.

**HYOSCYAMUS NIGER**
*Juice from the fresh plant is toxic and causes dizziness, mania, and hallucinations.*

**Common names**
Common henbane, black henbane, hog's bean.
**Source** Grows throughout Europe, in some parts of Asia, in Canada, and the US.
**Parts used** Juice, expressed from the whole plant in flower.

**AILMENTS TREATED**
*Hyoscyamus* is used for emotional problems, such as jealousy, suspicion, and paranoia. People who need this remedy may feel that they are being poisoned or watched, and that others are out to deceive or trick them. They may feel like outsiders and either be very talkative or silent for hours, just sitting and staring. There may be violent outbursts and a sexual element, even in children, with the use of foul language just to shock. The remedy is also given for dry,

spasmodic coughs, epilepsy, and other conditions, in which twitching, jerking, and cramps occur.
**Symptoms better** Sitting up.
**Symptoms worse** From emotional stress; if touched; lying down.

## IODUM

### IODUM

*Iodine is essential for the normal functioning of the human body. Iodine deficiency causes symptoms such as dry skin, hair loss, swollen face and thyroid gland, weak muscles, weight gain, mental sluggishness, and fatigue. This condition is rare in the West because potassium iodide (a salt of iodine) is added to table salt.*

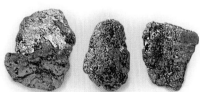

**IODUM** *In the past, iodine was used as a local antiseptic. It is still used in this way as povidine iodine (an iodine and alcohol mix).*

**Common name** Iodine.
**Source** Largely derived from seaweed, and saltpeter deposits particularly in Chile.
**Parts used** Iodine.

#### AILMENTS TREATED
*Iodum* is used mainly to treat symptoms associated with an overactive thyroid. These include eye pain, enlarged glands, and a ravenous appetite but a tendency to lose weight and to feel weak from hunger. The slightest physical exertion causes sweating.

People who require this remedy have an obsessive desire to keep frantically busy because they get persistent frightening thoughts when they have to sit and remain still. However, their excessive activity is not organized, making them extremely forgetful, and leads to constant rechecking, for example, to make sure that they have locked the doors at night. They are talkative and are excessively restless mentally.

*Iodum* is also used to treat disorders of the mucous membranes (particularly those of the larynx) and

the heart and blood vessels. It is also given for bone pain that comes on at night and deep, hacking coughs.
**Symptoms better** From eating; from fresh air; with movement.
**Symptoms worse** In hot rooms.

## KALI BROMATUM

### KALI BROM.

*Potassium bromide is a white crystalline salt that is used in photography. In orthodox medicine it was once used in large doses for severe epilepsy and other convulsive disorders. It was also given to men with excessive sexual desires and male prisoners were given potassium bromide to reduce their sexual urges.*

**Common name** Potassium bromide.
**Source** A crystalline solid that is prepared chemically.
**Parts used** Potassium bromide.

#### CONSTITUTIONAL TYPE
These types are continually in conflict between morality and immorality, and feel nervous and suspicious. They believe that they are the object of divine vengeance and worry that they have been singled out for punishment. They have a strong sense of helplessness and insecurity, particularly during puberty, when they may become obsessed by a guilty conscience about their sexual urges. This makes them restless, with a desire to keep continually busy.

#### AILMENTS TREATED
*Kali brom.* is used to treat conditions that affect the nervous system, such as epilepsy, and skin complaints, particularly acne that leaves unsightly scars. People who need this remedy are prone to acne, especially in puberty and during menstruation. They are warm-blooded but sometimes feel numb.

**KALI BROMATUM** *The Kali brom. remedy is made from white potassium bromide.*

## KALI CARBONICUM

### KALI CARB.

*Potassium carbonate is a compound that was used by the Egyptians more than 3,000 years ago to make glass. It occurs naturally as a vegetable alkali and is found in all plant structures. Potassium carbonate is either obtained from the ashes of burned wood and plants or prepared industrially.*

**Common name** Potassium carbonate.
**Source** Potassium carbonate, which is obtained from wood ashes.
**Parts used** Potassium carbonate.

#### CONSTITUTIONAL TYPE
People who need this remedy (along with other *Kali* types) have high moral standards, with a sense of duty and a strong fear of losing control. They are very possessive both in material and emotional terms. This can make life very difficult for those close to them. *Kali carb.* types are prone to react badly to emotional upsets and will usually feel these as a blow to the stomach.

#### AILMENTS TREATED
This remedy is used for disorders of the muscles and spine, such as backache, especially in the lumbar region; menopausal and menstrual problems; and complaints in the mucous membranes, especially in the chest, such as bronchitis and coughs. Pain tends to be stitchlike. People who need this remedy are very chilly and have a characteristic puffiness under their upper eyelids. They sweat profusely and the cooling that results may cause them to get chilled easily and make them more susceptible to colds and flu.
**Symptoms better** With warmth; in dry, warm weather.
**Symptoms worse** With rest; in cool surroundings; before menstruation; from exertion; between 2 a.m. and 3 a.m.; bending forward.

**Symptoms better** When busy.
**Symptoms worse** During menstruation.

**MAIN SELF-HELP USE**
Acne – see pp. 186–7.

*KALI IODATUM*

# KALI IOD.

*Potassium iodide is the compound added to table salt and animal feeds to protect against iodine deficiency (see Iodum on p. 131). The World Health Organization recommends that 1 part potassium iodide be added to every 100,000 parts salt. Potassium iodide was once used to treat syphilis.*

**Common name** Potassium iodide.
**Source** Prepared chemically from iodine and potassium hydroxide.
**Parts used** Potassium iodine.

## CONSTITUTIONAL TYPE

*Kali iod.* types have a very highly developed sense of what is right and what is wrong, and tend to see things in black and white. They are difficult to live with, irritable with a very bad temper, and may even be cruel to others. They prefer cool weather.

## AILMENTS TREATED

This remedy is used to treat glandular complaints, such as swollen glands associated with flu, sore throats, and prostate problems. Pains are diffuse rather than localized. People who need this remedy tend to get hay fever and sinus congestion, especially in hot weather, and they have thick green mucus or acrid watery discharges from the nose.
**Symptoms better** From fresh air; with movement.
**Symptoms worse** Between 2 a.m. and 5 a.m; with heat; if touched.

*KALI MURIATICUM*

# KALI MUR.

*Potassium chloride is a white crystalline solid or powder, and is the most abundant of the naturally occurring salts of potassium, found mainly in the mineral sylvine. It is a Schussler tissue salt (see p. 227), which is used for the secondary stage of inflammatory illnesses. A deficiency of this salt affects fibrin, which is an important component in bloodclotting in the body.*

**Common name** Potassium chloride.
**Source** Sylvine, which is found in Germany, Canada, and the US.
**Parts used** Potassium chloride.

## AILMENTS TREATED

*Kali mur.* is used to treat inflammation of the mucous membranes with a stringy discharge. It is very good for infections in the middle ear and the eustachian tubes (which connect the middle ear cavity to the back of the nose), particularly where secretions are white, thick, sticky, and slimy; it is also used for temporary deafness from eustachian tube mucus. This remedy is also given for glue ear (fluid inside the ear), mucus that drips down the back of the throat, and tonsillitis, when swallowing is only possible by twisting the neck and the tonsils have a white coating on them.
**Symptoms better** From cold drinks; from rubbing the affected part.
**Symptoms worse** From fresh air; in cold, damp weather; from rich, fatty foods; during menstruation.

 **MAIN SELF-HELP USE**
Phlegm – see pp. 170–1.

*LAC CANINUM*

# LAC CAN.

*Bitch's milk (from female dogs) is an ancient medicine and was recommended by Pliny to stimulate the expulsion of a dead fetus, and to treat ovarian pain, and cervical and uterine problems. Sextus, an ancient Greek physician, found it useful for light intolerance and inflammation of the inner ear.*

**Common name** Bitch's milk.
**Source** Mongrel bitch.
**Parts used** Bitch's milk.

## CONSTITUTIONAL TYPE

*Lac can.* types tend to be very sensitive (to the point of getting hysterical), lack self-confidence, and have an overactive imagination. They are also fearful, especially of snakes. They may be absentminded and aggressive.

## AILMENTS TREATED

Sore throats, tonsillitis, and cervical erosion (wearing away of the cells lining the cervix) are treated with this remedy. It is very helpful when symptoms alternate from one side of the body to the other. For example, with a sore throat the pain may start in the right side of the throat, then move to the left, then back to the right. It is also a common remedy for swollen breasts before menstruation and for breastfeeding problems. People who need this remedy may have a sensation of floating on air, and desire salty, pungent foods, and warm drinks.
**Symptoms better** From fresh air.
**Symptoms worse** If touched.

*LACTRODECTUS MACTANS*

# LACTRODECTUS MAC.

*The black widow has extremely toxic venom, which can be fatal to both humans and animals. Symptoms of poisoning include muscular cramps, vascular spasms, cold sweats, and chest pain that resembles angina. The homeopathic remedy, which is made from the venom of the female spider, is used to treat acute chest pain associated with angina and heart attacks.*

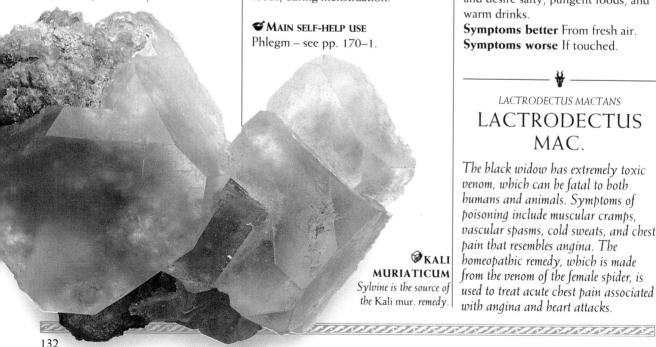

 **KALI MURIATICUM**
*Sylvine is the source of the Kali mur. remedy.*

**Common name** Black widow spider.
**Source** Found in warm areas in the world, especially the US.
**Parts used** Whole, live female spider.

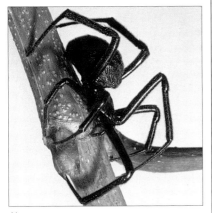

**⚕LACTRODECTUS MACTANS**
*The female black widow spider is the source of a remedy given for angina and anxiety.*

### AILMENTS TREATED
Severe, unremitting chest pain associated with heart attacks and angina is treated with this remedy. Angina may be accompanied by numbness, extending into the left arm and hand. This remedy is also given for collapse, anxiety, restlessness, and a fear of breathlessness.
**Symptoms better** Sitting quietly; after a hot bath.
**Symptoms worse** At night; in damp weather; before a thunderstorm.

---

*LILIUM TIGRINUM*
# LILIUM

*Tiger lily, an erect perennial plant with funnel-shaped flowers and capsule-shaped fruit, belongs to the Lilium genus, which comprises about 80 species. It is a popular cultivated plant and was introduced to the West from China and Japan. The homeopathic remedy was proved in 1869.*

**Common name** Tiger lily.
**Source** Native to China and Japan and now grown worldwide.
**Parts used** Fresh plant in flower.

### CONSTITUTIONAL TYPE
These types have a strong conflict between their intense sexual urges

**❦LILIUM TIGRINUM** *Orange spots mark the flowers of this lily, which is the source of an important remedy for uterine pain.*

and very high moral standards. This conflict may make them sensitive to criticism and easily offended.

They are hurried, impatient, and try to do too many different things at once, which results in a fear of insanity. *Lilium* types want to be the center of attention and get angry if this does not happen. At other times they are filled with remorse, especially of a religious nature, about their behavior, and torment themselves endlessly.

### AILMENTS TREATED
This remedy is mainly given for disorders of the female reproductive organs, such as swollen ovaries, vulval itching, and uterine prolapse. It is also used for women suffering from painful menstruation or fibroids (benign uterine tumors), with a bearing down pain in the pelvis and a constant urge to pass urine.

*Lilium* is also useful for angina in which symptoms include palpitations, a feeling that the heart is being clutched, and numbness in the right arm. Disorders of the rectum, bladder, and venous circulation are also eased by *Lilium*. People who need this remedy prefer cool weather and have a burning sensation in their hands.
**Symptoms better** From cool, fresh air; lying on the left side.
**Symptoms worse** With warmth; at night.

---

*LYCOPUS VIRGINICUS*
# LYCOPUS

*This plant has been used as a substitute for the herb Digitalis purpurea (see p. 127) to treat heart disease, and is said to be one of the mildest and best narcotics in existence. It was once used to encourage the spitting up of blood; for example, in tuberculosis, or heart failure due to disease of the heart valves.*

**Common name** Bugleweed, Virginia horehound.
**Source** Grows in the US.
**Parts used** Fresh plant in flower.

### AILMENTS TREATED
*Lycopus* is used as a heart remedy to treat aneurysms (swelling of the arteries, most commonly in the aorta and the arteries supplying blood to the brain), pericarditis (inflammation of the membrane that surrounds the heart), heart failure, and abnormal rhythms of the heartbeat. It is particularly useful when the heart itself is feeble but there are violent sensations such as heavy beats (palpitations). The pulse may be weak or very strong. This remedy is also given for protrusion of the eyeballs due to goiter.
**Symptoms better** From pressure.
**Symptoms worse** From excitement; with heat; from exertion; with sleep.

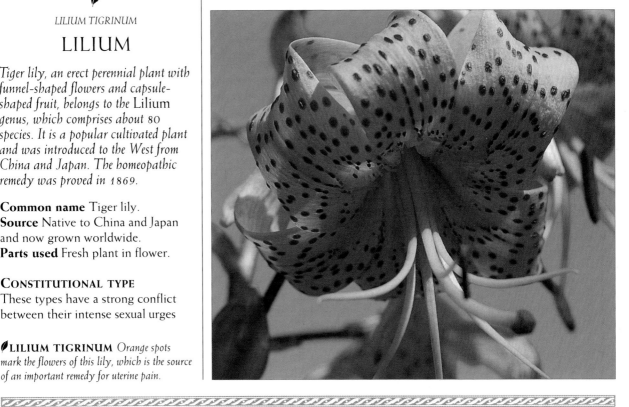

### MAGNESIA CARBONICA

# MAG. CARB.

*Magnesium carbonate has a long history of use as a laxative. It is still used in the pharmaceutical industry as a bulking compound in powder formulations and is an ingredient of some antacids. In industry it is used to make bricks, insulating compounds, and as a filler for paper and plastic paints. The remedy was proved by Hahnemann.*

**Common name** Magnesium carbonate.
**Source** Magnesite, which is found in Austria, China, and the US.
**Parts used** Magnesium carbonate.

#### CONSTITUTIONAL TYPE
*Mag. carb.* types need to be in peaceful surroundings and may feel abandoned or deserted. They tend to have a pale complexion and are intolerant of milk. Their body feels tired and painful, especially the legs and feet. They have a sour taste in the mouth, and their perspiration and other bodily secretions smell sour.

#### AILMENTS TREATED
*Mag. carb.* is used to treat taste disorders, for example a bitter taste in the mouth with thick, white mucus on the tongue. It is also effective for digestive complaints that are accompanied by a desire for acidic drinks, such as constipation, indigestion, diarrhea, and heartburn, where acid splashes back up into the gullet.

**MAGNESIA CARBONICA** *The mineral magnesite is magnesium carbonate.*

It is also given to infants who fail to thrive, with limited weight gain, a delay in muscle development, and an inability to hold up the head.
**Symptoms better** From fresh air; from walking.
**Symptoms worse** At night; with rest; in windy weather; if touched.

---

### MAGNESIA PHOSPHORICA

# MAG. PHOS.

*Magnesium phosphate is a Schussler tissue salt (see p. 227). He believed that the homeopathic remedy was good for diseases that affect nerve endings in muscles or muscular tissue itself. He was justified, for a lack of magnesium in the body does result in symptoms such as spasms and cramps.*

**MAGNESIA PHOSPHORICA** *A remedy is made from these two compounds.*

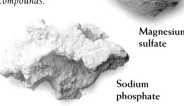

Magnesium sulfate

Sodium phosphate

**Common names** Magnesium phosphate, phosphate of magnesia.
**Source** Prepared chemically from magnesium sulfate and sodium phosphate.
**Parts used** Magnesium phosphate.

#### AILMENTS TREATED
This remedy is used for complaints that affect the nerves and muscles, such as aches and pain with cramps, neuralgic pain, and a constricting sensation. It is also an excellent remedy for colic, in which the pain is better from pressure, doubling over, and warmth, and worse with touch and cold. Complaints treated are often on the right-hand side of the body, and there is a tendency to be chilly. People who require this remedy may be very sensitive or intellectual.

---

**Symptoms better** With warmth; from hot compresses; from pressure.
**Symptoms worse** In cool surroundings; if touched; at night; if exhausted and run-down.

**☙ MAIN SELF-HELP USE**
Colic – see pp. 214–15.

---

### MATRICARIA RECUTITA

# CHAMOMILLA

*The use of chamomile in medicine is ancient, going back to the time of Hippocrates. In herbal medicine it has been used for conditions such as eczema, asthma, and insomnia, and in childbirth to strengthen the uterus. The herb is still widely used for skin diseases and as a calming remedy.*

**Common name** German chamomile.
**Source** Grows in Europe and the US.
**Parts used** Juice expressed from the whole, fresh plant in flower.

#### CONSTITUTIONAL TYPE
People who need this remedy have anxious dreams and moan or cry out in their sleep. They stick their feet out from the bedclothes at night to keep them cool and feel extremely angry if suddenly woken from sleep.

#### AILMENTS TREATED
*Chamomilla* is good for people with a very low pain threshold, who are often angry, impatient, and complain a great deal when ill. The slightest pain causes sweating and fainting, particularly in women and children.

It is especially good for children's teething complaints that are accompanied by a fever and where children insist on being carried and scream angrily when put down. It is also used for toothache that is better with cold but flares up with heat. One cheek is red and the other pale.

This remedy is also given for earache where there is a blocked feeling; heavy menstruation with severe cramps; sore, inflamed nipples in women who are breastfeeding; and colic and sleeplessness in children.
**Symptoms better** In warm, wet weather; from fasting.
**Symptoms worse** If angry; with heat; from cold winds; from fresh air.

**❧ MAIN SELF-HELP USES**
Breastfeeding problems – see
pp. 212–13
Colic – see pp. 214–15
Sleeplessness in children – see
pp. 216–17
Teething problems
– see pp. 216–17
Toothache –
see pp. 162–3.

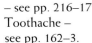

*MATRICARIA
RECUTITA
Chamomile, a
well-known
medicinal herb,
is the source of a
homeopathic remedy
that is good for
children's complaints.*

---

*MEDORRHINUM*

# MEDORRHINUM

*Gonorrhea is a sexually transmitted
infection caused by a bacterium. The
homeopathic remedy Medorrhinum,
which is made from gonorrheal
discharge, is used to treat a range
of ailments, including gynecological ones. The infection, named
gonorrhea by the Roman physician
Galen, was probably also known to the
ancient Chinese and Egyptians. It was
once treated with injections of silver
nitrate and was thought by
Hahnemann to be responsible for the
sycotic miasm, one of the three miasms,
or inherited traits (see p. 19).*

**Common name** Gonorrhea.
**Source** Patients suffering from
gonorrhea.
**Parts used** Urethral
discharge.

**AILMENTS TREATED**
Chronic and recurrent pelvic
diseases, such as pelvic
inflammatory disease, painful
menstruation, and ovarian pain are
treated with this remedy.
*Medorrhinum* is also used for
conditions that affect the nerves,
spine, kidneys, and mucous
membranes, or for problems of an
emotional nature. It may be given if a
person or their parents have a history
of gonorrhea, or a history of early
heart disease runs in the family.
Characteristically, their complaints
clear when they are near the seaside.
Psychologically, people who
require this remedy are hurried, with
a sense of anticipation. They feel
empty inside, forsaken, deserted, and
in a dreamlike state, as if everything is
unreal. Curiously, the soles of their
feet are extremely sensitive.
This remedy is used to treat people
who exhibit extremes of behavior;
those who are selfish, egotistical, and
self-centered on the one hand and yet
can be withdrawn, absentminded, and
very sensitive to beautiful things,
especially in nature.
**Symptoms better** In the evening;
lying on the abdomen or being on all
fours; near the sea.
**Symptoms worse** In damp; between
3 a.m. and 4 a.m.; after urinating; with
heat; with the slightest movement.

---

*MERCURIUS CORROSIVUS*

# MERC. COR.

*Mercuric chloride is a violent poison
that was used in the 17th and 18th
centuries as a local antiseptic. It is now
used as a fungicidal dip to treat bulbs
and tubers and in the chemical industry
for plastics manufacture. If swallowed,
it causes death of the cells and burning
pains in the throat and stomach.*

**Common name** Mercuric chloride, a
corrosive sublimate of mercury.
**Source** Mercuric chloride, which is a
salt that is found in Germany,
Mexico, the former Yugoslavia, and
the US.
**Parts used** Mercuric chloride.

**AILMENTS TREATED**
The remedy is used for ulcers,
particularly if they affect the gut as
in ulcerative colitis; where there is
diarrhea with bleeding, and great
straining to pass small amounts of
mucus or blood. Similar urging, and
possibly bleeding and discharge of
mucus, occurs in the bladder. *Merc.
cor.* is also given for ulcers associated
with exhaustion, in the throat,
mouth, and on the front of the eyes.
Symptoms may include sharp pain in
the back of the nose that extends out
to the ears, excessive saliva, and a
sensation that the teeth are loose.
**Symptoms better** From eating
breakfast; with rest.
**Symptoms worse** From eating
acidic or fatty foods; in the evening.

---

*MERCURIUS DULCIS*

# MERC. DULC.

*The use of calomel as a laxative dates
back to the 16th century. It was used
in orthodox medicine for any complaint
where a liver imbalance was thought to
be the cause. Today, it is used in a
number of insecticides and fungicides.*

**Common names** Calomel,
mercurous chloride.
**Source** Calomel, which is found in
Germany, Mexico, the US, and the
former Yugoslavia.
**Parts used** Mercurous chloride.

MERCURIUS DULCIS continued on page 136

**MERCURIUS DULCIS** *continued*

Black deposits of calomel

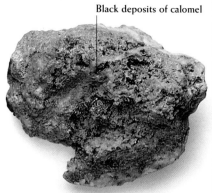

**MERCURIUS DULCIS** *Calomel, or mercurous chloride, is the source of a remedy used for glue ear in children.*

**AILMENTS TREATED**
*Merc. dulc.* is used to treat pale, thin children who have swelling in the neck glands and tend to produce a thick, white, sticky discharge from their mucous membranes, particularly in the middle ear and the eustachian tubes (which connect the middle ear cavity to the back of the nose). It is one of the main remedies for glue ear (fluid in the ear) and is also used for phlegm. *Merc. dulc.* is also given for dry, red eyes.
**Symptoms better** No specific factors.
**Symptoms worse** At night; from exercise.

---

*MOSCHUS MOSCHIFERUS*

## MOSCHUS

*The male musk deer secretes musk to attract a female. The odor of musk is so strong that some people may faint just from smelling it. It has been used in perfume for centuries and in the past an aromatic scent made from musk was given to people who were dying. Hahnemann warned that people who wore musk as a perfume were weakening their resistance to disease. He stressed that the smell of musk remained for many years and that those affected by chronic disease should avoid it.*

**Common name** Musk deer.
**Source** Musk contained in a hairy bag just behind the navel of the male musk deer, which is found in the mountainous parts of Asia.
**Parts used** Dried musk.

**AILMENTS TREATED**
*Moschus* is given to people suffering from hysterical excitement and who are hypochondriacs. It is used to treat fainting, dizziness, exhaustion, and vertigo, and is a remedy for neurotic illness. People who benefit from this remedy feel opposed by everyone, talk excitedly, and are hurried and clumsy. They are chilly (but may have a feeling of warmth inside) and often need to take a deep breath. They feel more exhausted resting than when moving around, and one side of the body may feel hot and the other cold.
**Symptoms better** With warmth; after burping.
**Symptoms worse** From excitement; in cool surroundings; from fresh air.

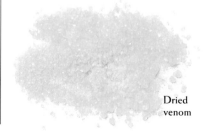

**NAJA NAJA** *The cobra expands its neck ribs to form a hood before it strikes.*

---

*MYGALE LASIODORA / M. AVICULARIA / ARANEA AVICULARIA*

## MYGALE LAS.

*The effects of a bite from this large spider include inflammation and a violet discoloration that turns green and spreads from the bite along the lymphatic drainage system. Other symptoms include chills followed by a fever, dry mouth, great thirst, trembling, difficulty in breathing, despondency, and fear of death.*

**Common name** Cuban spider.
**Source** Native to Cuba.
**Parts used** Whole live spider.

**AILMENTS TREATED**
*Mygale las.* is used to treat nervous disorders, such as chorea, in which there are jerking and convulsive movements of the limbs, particularly in the upper part of the body. The body is in constant motion and the muscles twitch. *Mygale las.* has also been used to treat venereal disease.
**Symptoms better** During sleep.
**Symptoms worse** In the morning.

---

*NAJA NAJA/N. TRIPUDIANS*

## NAJA

*This is a highly venomous snake, and bites are fatal in about 10 percent of human cases. The venom can be accurately directed into a victim's eyes at distances of more than 6 feet (2 meters) and may cause temporary or even permanent blindness unless promptly washed out. In India the venom was once used for nervous and blood disorders.*

**Common name** Cobra.
**Source** Found in Africa and Australasia.
**Parts used** Fresh venom.

Dried venom

## CONSTITUTIONAL TYPE

These types are nervous, excited, depressed, suicidal, and brood over imagined problems of their sexual organs. They have fears of being alone, the rain, and failure.

## AILMENTS TREATED

*Naja* acts mainly on the heart, lungs, nerves, and left ovary. Its main use is for vascular problems in the heart, with anginal type pains extending to the left shoulder blade and left hand. There may also be pain in the left ovary, which radiates to the heart region. *Naja* is also used to treat asthma that follows hay fever.

**Symptoms better** From sneezing.
**Symptoms worse** Lying on the left side; from wearing tight clothes; with sleep; from alcohol; in cold air and in a draft; after menstruation.

*NATRUM CARBONICUM*

# NAT. CARB.

*Sodium carbonate is used to make glass, soaps, and detergents, and to soften water. It was used in orthodox medicine externally to treat burns and eczema, and for nasal mucus and vaginal discharge.*

**Common names** Sodium carbonate, soda ash.
**Source** Once extracted from seaweed ashes, but now prepared chemically.
**Parts used** Sodium carbonate.

## CONSTITUTIONAL TYPE

These types are extremely dignified, delicate, unselfish, and devoted to their loved ones. They are sympathetic and suffer in silence, always trying to appear cheerful even when they feel sad. They are extremely sensitive to noise, music, and thunderstorms. Physically, they have a weak digestive system with a strong intolerance of milk. Their ankles are weak and are constantly giving way.

## AILMENTS TREATED

*Nat. carb.* is used for digestive problems such as indigestion, nervous disorders including headaches, and skin complaints such as herpes, warts, moles, blisters, and corns.

**Symptoms better** From eating.
**Symptoms worse** With heat; in hot sun; in humid weather.

*NATRUM PHOSPHORICUM*

# NAT. PHOS.

*Sodium phosphate is a Schussler tissue salt (see p. 227). It occurs naturally in the tissue cells and helps to regulate the body's acidity level and to break down fatty acids. The remedy Nat. phos. is used for conditions arising from an excess of lactic or uric acid, such as gout and also for indigestion caused by an excessive intake of fatty, sour foods.*

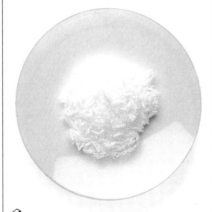

**NATRUM PHOSPHORICUM**
*Indigestion and gout are treated with a remedy made from sodium phosphate crystals.*

**Common name** Sodium phosphate.
**Source** Chemically prepared from phosphoric acid and sodium carbonate.
**Parts used** Sodium phosphate.

## CONSTITUTIONAL TYPE

*Nat. phos.* types are refined, fearful, and flush easily. They dislike being given advice, even if it is well-meaning and tend to be rather restless and fidgety despite their weariness and nervous weakness.

## AILMENTS TREATED

This remedy is used to treat indigestion, with sour burping caused by fatty, sour foods, or from excess stomach acid, especially in children who have been given too much milk and sugar. It is also good for gout and stiffness after exertion.

**Symptoms better** In cool surroundings; from fresh air.
**Symptoms worse** From milk, sour and sweet foods; in a thunderstorm.

*NATRUM SULFURICUM*

# NAT. SULF.

*Sodium sulfate is a white crystalline solid or powder used in the manufacture of paper, paperboard, glass, and detergents. A Schussler tissue salt (see p. 227), it occurs naturally in the body in the tissue cells and helps to maintain water balance. The homeopathic remedy is good for flabby people who feel worse in damp weather, near water, and in damp rooms.*

**Common name** Sodium sulfate, sal mirabile, Glauber's salt.
**Source** Sodium sulfate, which is found in saltwater lakes and in the Kalunda steppe in Russia.
**Parts used** Sodium sulfate.

## CONSTITUTIONAL TYPE

These types can be too serious and responsible, closed and depressed, and may even be suicidal. Although they tend to be quite materialistic, they may be very sensitive, crying when they hear music. Some are less restrained and more artistic, needing stimulation. *Nat. sulf.* people are flabby, prefer cool weather, and feel worse in damp and humidity. They tend to suffer from asthma brought on by dampness, and generally have profuse discharges with thin or thick yellowish green mucus.

## AILMENTS TREATED

Complaints treated with this remedy include liver ailments such as jaundice, chest problems such as asthma and bronchitis, and head injuries in which the person may become depressed, suicidal, or suffer other emotional changes.

**Symptoms better** From fresh air; from a change in position; in dry surroundings.
**Symptoms worse** In the late evening; in the morning; lying on the back; in damp surroundings.

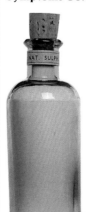

**NATRUM SULFURICUM**
*Sodium sulfate has long been used to make Nat. sulf.*

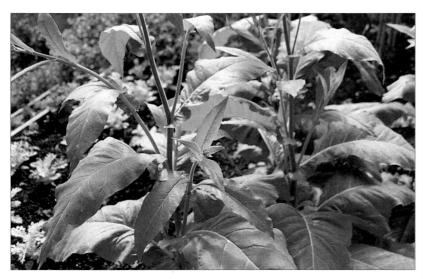

*NICOTIANA TABACUM Medicinally, tobacco was said to have painkilling effects. Herbalists used it for bites and stings.*

---

*NICOTIANA TABACUM*

# TABACUM

The tobacco plant was given its name by Jean Nicot, a French ambassador to South America who introduced it into Europe around 1560. However, the plant was used by Native Americans long before this date. Tobacco contains nicotine, which is a poison that can cause severe nausea, vomiting, sweating, dizziness, and palpitations. The homeopathic remedy is used to treat such symptoms.

**Common name** Tobacco.
**Source** Native to the US, South America, and the West Indies.
**Parts used** Fresh leaves.

### AILMENTS TREATED
*Tabacum* is mainly given for nausea, vomiting, and motion sickness. Symptoms come on suddenly and include excessive saliva, pain, chillinesss with perspiration, anxiety, and vertigo. The least motion aggravates the nausea and vomiting. It is also good for severe nausea that accompanies other ailments.
**Symptoms better** From being cold; from fresh air; after vomiting; from cold compresses.
**Symptoms worse** With movement; with heat; from opening the eyes; with the smell of tobacco smoke.

### 🍃 MAIN SELF-HELP USE
Motion sickness – see p. 222.

---

*NITRIC ACIDUM*

# NITRIC AC.

This colorless, volatile, highly corrosive liquid has been used to burn off warts and in a dilute form it was given for fevers, bronchitis, and other chest infections, for syphilis, and to dissolve kidney and bladder stones. Commercially, it is mainly used in the manufacture of explosives and fertilizers. The fumes are highly irritating and cause death if inhaled.

**Common names** Nitric acid, aqua fortis.
**Source** Prepared chemically from sodium nitrate and sulfuric acid.
**Parts used** Nitric acid.

### CONSTITUTIONAL TYPE
These types are selfish, bitter, critical, and unforgiving of others. They are easily offended and can explode in anger. There is a tendency to dwell on unpleasant past experiences. They are oversensitive, convinced that they have offended everybody, and that others are out to deceive them. They may become ill if they have undergone a long period of suffering. When ill, they are anxious about their health and fearful of death.

### AILMENTS TREATED
This remedy is used to treat splinter-like pain which may appear and disappear suddenly, for example, in sore throats, mouth ulcers and thrush. It is also good for piles with sharp, stitchlike pains in the rectum. Discharges are burning and offensive. Urine is strong smelling.

People who require *Nitric ac.* are chilly and often suffer from warts, broken skin, and ulcers in the stomach, vagina, and rectum.
**Symptoms better** With movement; in mild weather; from hot compresses.
**Symptoms worse** At night; with the slightest touch or movement; in cold and damp; from fresh air; from milk.

---

*NUX MOSCHATA / MYRISTICA FRAGRANS*

# NUX MOSCH.

*Nutmeg has been widely used since AD 540 when it was brought from India to Constantinople. It was used as a cosmetic to remove freckles. Medicinally, it was first mentioned by Avicenna in the 11th century, who called it "the nut of Banda." It was given for stomach upsets, headaches, and to ease gas. It has also been taken as a hallucinogen. The essential oil is good for rheumatic pain.*

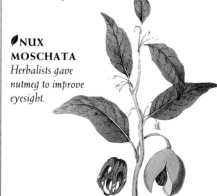

*NUX MOSCHATA Herbalists gave nutmeg to improve eyesight.*

**Common name** Nutmeg.
**Source** Mainly Banda in the Molucca Islands, which are part of the Indonesian Republic, India, and the Far East.
**Parts used** Seed without the mace (outer covering).

### AILMENTS TREATED
*Nux mosch.* is given for mental illness, hysteria, problems of the nervous system, and digestive complaints. It also treats the same hallucinogenic symptoms that are caused by large doses of nutmeg, such as drowsiness, with dizziness, fainting, and lack of coordination. Such symptoms may occur after a stroke or in epilepsy.

It is also good for gas with constipation and bloating in the digestive tract associated with

indigestion and gastritis (inflammation of the stomach lining). People who need this remedy are markedly dehydrated, but are not thirsty.
**Symptoms better** In humidity; in warm rooms; wrapping up warmly.
**Symptoms worse** From seasonal change; in cool surroundings; when jarred; from emotional problems.

---

*OLEUM PETRAE*

# PETROLEUM

*Petroleum is a liquid crude oil that comes from beneath the earth's surface. In the past it was used in shipbuilding and roadbuilding and was burned as a fuel. Today, petroleum is one of the most important of the earth's resources for fuel. In orthodox medicine, petroleum was used to treat wounds, but it is only in homeopathy that it has become a widely used medicine.*

**Common names** Petroleum, rock oil, coal oil.
**Source** Petroleum, which is formed from decomposed plant and animal material.
**Parts used** Purified crude oil.

**AILMENTS TREATED**
This remedy is mainly used to treat skin complaints, such as eczema, in which the skin is dry with deep, bloody cracks, especially on the hands and fingertips. The splitting of the skin is very bad in cold weather. It is also used for nausea, diarrhea, and vomiting, particularly when associated with motion sickness. Despite nausea and vomiting there may be constant hunger.
   People who require this remedy may have offensive-smelling sweat and dislike fatty foods. They suffer indigestion from gas-inducing foods. Mentally, they may become excitable, quarrelsome, and confused.
**Symptoms better** From warm air; in dry weather; from eating.
**Symptoms worse** With movement; in cold weather, particularly in winter; during a thunderstorm.

**♥ MAIN SELF-HELP USE**
Eczema – see pp. 186–7.

---

*PAEONIA OFFICINALIS*

# PEONY

*Today, the peony is mainly grown as an ornamental plant. It is thought to have been named after Paeon, who was a physician during the Trojan wars. In AD 77, Pliny recorded that peony was used to prevent nightmares. The herbalist Culpepper (1616–54) claimed that the root of the male herb hung around the neck of a child would prevent epilepsy. The herb was also given after childbirth. Peony is still used by herbalists as an antibacterial, an antispasmodic, a sedative, and to reduce blood pressure and swelling.*

**Common name** Peony.
**Source** Native to Europe and Asia.
**Parts used** Fresh root.

---

**AILMENTS TREATED**
*Peony* is mainly used for hemorrhoids that itch severely, causing the anus to swell slightly. There may be anal fissures. As in herbalism, the homeopathic remedy is used for sleep problems, such as sleepiness in the afternoon, nightmares, and insomnia due to digestive upsets.
**Symptoms better** Temporarily, from rubbing and scratching.
**Symptoms worse** At noon; at night.

---

*PAPAVER SOMNIFERUM*

# OPIUM

*Opium has been used as a painkiller since Greek and Roman times. It mimics the action of naturally occurring chemicals in the brain, called endorphins, which help to induce sleep and a state of well-being. Derivatives, such as morphine and codeine, are used in orthodox medicine.*

**Common name** Opium poppy.
**Source** Grows in Asia, Turkey, Iran, and India.
**Parts used** Dried milky juice from unripe green seed capsules.

**AILMENTS TREATED**
*Opium* is used for two types of mental state that can occur after a severe scare or shock, such as the death of a loved one. One is apathy and indifference as if the senses have been dulled – the person does not complain; the second is a state of overexcitement, with severe insomnia. The hearing is so acute that it is possible to hear things like crawling insects.
   The remedy is also given for constipation and respiratory problems, such as irregular breathing. It is very good after strokes and for delirium tremens caused by alcohol withdrawal.
**Symptoms better** In cool surroundings; with movement.
**Symptoms worse** With warmth; during sleep; from sleep.
**Caution** Not available in the US and Canada.

**♥ PAPAVER SOMNIFERUM** *Flowers vary from white to reddish purple. A milky juice is extracted from the unripe seed capsules.*

*PHOSPHORICUM ACIDUM*

## PHOS. AC.

*Phosphoric acid is used in the manufacture of pharmaceutical drugs, fertilizers, and detergents. It is also used in sugar refining and to give soft drinks a fruity, acidic flavor. In orthodox medicine, phosphoric acid was once used to stimulate digestion. Now it is used to reduce calcium levels in the blood of people with cancerous or benign tumors in the parathyroid glands (which lie in the neck).*

**Common name** Phosphoric acid.
**Source** Phosphoric acid is a trans-parent, crystalline solid, which is prepared chemically from phosphate minerals, such as apatite.
**Parts used** Dilute phosphoric acid.

### AILMENTS TREATED
This is one of homeopathy's most effective remedies for people who are apathetic and listless. This may be a result of too much studying or stress. Sluggishness and lethargy may also occur after a severe loss of fluids from dysentery or stomach flu.

Physical symptoms associated with listlessness and apathy include chilliness, loss of appetite, a craving for juicy fruits or refreshing fruit drinks, perspiration, the sensation of a crushing weight on the top of the head, and dizziness that occurs in the evening, after prolonged standing or when walking. *Phos. ac.* is suitable for children who grow too quickly and suffer from bone pain as a result, or who are distressed about masturbation and wet dreams.
**Symptoms better** With warmth; after a short sleep.
**Symptoms worse** If cold and in a draft; near noise.

*PHYTOLACCA DECANDRA*

## PHYTOLACCA

*Pokeweed was used in European folk medicine for glandular problems such as mastitis (inflammation of breast tissue) and small, hard breast tumors. Native Americans used it to treat skin problems, to cause vomiting, and as a heart stimulant, and a purgative.*

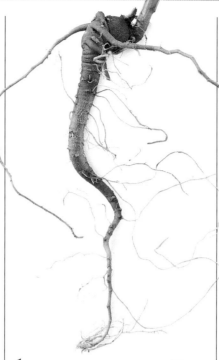

**PHYTOLACCA DECANDRA** *The root of this herb is still used today by herbalists for its anti-inflammatory properties.*

**Common names** Virginian poke-weed, reading plant, garget, pocon.
**Source** Grows in the US, Canada, the Azores, North Africa, and China.
**Parts used** Fresh, thick root.

### AILMENTS TREATED
*Phytolacca* is mainly used for glandu-lar problems, especially in the breasts, such as a tumor (either cancerous or benign) or mastitis with stitchlike pain. The breasts are swollen and hard and the pain can spread throughout the body. It is also given for tonsillitis and pharyngitis where the throat is dark red and the pain extends to the ear on swallowing.
**Symptoms better** From cold drinks; with rest; warmth; in dry weather.
**Symptoms worse** On starting to move; with prolonged movement; from swallowing; from hot drinks; in cold, damp weather.

*PICRICUM ACIDUM*

## PICRIC AC.

*This poison was first discovered in 1788. It acts powerfully on the liver, causing jaundice and weight loss. The homeopathic remedy, which was proved in 1868, is used to treat severe mental fatigue and degenerative conditions of the spinal cord.*

**Common name** Picric acid.
**Source** Picric acid is chemically prepared from carbolic acid, nitric acid, and sulfuric acid.
**Parts used** Picric acid.

### AILMENTS TREATED
The remedy's key use is for severe mental fatigue after prolonged mental strain, where indifference and a lack of willpower develop with an inability to undertake new things or to talk or think clearly. This condition, which may cause a burning, numb sensation along the spine, is common among students who have been studying constantly for exams.

There is a general sense of heaviness in all parts of the body. There may be associated headaches and boils in the external ear. The severe mental fatigue may also be brought on by grief.
**Symptoms better** With rest; in cool surroundings; in the sun.
**Symptoms worse** From mental or physical exertion; with heat.

*PLATINUM METALLICUM*

## PLATINUM

*Platinum, which means "like silver," was first discovered in the 18th century in South America. It is used to make jewelry and dental alloys and is also used in surgical pins and electrical contacts. In the 19th century, platinum was briefly used as a treatment for syphilis. In homeopathy it has been, and still is, used largely for the treatment of women's complaints.*

**Common name** Platinum.
**Source** Found mainly in South America.
**Parts used** Platinum.

### CONSTITUTIONAL TYPE
*Platinum* types tend to be women who are very idealistic and set impossibly high standards for them-selves and their partners. As neither can measure up to such exalted stan-dards, these women become either disappointed, dwelling on the past and feeling deserted, or arrogant with a contempt of others.

### AILMENTS TREATED
This is essentially a remedy for ailments of the female reproductive

organs and nervous system. It is used for absent or heavy menstruation, vulval itching, ovarian pain, an inability to have sexual intercourse because of vaginismus (spasms in the vaginal muscles), and neuralgia.

Physical symptoms include numbness of the skin, a constricted feeling, and coldness. Women who require this remedy have a particular sensitivity in the sexual organs; they may have a horror of pelvic examination because of this increased sensitivity.

**Symptoms better** From fresh air.
**Symptoms worse** From emotional stress; if touched; from nervous exhaustion; in the evening.

---

*PLUMBUM METALLICUM*

# PLUMBUM MET.

*The Romans used lead in pipes for plumbing and to make hairpins and tokens for entry into arenas. Symptoms of lead poisoning include wrist drop (a weakness in the muscles controlling the wrist) and colicky, abdominal pain. These symptoms were observed in those who drank water with a high lead content. The homeopathic remedy is used to treat colicky pain and nerve damage.*

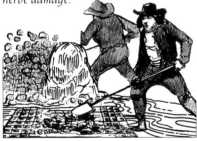

**PLUMBUM METALLICUM** *Lead has been mined for centuries. The remedy made from it is given for diseases with hardened tissue.*

**Common name** Lead.
**Source** Found in the US, Africa, Australia, and parts of Europe.
**Parts used** Lead, the acetate or the carbonate.

### CONSTITUTIONAL TYPE
The mental characteristics of *Plumbum met.* types are similar to those of people suffering from arteriosclerosis. The ability to express thoughts is slowed, there is memory loss, and perception is difficult. These types may be apathetic and irritable.

### AILMENTS TREATED
*Plumbum met.* is an important remedy for diseases that take a long time to appear, for example, sclerotic conditions or those with hardened tissue, including arteriosclerosis, multiple sclerosis, and Parkinson's disease. The remedy has wide-reaching effects on the tissues, especially on muscles and nerves. It is given for weakness, spasm, and trembling in the muscles. Symptoms of muscle weakness include urinary retention and constipation with colicky pain.
**Symptoms better** With warmth; from massage; from pressure.
**Symptoms worse** At night; with movement.

---

*PODOPHYLLUM PELTATUM*

# PODOPHYLLUM

*Native Americans used the root of this plant to expel worms and to cure deafness. The first homeopathic proving was made in the 19th century and the remedy is used to treat digestive problems.*

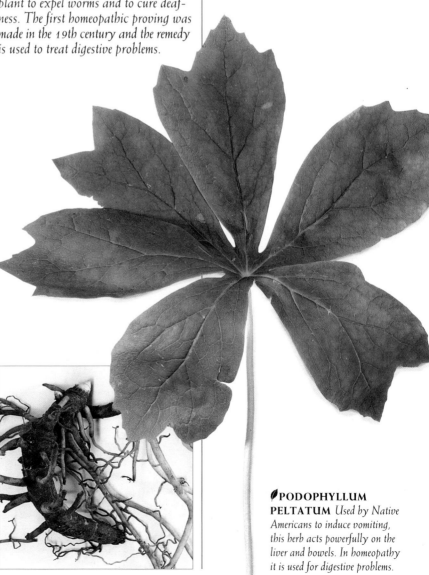

**PODOPHYLLUM PELTATUM** *Used by Native Americans to induce vomiting, this herb acts powerfully on the liver and bowels. In homeopathy it is used for digestive problems.*

**Common name** May apple.
**Source** Found throughout Canada and the US.
**Parts used** Roots gathered after the fruit has ripened, or the whole, fresh plant.

### AILMENTS TREATED
*Podophyllum* acts mainly on the duodenum, the small intestine, the liver, and rectum. It is given for stomach flu with colicky pain, bilious vomiting, and diarrhea, or if the liver region is sensitive due to inflammation or gallstones. People who need *Podophyllum* tend to clench and grind their teeth, and it is a useful remedy for difficult teething. Complaints typically alternate, for example, constipation and diarrhea.
**Symptoms better** Lying on the abdomen; from rubbing the abdomen.
**Symptoms worse** In hot weather; in the early morning; when teething.

PSORINUM

# PSORINUM

The remedy Psorinum, derived from scabies, was proved by Hahnemann. He believed that in some people the blisters produced by the scabies mite were a reflection of a deeper "dis-ease." Although the blisters might disappear, the person was not completely cured and the disease continued to attack deeper organs. This phenomenon of a suppressed disease became known as a miasm, and "psora" was the first of the three basic miasms (see p. 19).

**Common name** Scabies.
**Source** Scabies infection, which produces blisters or weals on the skin.
**Parts used** Fluid from scabies blisters.

### CONSTITUTIONAL TYPE
Psorinum types are anxious, lack stamina and ambition, and have a rather pessimistic view of life with a fear of failure, poverty, and death. They feel forsaken and abandoned. Even in summer, they are extremely sensitive to cold and drafts. They sweat readily and are constantly hungry, with an associated headache that is relieved by eating. They have an increased sense of well-being just before the onset of illness, which may recur at regular intervals.

### AILMENTS TREATED
This remedy acts mainly on the skin and to a lesser extent the bowels and respiratory tract. It is used to treat skin complaints that suppurate easily, such as eczema, ulcers, acne, and boils. All these conditions are worse in winter weather but are aggravated by heat, for example, from a warm bed, being overdressed, and physical exertion. Bowel problems treated include diarrhea associated with irritable bowel syndrome, stomach flu, and diverticulitis. Psorinum is also given for complaints of the respiratory tract, including hay fever and asthma and can be useful for debility from an acute illness.
**Symptoms better** In warm rooms; in summer; lying down with the arms stretched wide.
**Symptoms worse** From coffee; in winter; from changes in weather.

PYROGENIUM

# PYROGENIUM

Pyrogenium was introduced to homeopathy in 1880 by Dr. Drysdale. It was made by mixing beef with water and leaving it to stand for three weeks. The mixture was strained to leave a clear amber liquid called sepsin. Sepsin was mixed with glycerine and called pyrogen. Drysdale concluded that if pyrogen was given in a large dose it produced changes in the blood and tissues analogous to those of blood poisoning after wounds, whereas smaller doses resulted in a full recovery.

**Common name** Pyrogenium.
**Source** Beef.
**Parts used** Solution left after straining, evaporating, and diluting a mixture of lean beef and water.

### AILMENTS TREATED
Pyrogenium acts mainly on the blood and is used to treat the symptoms of blood poisoning. These include cold sweats and a high fever, where the pulse is abnormally rapid in relation to the fever. The bones ache severely and the entire body feels bruised. There is great restlessness, and the tongue is dry, cracked, red, and shiny.

This remedy is often given for septic conditions or where there is a history of sepsis from which there has never been a full recovery. There may be violent burning sensations, for example in association with an abscess. All bodily discharges are highly offensive.
**Symptoms better** With movement; changing position; from hard rocking.
**Symptoms worse** From cold.

RADIUM BROMATUM

# RADIUM BROM.

Radium is used in orthodox medicine in radiotherapy for the treatment of cancer. It was discovered in 1898 by Pierre and Marie Curie in the mineral uraninite. Pierre Curie identified the active disintegration property of radium when he put a little radium salt into a capsule and fastened it to his arm. When he took it off the skin was red, the resulting wound took months to heal, and left puckered skin around a white scar.

**Common name** Radium bromide.
**Source** Prepared chemically from radium.
**Parts used** Radium bromide.

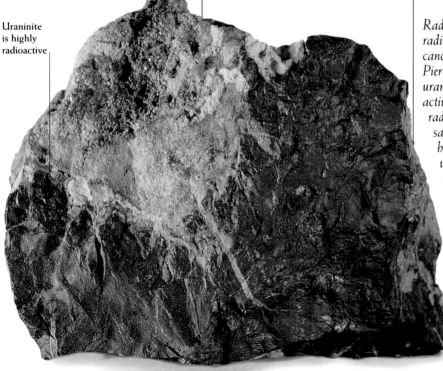

Uraninite is highly radioactive

**RADIUM BROMATUM** The radioactive element radium, which is used to make the Radium brom. remedy, is found in uraninite.

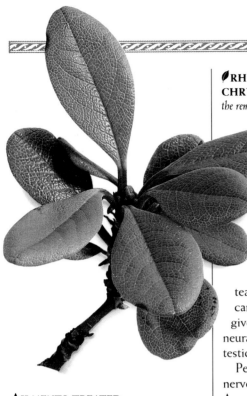

## AILMENTS TREATED

*Radium brom.* is used for skin complaints such as acne, moles, skin cancer, ulcers, eczema, dermatitis, and acne rosacea (flushed face and acnelike symptoms that occur in middle age). Symptoms include burning, itchy skin, with possible ulceration and an associated craving for cool air. Pain affects alternate sides of the body. This remedy is also used for bone cancer, lumbago, and arthritis with a dull aching pain in the bones and joints.

**Symptoms better** From fresh air; with continued movement; after a hot bath; lying down.

**Symptoms worse** From getting up after lying down; at night.

---

*RHODODENDRON CHRYSANTHEMUM*

# RHODODENDRON

*This plant was introduced to Europe from Siberia, where it had traditionally been used as a herbal treatment for rheumatism and gout. The homeopathic remedy was proved in 1831. People who need the remedy, which is used for a variety of ailments, are affected badly by the approach of a thunderstorm.*

**Common names** Siberian rhododendron, yellow snow rose.
**Source** Mountainous regions of Siberia, Europe, and Asia.
**Parts used** Fresh leaves.

*⟋*RHODODENDRON CHRYSANTHEMUM *Gout is a key use of the remedy made from the leaves.*

## AILMENTS TREATED

Gout, arthritis, and rheumatism are the main complaints treated by *Rhododendron*. Symptoms include swelling and rheumatic, tearing pain in the ligaments, cartilage, and joint tissue. It is also given for fever, delirium, headaches, neuralgic pain in the eyes, and testicular inflammation.

People who need the remedy are nervous and dread thunderstorms. Any symptoms they may have are worse before a thunderstorm, and improve when it breaks.

**Symptoms better** With warmth; from eating; after a thunderstorm.
**Symptoms worse** At night; before a thunderstorm; from rest; from starting to move; from prolonged standing.

---

*SABADILLA OFFICINARUM/ ASAGRAEA OFFICINALIS*

# SABADILLA

*This uses of this plant were first described in the 16th century. It was used almost exclusively for destroying lice and for killing intestinal worms. Sabadilla produces symptoms similar to those of a cold or hay fever, which it is used to treat homeopathically.*

**Common names** Cebadilla, cevadilla.
**Source** Grows in Mexico, Venezuela, Guatemala, and the US.
**Part used** Seeds.

## AILMENTS TREATED

This remedy acts on the mucous membranes of the nose and tear glands and is used to treat colds and hay fever, with spasmodic sneezing, a runny, itchy nose, tingling in the soft palate, and burning, watery eyes with a splitting headache across the eyes. The throat feels dry and sore, and swallowing is painful. Hot drinks are soothing. *Sabadilla* is also used for threadworms in children.

**Symptoms better** With warmth; from wrapping up warmly.
**Symptoms worse** From cold air.

*⟊* **MAIN SELF-HELP USE**
Hay fever – see pp. 168–9.

---

*SABAL SERRULATA*

# SABAL

*In 1885, Dr. Hale, an American homeopath, observed that during the summer when food was scarce, wild animals ate raw saw palmetto berries and rapidly regained weight. In the 19th century, another American homeopath claimed that if eaten regularly the berries could increase the weight and size of the breasts.*

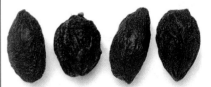

*⟋*SABAL SERRULATA *The remedy made from the berries and seeds is given for prostate disorders and mastitis.*

**Common name** Saw palmetto.
**Source** Grows in the US.
**Parts used** Fresh, ripe berries and seeds.

## AILMENTS TREATED

*Sabal* is used to treat enlargement of the prostate gland, with sharp stinging pain in the urethra, difficulty urinating, a cold feeling in the genitals with a lack of libido, weakness, and nervous irritability. It is also given for testicular inflammation.

In women, the remedy is helpful for mastitis (inflammation of breast tissue), which may occur from breast-feeding, and for pain and tenderness of swollen breasts before menstruation. It is also given for breasts that become small and shrunken due to a hormonal imbalance.

People who need this remedy are afraid of falling asleep.

**Symptoms better** With warmth.
**Symptoms worse** In cold, damp weather; from sympathy.

*⟊* **MAIN SELF-HELP USE**
Prostate enlargement – see pp. 200–1.

## SANGUINARIA CANADENSIS

# SANGUINARIA

*This plant contains a powerful alkaloid called sanguinarin, which can cause nausea and vomiting, and burning pains in the stomach. It is fatal in large doses. The burning quality of the plant is of most significance in the homeopathic remedy.*

**Common names** Sanguinaria, blood root, red puccoon.
**Source** Native to the US and Canada.
**Parts used** Fresh root, leaves, seeds, expressed juice, or powdered fruit.

### SANGUINARIA CANADENSIS
*Native Americans dyed clothes and painted their bodies with the red juice of the root.*

Fresh leaf

Bulbous, thick root contains orange-red juice

### AILMENTS TREATED
*Sanguinaria* is used for respiratory problems, such as asthma, bronchitis, inflammation of the pharynx (which is between the tonsils and the larynx), and nasal or laryngeal polyps. The first symptoms include dryness, rawness, and burning in the mucous membranes, and later phlegm. The remedy is also given for indigestion, coughs that are typically dry and spasmodic, for example, after whooping cough or flu, and hay fever with burning and dryness in the nose and throat. A key symptom of all these ailments is a burning chest pain that extends to the right shoulder; it may make it difficult to raise the arm.

*Sanguinaria* is also used for rheumatism in the right shoulder, menopausal hot flashes, and throbbing headaches and migraines that settle over the right eye.

Symptoms are mostly right-sided.
**Symptoms better** Lying on the left side; with sleep; in the evening.
**Symptoms worse** From cold and damp; with movement and touch; lying on the right side; from sweet foods.

### MAIN SELF-HELP USE
Migraine – see pp. 160–1.

### SANICULA AQUA

# SANICULA

*Sanicula is the name of a spring in the state of Illinois. In 1890, the homeopathic remedy was unintentionally proved by a family who drank the spring water for a year and suffered various side effects. The water has naturally occurring salts and a rare combination of minerals, many of which are used to make individual homeopathic remedies. The remedy Sanicula is a mixture of such remedies.*

**Common name** Spring water.
**Source** Ottawa, in the state of Illinois.
**Parts used** Evaporated salt.

### CONSTITUTIONAL TYPE
*Sanicula* is predominantly a childhood remedy. Children who benefit from it are likely to appear emaciated despite a good appetite and tend to have sweaty heads and feet. They may have a marked fear of downward movement and a tendency to abrupt mood changes from laughter to anger.

### AILMENTS TREATED
The main uses of this remedy are for the following: bedwetting; constipation with painful straining that results in a stool which slips back into the rectum; diarrhea immediately after eating; and motion sickness with nausea, vomiting, and a pronounced thirst. There is a tendency to vomit when fluids reach the stomach.
**Symptoms better** With rest; from being uncovered.
**Symptoms worse** With the arms held backward and downward; from downward movement.

### SECALE CORNUTUM

# SECALE

*Ergot is produced by a fungus that grows on rye and other cereals. It has several alkaloids with medicinal and poisonous effects. Outbreaks of ergot poisoning (caused by eating contaminated flour) occurred as far back as AD 857. Symptoms include a sensation of ants crawling on the skin, delirium, severe burning, gangrene, convulsions, and uterine spasms. Today, ergot is used in a drug that controls blood loss following childbirth or miscarriage.*

**Common names** Ergot, spurred rye.
**Source** A fungus that grows on rye grains and other cereals that grow in Europe, Asia, Canada, and the US.
**Parts used** Immature ergot collected before the grain is harvested.

### AILMENTS TREATED
This remedy is used for circulatory disorders, in which the muscle fibers of the arteries constrict to cause spasms. This leads to severe blanching and coldness of the extremities with numbness, similar to Raynaud's syndrome, intermittent cramp in the calf muscles, and, in severe cases, gangrene. Typical symptoms include skin that feels ice-cold to the touch but with an internal sensation of burning heat.

The remedy is also given to treat constriction of the muscle fibers in

the uterus, resulting in pain and hemorrhage. Symptoms include menstrual cramps with irregular, dark, copious bleeding and continuous oozing of watery blood until the next menstrual period. Other symptoms treated include weak contractions in labor.
**Symptoms better** From cool air.
**Symptoms worse** With heat; from covering the affected parts.

🥣 **Main self-help use**
Cold hands & feet – see pp. 198–9.

Ergot

✦**SECALE CORNUTUM** *Ergot is caused by a fungus that grows on cereals, including rye. It is used to make the Secale remedy, which is good for circulatory problems.*

SMILAX OFFICINALIS / S. MEDICA

# SARSAPARILLA

*The word sarsaparilla is of Spanish origin from* sarza, *meaning "bramble," and* parilla, *meaning "vine." The plant is thought to have been brought as a medicine to Spain from South America around 1573. One of its earliest uses was in the treatment of syphilis. It was also used to treat chronic rheumatism and skin diseases.*

**Common name** Red-bearded sarsaparilla.
**Source** Grows on the slopes of the Mexican Sierra Madre and in the US.
**Parts used** Fresh root.

**AILMENTS TREATED**
*Sarsaparilla* is mainly used for the urinary system and is an important remedy for cystitis and renal colic from kidney stones. Symptoms of cystitis include a constant urge to urinate and pain in the bladder as the last few drops of urine are passed. In addition, there may be dribbling and incontinence, especially when sitting. The urine is cloudy and may be bloody and contain gravel or small kidney stones.

This remedy is also good for eczema with deep, bloody cracks on the hands, especially on the sides of the fingers. Rheumatic pain that is worse in damp weather and at night is also treated with *Sarsaparilla*. People who need this remedy feel very chilly and tend to have itchy, scaly spots, which become crusty, especially in the spring.
**Symptoms better** Standing; from uncovering the neck or chest.
**Symptoms worse** During the night; in cold, damp weather.

SOLANUM DULCAMARA

# DULCAMARA

Solanum dulcamara *has a long history in medicine, dating back to ancient Rome. It was used to treat pneumonia, absent menstruation, jaundice, rheumatism, cramps, eczema, psoriasis, asthma, and phlegm. In homeopathy, it is similar to the* Belladonna, Capsicum, Hyoscyamus, *and* Stramonium *remedies, which are also given to people who are very sensitive to cold and damp.*

**Common name** Woody nightshade.
**Source** Grows throughout Europe.
**Parts used** Young, green shoots and leaves of the fresh plant in flower.

**AILMENTS TREATED**
Complaints that result from exposure to cold, wet weather, or sudden temperature changes, or cooling down too quickly after sweating are helped by this remedy. People who need *Dulcamara* are strong-minded, domineering, and possessive. They are extremely sensitive to cold, wet weather, and are susceptible to colds, which may lead to other ailments, for example, conjunctivitis, cystitis, a wheezy cough, or diarrhea. They have excessive, thick, yellow mucus.

This remedy is also used for skin conditions such as hives (urticaria), ringworm, itchy, crusting eruptions on the scalp and face with a tendency to bleed when scratched, and large, smooth, flat warts.

**Symptoms better** With warmth; with movement.
**Symptoms worse** In cold and damp; from extremes of temperature.

🥣 **Main self-help use**
Sore throats – see pp. 176–7.

SPIGELIA ANTHELMIA

# SPIGELIA

*This plant was first introduced as a medicine in 1751 by Dr. Browne, who commented, "it produces sleep almost as certainly as opium." It was also known to have poisonous properties similiar to those of strychnine and was used in the 17th century as a key ingredient of poisons. The fresh plant has an offensive odor, which may have a narcotic effect in an enclosed space.*

**Common names** Pink root, annual worm grass.
**Source** Grows in the US, South America, and the West Indies.
**Parts used** Dried plant.

**AILMENTS TREATED**
The main uses of this remedy are to treat heart disorders with anginal pain, such as coronary artery disease, as well as migraines, neuralgia, and iritis (inflammation of the iris), the symptoms of which include violent, radiating, sharp or throbbing pain, typically affecting the left temple and left eye. When ill, people who need this remedy have a fear of sharp, pointed objects, such as needles.
**Symptoms better** In dry weather; with rest; after sunset; lying on the right side with the head raised.
**Symptoms worse** If touched; lying on the left side; with movement; from changes in weather, especially before a thunderstorm.

✦**SPIGELIA ANTHELMIA**
*The remedy made from this dried plant is used for anginal pain that is often left-sided.*

## SPONGIA

### *SPONGIA TOSTA*

*Sponge first came to prominence medicinally in the 14th century, when it was used as a treatment for goiter, which results from iodine deficiency (see p. 131). Some 500 years later it was concluded that sponge contains significant amounts of iodine and bromine, which explain its success in treating goiter and other thyroid complaints.*

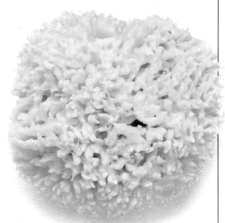

**♥SPONGIA** *Roasted sponge is used to make the homeopathic remedy which is given for swelling of the thyroid gland and coughs.*

**Common name** Sponge.
**Source** The Mediterranean and other seas.
**Parts used** Roasted sponge.

### CONSTITUTIONAL TYPE
People who benefit from this remedy have fair hair and a pale complexion, blue eyes, and a lean build. When ill, they fear dying.

### AILMENTS TREATED
Typically, this remedy is used to treat toxic symptoms that result from goiter, such as palpitations, breathlessness, and flushing. It is also used for acute, dry, croupy coughs, asthma, and heart disease. Symptoms associated with these conditions include: a sense of exhaustion and heaviness after minimal exertion; violent palpitations with anginal chest pains; a flushed face or neck; and a sense of suffocation that often wakes the person shortly after midnight.

It is also given for laryngitis with a raw, dry, burning sensation in the throat, which is extremely sensitive to touch. It is particularly useful when there is a family history of tuberculosis or chest conditions.
**Symptoms better** Sitting up; from warm food and drinks.
**Symptoms worse** With movement; from touching the affected areas; from talking; lying with the head lowered; from sweet foods and cold drinks.

## STANNUM MET.

### *STANNUM METALLICUM*

*Tin is a soft, silvery-white metal with a bluish tinge. In folk medicine it was used to treat tapeworm and was given in the form of tin filings, which were thought to expel the tapeworm by means of their weight and sharp points, or by stupefying the worm. Later, however, it was realized that any likely benefit was due to the purgative given to the patient after the tin filings.*

**Common name** Tin.
**Source** Found in the mineral cassiterite in Europe, Africa, China, and the Far East.
**Parts used** Pure tin.

### AILMENTS TREATED
This remedy is used to treat chest ailments such as bronchitis, asthma, and tracheitis (inflammation of the trachea with symptoms such as a dry cough and hoarseness). Symptoms include a wracking cough with green sweetish-tasting sputum, weakness of the chest, and associated tearfulness. People who need this remedy may suffer from hoarseness or a cough from talking, laughing, or singing.

Other ailments treated with this remedy are left-sided headaches and neuralgia. Symptoms usually come on gradually and resolve slowly.

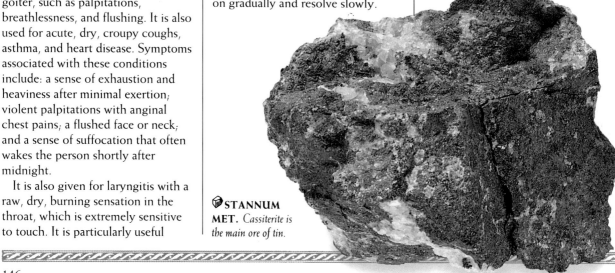

**⬢STANNUM MET.** *Cassiterite is the main ore of tin.*

**Symptoms better** From hard pressure; from coughing up phlegm.
**Symptoms worse** Lying on the right side; from warm drinks.

## SYPHILINUM

### *SYPHILINUM*

*Syphilis, the bacterium from which this remedy is made, is a sexually transmitted infection that first appeared in Europe in the 15th century. It was thought to have been brought from the North American continent by early explorers. Original treatments, made with mercury and arsenic preparations, were almost as dangerous as the disease itself. According to Hahnemann, syphilis was responsible for the third miasm or inherited trait (see p. 19).*

**Common name** Syphilis.
**Source** Syphilitic lesion or chancre.
**Parts used** Secretion from chancre.

### CONSTITUTIONAL TYPE
Individuals likely to benefit from *Syphilinum* typically exhibit mental fogginess with poor concentration and memory, high levels of anxiety, and a tendency toward compulsive thought or behavior, for example, checking and rechecking things or obsessively washing their hands. There is often an associated dependency on alcohol, tobacco, or drugs.

### AILMENTS TREATED
This remedy is used to treat chronic, although relatively painless, ulceration with recurrent abscesses typically in the groin. It is also used

for chronic conditions such as asthma, constipation, painful menstruation, iritis (inflammation of the iris), and neuralgia. Symptoms appear gradually and resolve slowly.
**Symptoms better** During the day; in a mountain environment; from walking slowly.
**Symptoms worse** At night; by the sea; with extreme heat or cold; during a thunderstorm.

---

*TARENTULA CUBENSIS*

# TARENTULA CUB.

*When this spider bites, the victim does not realize it until the next day, when an inflamed spot outlined in red develops. The spot swells and spreads and is followed by a fever and an abscess. The delay between the spider's bite and the onset of symptoms indicates blood poisoning. The homeopathic remedy is used to treat similar symptoms associated with septic conditions.*

**Common name** Tarentula.
**Source** Found in Cuba and the southern states of the US.
**Parts used** Whole, live spider.

### AILMENTS TREATED
Septic conditions, such as intensely burning abscesses or carbuncles with a bluish hue are treated with this remedy. It is also given for vulval itching and persistently restless feet.
**Symptoms better** Curiously, from smoking.
**Symptoms worse** At night; from cold drinks; from exertion.

---

*TEREBINTHINAE OLEUM*

# TEREBINTH.

*Turpentine is used in the manufacture of paint thinners, synthetic pine oil, and camphor. When it is splashed on the skin and left for any length of time, turpentine causes a burning and blistering sensation. When inhaled, it results in sneezing and breathlessness, and if swallowed causes burning in the mouth and stomach, vomiting, and diarrhea. It was used in orthodox medicine to treat gonorrhea, vaginal discharge, and discharge from the*

bladder. *The homeopathic remedy was proved in the 19th century.*

**Common name** Turpentine.
**Source** Coniferous trees, particularly the pine found in the Northern Hemisphere.
**Parts used** Oil distilled from oleoresin (turpentine).

### AILMENTS TREATED
The mucous membranes of the bladder and kidneys are mainly affected by this remedy. It is used for infection or inflammation of the urethra or kidneys, or cystitis with violent burning and drawing pains in the urethra, bladder, or kidneys, together with cloudy or dark, sweet-smelling urine. There is associated pain in the back and a sense of contraction and coldness in the umbilical region. Terebinth. is also used for edema (fluid retention in the tissues), associated with kidney disease.

**Symptoms better** From walking in fresh air.
**Symptoms worse** In damp surroundings; at night.

---

*TEUCRIUM MARUM VERUM*

# TEUCRIUM MAR. VER.

*Despite its common name, cat thyme belongs to the same genus as the mint family. This highly aromatic plant has long been used by herbalists because it is astringent and acts as a stimulant. The homeopathic remedy is given for conditions with excess mucus and polyps (growths in the mucous membranes). Dr. Stapf, a close friend of Hahnemann, proved the remedy in 1846.*

**Common name** Cat thyme.
**Source** Found worldwide.
**Part used** Whole fresh plant.

### AILMENTS TREATED
This remedy is mainly used where polyps are present, for example, in the nose, ear, bladder, or rectum. It is effective for threadworms. It is also used to treat chronic, excessive nasal discharge and a blocked nose with a poor sense of smell and frequent discharge of green crusts, which makes the nostrils feel raw. Blowing the nose or sneezing fails to relieve the sense of obstruction.
**Symptoms better** From fresh air.
**Symptoms worse** From changes of weather; with damp and cold; from being too hot in bed.

When rubbed, the leaves and deep pink flowers give off an aromatic smell

**TEUCRIUM MARUM VERUM** *This pungent-smelling herb is used to make a remedy that is given for ailments with excess mucus.*

*THERIDION CURASSAVICUM*

# THERIDION

*This spider is about the size of a cherry pit; it has orange spots on its back, and a large yellow spot on its belly. Its venom is particularly virulent, causing nervousness, weakness, trembling, coldness, anxiety, fainting, and a cold sweat. The homeopathic remedy was proved and introduced by Dr. Hering (see p. 19) in 1832.*

**Common name** Orange spider.
**Source** Native to the West Indies, particularly Curaçao.
**Parts used** Whole, live spider.

### AILMENTS TREATED
*Theridion* acts mainly on the nerves, spine, and bones. It is given for conditions such as spinal inflammation, toothache, vertigo, motion sickness, bone decay, and Ménière's disease (a disorder of the inner ear). All these conditions are characterized by extreme sensitivity to noise and vibration that penetrate the body and cause pain. The spine is especially sensitive. People who need this remedy cannot bear the repeated jarring of walking. They will sit sideways on a chair to avoid pressure on the lower spine. Due to this hypersensitivity, travel or movement causes nausea or vertigo, which is worse from closing the eyes.

**Symptoms better** With rest; with warmth; from drinking warm water.
**Symptoms worse** Near noise; if touched; from pressure; with travel; with jarring or movement; closing the eyes; bending forward; at night.

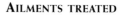

*TUBERCULINUM KOCH & T. BOVUM*

# TUBERCULINUM

*In 1882, Robert Koch discovered that a preparation of dead tuberculinum bacillus could be used to prevent and treat tuberculosis (TB). Between 1885 and 1890, Burnett conducted a series of experiments using lung tissue from TB patients and proved the homeopathic remedy, which is used to treat ailments that affect the respiratory tract.*

**Common name** Tuberculosis.
**Source** Human or animal tuberculous tissue rendered sterile.
**Parts used** Bacterium.

### CONSTITUTIONAL TYPE
In typical *Tuberculinum* individuals there is a constant need for change, for example, of jobs, partners, or home interiors, a love of travel, and often a deep romantic longing but lack of fulfillment. These types often have fair hair with blue eyes, are tall and lean, and tend to lack stamina. They may have a strong fear of dogs or cats and a craving for smoked foods and cold milk.

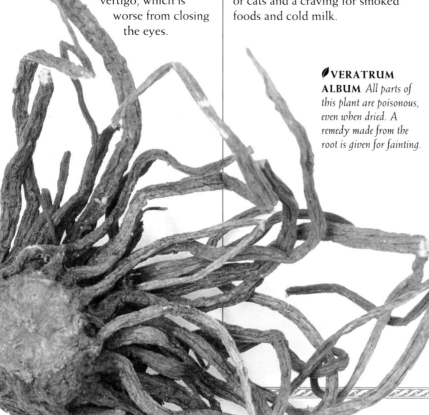

**🖊 VERATRUM ALBUM** *All parts of this plant are poisonous, even when dried. A remedy made from the root is given for fainting.*

### AILMENTS TREATED
People with a marked susceptibility to colds, and in whose family history there is evidence of tuberculosis, allergies, or a chronic respiratory disorder, are helped by this remedy. They may have an inherited weakness in the immune system. *Tuberculinum* is given mainly for coughs, and fever with night sweats, emaciation, and sharp pains that may be felt through the left upper lung. The lymph glands in the neck are enlarged. Symptoms change and move from one part of the body to another, or start and end abruptly.
**Symptoms better** From fresh air; in cold, dry surroundings.
**Symptoms worse** In cold, damp, and humidity; from exertion.

*VERATRUM ALBUM*

# VERAT. ALB.

*Mania, melancholia, and epilepsy were treated with this plant, and it was used by Hippocrates to cure a case resembling Asiatic cholera. The homeopathic remedy was first proved by Hahnemann between 1826 and 1830.*

**Common name** White hellebore.
**Source** Grows in mountainous regions of Europe.
**Parts used** Fresh root.

### CONSTITUTIONAL TYPE
These types are ambitious and ruthless, yet fearful regarding their position in society, which leads to deceitful manipulation.

### AILMENTS TREATED
This remedy is given for fainting or collapse where the person is pale, ice-cold, sweaty (particularly on the forehead), and dehydrated. Such a state of collapse may result from an acute fright, from violent vomiting with diarrhea and cramps, especially in pregnancy, or may be associated with severe menstrual pain.
**Symptoms better** From hot drinks and food; lying down.
**Symptoms worse** From cold drinks; with movement; at night.

**🥄 MAIN SELF-HELP USE**
Cramps in pregnancy – see
pp. 210–11.

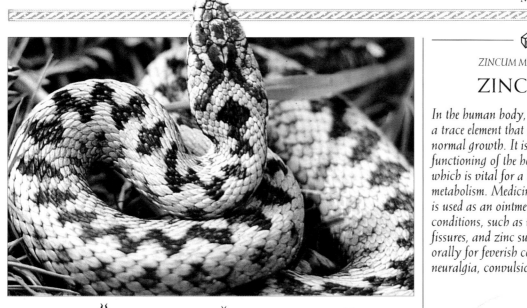

*ZINCUM METALLICUM*

# ZINC MET.

*In the human body, zinc occurs as a trace element that is essential for normal growth. It is involved in the functioning of the hormone insulin, which is vital for a healthy metabolism. Medicinally, zinc oxide is used as an ointment for local conditions, such as ulcers and skin fissures, and zinc supplements are taken orally for feverish conditions, hysteria, neuralgia, convulsions, and tetanus.*

*VIPERA COMMUNIS*

# VIPERA

*This stout-bodied viper eats lizards and small mammals. Although rarely fatal to humans, its bite causes inflammation and bleeding in the blood vessels. The veins become swollen and painful, especially when the affected limb hangs down. The homeopathic remedy is used for similar symptoms.*

**Common names** Common viper, adder.
**Source** Widely found across Europe and Asia.
**Parts used** Fresh venom.

**AILMENTS TREATED**
Painful swelling of the veins, such as varicose veins and phlebitis (inflamed veins) are mainly treated with this remedy. Typically, when the legs hang down they feel so full there is a sensation that they will burst.
**Symptoms better** Raising the affected limb.
**Symptoms worse** From a change in weather; from pressure; if touched.

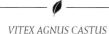

*VITEX AGNUS CASTUS*

# AGNUS CASTUS

*The twigs of this aromatic shrub are very flexible and are used in basket-making, while the red fruits are used as a flavoring. Herbalists still use the berries to increase hormone production during PMS or menopause. The remedy was proved by Hahnemann between 1826 and 1830.*

**VIPERA COMMUNIS** *The viper is usually gray with a black zigzag on its back and brown spots on its sides. Its venom is the source of a remedy used for inflamed veins.*

**Common names** Chaste-tree, monk's pepper, wild lavender.
**Source** Native to Europe and Asia, particularly the shores of the Mediterranean, now naturalized in the US.
**Parts used** Fresh, ripe berries.

**AILMENTS TREATED**
This remedy is most effective during menopause and for treating physical breakdown that results from the abuse of alcohol or drugs, or from excessive sexual intercourse. It is given for depression, anxiety, and fatigue, with mental dullness and despair. Symptoms include premature ejaculation, particularly in men with a previously high sex drive, and loss of libido in women, for example, around menopause. *Agnus castus* is also good for loss of breast milk after childbirth and associated postpartum depression.
**Symptoms better** From pressure.
**Symptoms worse** With movement; in the morning; after urinating.

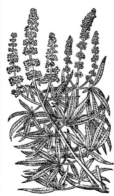

**VITEX AGNUS CASTUS** *Herbalists use this shrub to stimulate the pituitary gland.*

**ZINCUM METALLICUM** *To make the Zinc met. remedy this bluish white metal is triturated (see p. 20).*

**Common name** Zinc.
**Source** Zinc sulfide, which is common in nature, is found in the US, South America, Australia and Asia.
**Parts used** Zinc.

**AILMENTS TREATED**
*Zinc met.* is mainly used for conditions of extreme mental or physical weakness, or exhaustion with restless, fidgety movements, such as restless legs. These symptoms may develop from too much stress and lack of sleep. In addition to being run-down and generally exhausted, the person may have brain fatigue with a tendency to repeat a question before answering it, and associated irritability and jumpiness, especially in response to noise or touch.
  Symptoms worsen if discharges are suppressed, for example by using cough suppressants.
**Symptoms better** From the onset of discharge such as menstruation, urination, and bowel movements.
**Symptoms worse** From drinking alcohol, especially wine; near noise.

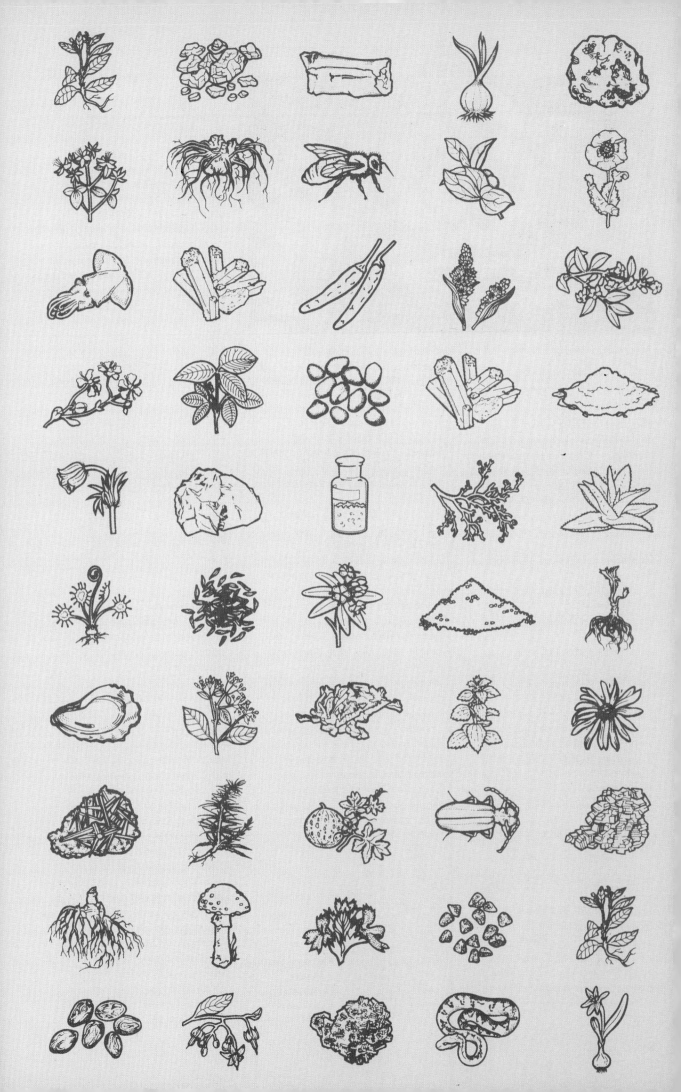

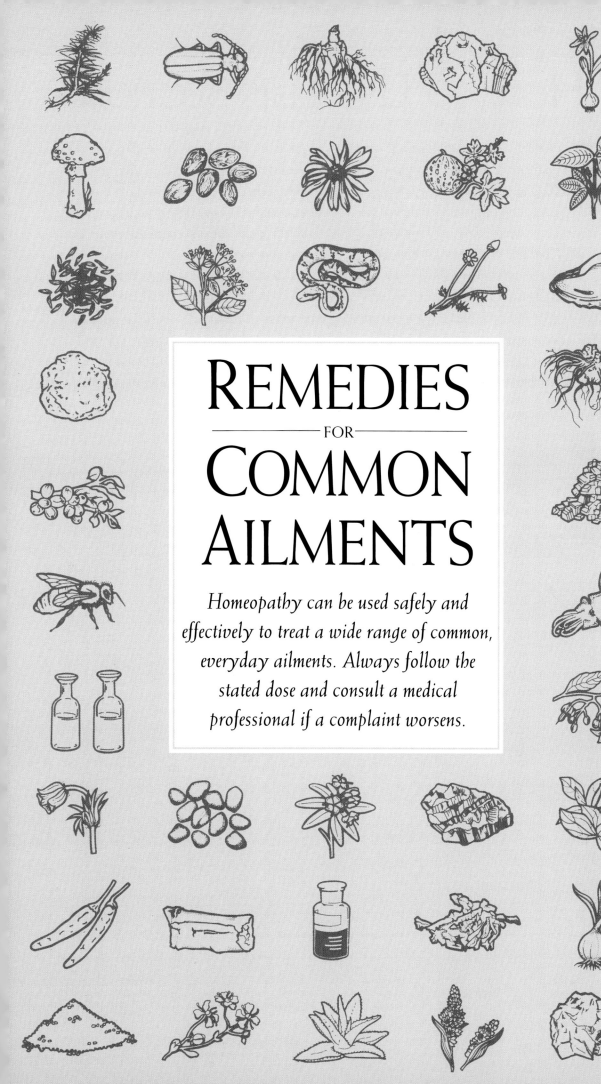

# REMEDIES

## —FOR—

# COMMON AILMENTS

*Homeopathy can be used safely and effectively to treat a wide range of common, everyday ailments. Always follow the stated dose and consult a medical professional if a complaint worsens.*

# HOW TO USE THIS SECTION

The common ailments in this section can be safely treated with homeopathy at home. They are grouped according to parts of the body, body systems, or special problems, such as women's health. For each group of ailments, for example, colds, coughs, and flu, there is an introduction with information about general causes, symptoms, and other characteristics. Specific ailments are featured in charts. For each ailment, for example, a cold that comes on slowly, there is detailed information about the symptoms, cause, and onset, and factors that improve or worsen the condition.

To pinpoint the best remedy to take, find the closest match between the information given in the ailment chart and the cause and onset of your ailment and its symptoms. If your symptoms change, consult the ailment chart again and try another remedy.

For ailments that are not covered in this section or for chronic, long-term conditions or for ailments that deteriorate, consult a medical professional. Recurrent ailments may need constitutional treatment and should be referred to a qualified homeopath (see pp. 24–5).

## SAMPLE ENTRY

General information about complaints

Precautions

Self-help treatments

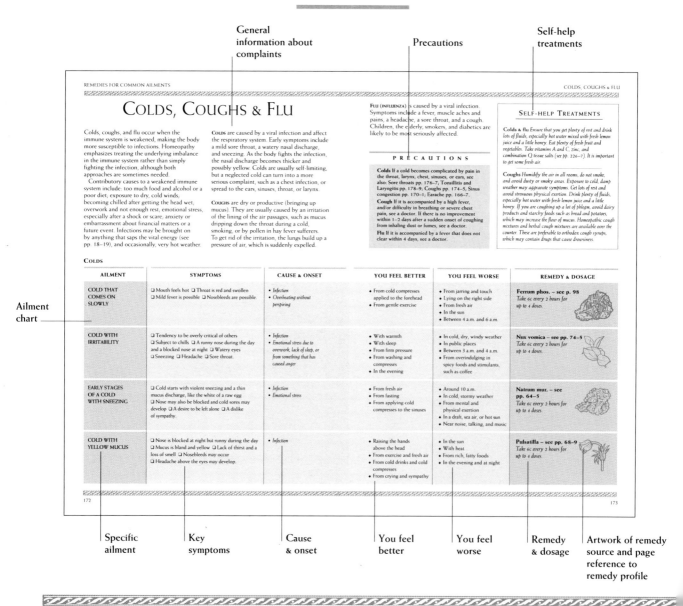

Ailment chart

Specific ailment

Key symptoms

Cause & onset

You feel better

You feel worse

Remedy & dosage

Artwork of remedy source and page reference to remedy profile

## KEY TO THE SAMPLE ENTRY

### IMPORTANT NOTE

**To select the best remedy, try to match, as closely as possible, the cause and onset and the symptoms with yours. You do not have to have all the symptoms listed, nor match all the "you feel better" or "you feel worse" information. If there is no improvement within the recommended time for taking the remedy, see a medical professional.**

**Introduction** Information about the general causes and symptoms of complaints. (Not all the symptoms mentioned here will necessarily be in the symptoms listed for specific ailments featured in the ailments chart.)

**Ailment** Brief description of a specific type of ailment.

**Symptoms** Key physical symptoms and emotional symptoms for specific ailments.

**Cause & onset** Specific causes of the ailment, for example, viral infection, and other factors that bring about the onset of an illness, such as being exposed to a sudden change in temperature or emotional stress.

**You feel better** Factors that improve the symptoms of an illness or make you feel better when ill.

**You feel worse** Factors that worsen the symptoms of an illness or make you feel worse when ill.

**Remedy & dosage** The appropriate remedy, along with the potency (either 6c or 30c), and frequency of dosage. There is also a page reference to the *Index of Homeopathic Remedies*, which provides a full remedy profile.

**Precautions** Always read the precautions before treating an ailment. Professional help is recommended if complaints become complicated or if symptoms worsen.

**Self-help treatments** Nutritional supplements, herbal remedies, and other self-help measures that may help an illness.

## GUIDELINES FOR USING HOMEOPATHIC REMEDIES

### POTENCY & DOSAGE

Under the heading *Remedy & dosage* in the ailment charts there are guidelines on how long and how often to take a remedy. As a general rule, homeopathic remedies, like orthodox medicines, should be taken only when needed and stopped as soon as they are no longer needed. The efficacy of remedies depends on matching the symptoms experienced to the remedy information as precisely as possible.

If the symptoms worsen (what homeopaths call an aggravation) it may be a sign that a remedy is working and has prompted your vital force into action (see pp. 18–19). This worsening should last only a few hours and then you should begin to feel better. If you experience an aggravation, stop taking the remedy and allow your immune system to fight the illness on its own. If the original symptoms recur, take the remedy again. If there is still no improvement, stop taking the remedy and consult a medical professional.

### HOW SAFE ARE REMEDIES?

• Homeopathic remedies are completely safe because they are repeatedly diluted. If a child were to swallow a bottle of tablets, he or she might suffer transient diarrhea from the lactose (milk sugar) but no adverse long-term effects.

• Remedies are safe to be taken by the elderly and lactating mothers. They are also safe to use in pregnancy, although it is best to take them only if absolutely necessary (see p. 208–9).

• Remedies can be safely given to babies and children. The dosage information in the ailment charts is suitable for babies and children.

• Orthodox or herbal medicines can be taken in addition to homeopathic remedies. Do not undertake self-treatment with homeopathic remedies while you are undergoing a prescribed course of medical treatment without first seeking professional advice.

### HOW TO TAKE THE REMEDIES

• Do not touch or handle the remedies. Use a clean, dry teaspoon to drop them onto a clean tongue.

• Do not take the remedies with food or drink. Wait at least 30 minutes after eating before taking them.

• Avoid the following, which may antidote a remedy: coffee, alcohol, tobacco, spicy foods, and anything with a minty flavor, especially toothpaste. (Toothpastes without mint flavoring are available from health food stores.)

• Do not wear strong perfumes or use strong-smelling household cleaners when taking a remedy.

• Some essential oils have an antidoting effect, in particular, camphor, eucalyptus, peppermint, rosemary, and all thyme oils. Lavender essential oil should be used only at less than 2% solution.

• It is best not to take more than one remedy at a time.

### TYPES OF REMEDY AVAILABLE

Remedies commonly are made by impregnating lactose (milk sugar) with the potency. They are available as tablets, pillules, granules, and powders. If you are allergic to lactose, use liquid remedies (available from homeopathic pharmacies). Granules and powder are good for babies and children because they dissolve quickly on the tongue and cannot be spat out. Alternatively, dissolve pillules in a little boiled, cooled water and give a teaspoonful of the resulting solution.

### STORAGE

Remedies should be stored in a cool, dark place well away from food or other products with a strong smell. Ensure that the tops of the containers are screwed on tightly. If stored properly, remedies will last for many years. As with all medicines, keep remedies out of the reach of children.

# ACHES & PAINS

Pain in the bones, joints, muscles, tendons, and ligaments is very common and accounts for a large number of lost working hours. A common cause of bone pain is flu. Other causes, such as a fracture, may have to be ruled out by a doctor. Muscle and joint pain can be the result of a poor working position, inactivity, bad posture, or aging, or symptomatic of an underlying emotional problem such as anxiety. Acute pain in the muscles, joints, tendons, and ligaments can be due to an injury that damages the muscle fibers, tendons, and ligaments and causes stiffness, swelling, and loss of movement.

**OSTEOARTHRITIS** is caused by the wearing away of the cartilage that lines the joints due to age, obesity, injury, or overuse. It results in limited movement, pain, and occasionally acute inflammation. Many people over the age of 40 have some degree of osteoarthritis, often in the weight-bearing joints such as the hips, knees, and spine. Osteoarthritis often starts in the fingers, particularly during menopause.

**RHEUMATISM** is a general term for muscle aches and pains. The symptoms can be the result of a viral infection or food allergy, or may indicate an underlying joint disease. The pain may be constant or may vary in intensity according to the weather or with hormonal changes. Tensing the muscles because of emotional stress, upset, and anxiety also aggravates rheumatism.

**CRAMPS** are spasms in the muscles due to a lack of oxygen and a buildup of waste products. Lying in an unusual position, too much exercise, or prolonged sitting or standing are common causes. Extreme sweating can also cause cramps due to a loss of sodium in sweat. Cramps also occur in pregnancy.

## OSTEOARTHRITIS

| AILMENT | SYMPTOMS | CAUSE & ONSET |
|---|---|---|
| **PAIN WITH STIFFNESS** | ❑ Restlessness and irritability ❑ A tendency to dream of doing exercise ❑ Great stiffness and aching pain in the affected joints, especially on waking in the morning. | • *Inactivity*<br>• *Cold, wet weather* |
| **SEVERE PAIN ON MOVEMENT** | ❑ Hot, swollen joints that are excruciatingly painful with the slightest movement. | • *Overuse or injury* |
| **PAIN ACCOMPANIED BY TEARFULNESS** | ❑ A tendency to be emotional and tearful ❑ Pain in the joints flits from place to place ❑ A desire for sympathy and consolation. | • *Hormonal changes associated with the menstrual cycle* |
| **PAIN AGGRAVATED BY INJURY** | ❑ Bruising pain that is sore to the touch ❑ Movement is difficult ❑ Whole system feels in a mild state of shock from the injury ❑ A desire to be alone ❑ A tendency to have bad dreams. | • *Injury such as a fall or a severe wrench* |

**RESTLESS LEGS** include symptoms such as tickling, prickling, burning, or aching sensations, especially in the lower legs, which may cause the legs to twitch or jerk. The condition is usually due to problems with the nervous system and may be partly inherited. It is more common in older people and smokers, and if the muscles are overexerted and fatigued, particularly in cold and damp weather. Restless legs can be the result of diabetes, vitamin B deficiency, excess caffeine, drug withdrawal, or food allergy. Orthodox medicine has not yet identified the exact cause of this condition, but it has been shown that a majority of sufferers have an iron deficiency.

## PRECAUTIONS

If muscle, bone, or joint pain becomes severe and persistent, contact a doctor within 12 hours. If there is no deterioration, but the pain does not respond to the appropriate homeopathic remedy within 14 days, see a doctor.

## SELF-HELP TREATMENTS

**Osteoarthritis** *Many sufferers find that an alkaline diet is helpful (see p. 228). If a joint is inflamed, take your weight off it, using a cane if necessary. If overweight, try to lose some weight. Sleep on a firm bed. There are a number of nutritional and herbal supplements that may be beneficial, including cod liver oil, copper, devil's claw, green mussel extract, iron, kelp, manganese, selenium, vitamins A, B complex, C, and E, and zinc (see pp. 224–7).*

**Rheumatism** *Try an alkaline diet (see p. 228) and take calcium, magnesium, and vitamin $B_6$ (see pp. 224–6).*

**Cramps** *Stretch the muscles and massage them to increase the blood supply. Raise the foot of the bed about 4 in (10 cm). Take magnesium supplements (see p. 225).*

**Restless legs** *Wear warm socks in bed or use a hot-water bottle. Make sure your diet contains enough folic acid and vitamin E, and take extra iron and vitamin B complex (see pp. 225–6). Cut out caffeine (tea, coffee, and cola drinks).*

| YOU FEEL BETTER | YOU FEEL WORSE | REMEDY & DOSAGE | |
|---|---|---|---|
| ◆ With heat<br>◆ With sustained movement<br>◆ In dry weather | ◆ On starting to move<br>◆ From getting cold on undressing<br>◆ In wet, cold, windy, stormy weather<br>◆ At night | **Rhus tox. – see p. 108**<br>*Take 6c 4 times a day for up to 14 days.* | 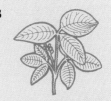 |
| ◆ From cold compresses and firm pressure applied to the affected part | ◆ With heat<br>◆ With the slightest movement<br>◆ Around 9 p.m. and 3 a.m.<br>◆ If lightly touched | **Bryonia – see p. 88**<br>*Take 6c 4 times a day for up to 14 days.* |  |
| ◆ From crying<br>◆ From gentle exercise<br>◆ From cold compresses<br>◆ From sympathy | ◆ With heat<br>◆ From rich, fatty foods<br>◆ Lying on the painful side<br>◆ In the evening and at night | **Pulsatilla – see pp. 68–9**<br>*Take 6c 4 times a day for up to 14 days.* |  |
| ◆ With gentle movement, for a short period | ◆ With prolonged movement<br>◆ With heat<br>◆ With rest<br>◆ From light pressure | **Arnica – see p. 85**<br>*Take 6c 4 times a day for up to 14 days.* |  |

# RHEUMATISM

| AILMENT | SYMPTOMS | CAUSE & ONSET |
|---|---|---|
| PAIN BROUGHT ON BY MOVEMENT | ❑ Aches and pains are aggravated by the slightest movement, and are better with rest ❑ Pressure on the affected joint helps ❑ Pain is associated with a dull feeling ❑ A tendency to dream about work. | • Movement<br>• Worry about job or finances |
| PAIN WITH TEARFULNESS | ❑ Pain flits from one joint to another and is associated with depression and emotional stress ❑ A desire for lots of sympathy and consolation. | • Hormonal changes associated with the menstrual cycle |
| STIFFNESS DUE TO CONTRACTED TENDONS | ❑ Pain with muscle spasms, especially in the jaw and neck, is due to contracted tendons ❑ Stiff neck after being in a draft ❑ Sharp, tearing pain in the muscles, often on the right side. | • Exposure to cold, dry weather |
| PAIN EASED BY PROLONGED GENTLE MOVEMENT | ❑ Aching and stiffness is worse first thing in the morning on waking ❑ Pain worsens on starting to move, and then eases after sustained movement ❑ Extreme restlessness. | • Immobility |
| PAIN IN THE TENDONS | ❑ Pain appears after injuries to the tendons, or where the lining of the bone has become bruised and sore. | • Injury |

# CRAMPS

| AILMENT | SYMPTOMS | CAUSE & ONSET |
|---|---|---|
| SEVERE CRAMPS IN THE FEET OR LEGS | ❑ Cramps start with a twitching of the muscles, leading to violent muscle spasms in the toes, ankles, and legs. | • Loss of body salt after sweating or vomiting<br>• Sudden chills, for example, after swimming |
| CRAMPS FROM MUSCLE FATIGUE | ❑ Cramps come on as a result of overexertion ❑ Limbs feel as if they have been beaten. | • Muscle fatigue from too much exercise |

# RESTLESS LEGS

| AILMENT | SYMPTOMS | CAUSE & ONSET |
|---|---|---|
| SYMPTOMS BETTER WITH CONTINUED MOVEMENT | ❑ Restlessness that is better with sustained movement ❑ Tickling feeling like ants under the skin ❑ Burning, prickling sensations. | • Overexertion, muscle sprain<br>• Exposure to cold, damp weather |

| YOU FEEL BETTER | YOU FEEL WORSE | REMEDY & DOSAGE |
|---|---|---|
| ◆ From pressure applied to the affected part<br>◆ With rest | ◆ In cold, dry, windy weather<br>◆ In a draft<br>◆ With movement<br>◆ Around 3 a.m. | **Bryonia – see p. 88**<br>*Take 6c 4 times a day for up to 14 days.* 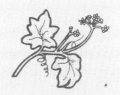 |
| ◆ From crying and sympathy<br>◆ From gentle exercise<br>◆ From fresh air<br>◆ From cold compresses | ◆ With heat<br>◆ From rich, fatty foods<br>◆ Lying on the painful side<br>◆ In the evening and at night<br>◆ From emotional stress | **Pulsatilla – see pp. 68–9**<br>*Take 6c 4 times a day for up to 14 days.*  |
| ◆ In warm, damp weather | ◆ In cold, dry, windy weather<br>◆ In a draft<br>◆ After a scare or grief<br>◆ From sweet foods and coffee | **Causticum – see p. 123**<br>*Take 6c 4 times a day for up to 14 days.*  |
| ◆ With sustained movement<br>◆ With heat | ◆ In the morning<br>◆ From sleeping or resting<br>◆ In cold, damp weather | **Rhus tox. – see p. 108**<br>*Take 6c 4 times a day for up to 14 days.* 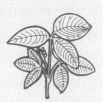 |
| ◆ With movement | ◆ In cold, damp weather<br>◆ From resting | **Ruta grav. – see p. 109**<br>*Take 6c 4 times a day for up to 14 days.*  |
| ◆ From firm pressure applied to the affected part | ◆ With movement and from light pressure | **Cuprum met. – see p. 95**<br>*Take 6c 4 times a day for up to 14 days.* 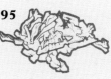 |
| ◆ On starting to move | ◆ With heat and from light pressure<br>◆ With prolonged movement | **Arnica – see p. 85**<br>*Take 6c 4 times a day for up to 14 days.*  |
| ◆ With continuous movement | ◆ With rest<br>◆ On starting to move<br>◆ In cold, damp weather | **Rhus tox. – see p. 108**<br>*Take 6c 4 times a day for up to 14 days.* 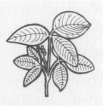 |

# HEADACHES & MIGRAINES

Unless caused by injury, headaches and migraines, particularly persistent ones, are viewed by homeopaths as symptomatic of an underlying imbalance in the body as a whole. To treat chronic headaches and migraines successfully, homeopaths look at the whole person. In addition to immediate symptoms, environmental and general factors such as diet, physical fitness, and emotional makeup are assessed to see what may predispose a sufferer to headaches. A homeopath will use this information to prescribe a remedy to match a person's constitutional type (see pp. 24–5).

The homeopathic remedies recommended here are effective for treating many types of headaches and migraines.

**HEADACHES** are an extremely common complaint. Most are due to muscular tension in the head, neck, or shoulders, or congestion of the blood vessels supplying blood to the brain or the muscles. Although headaches can be a symptom of a serious underlying disorder, they usually have more mundane causes. These include lack of sleep; too much caffeine or abrupt withdrawal from caffeine; food allergy; eyestrain; fever; low blood sugar (accompanied by a drop in energy if some time has passed since eating); anxiety, stress, and fright. Rheumatism in the neck, sinus congestion, or premenstrual tension may also be causes.

**MIGRAINES** are severe headaches. They are often one-sided, and may be accompanied by symptoms such as light intolerance, vision difficulty, nausea or vomiting, and occasionally, numbness or tingling in the arms. Pain is due to the blood vessels supplying the brain being narrowed and then dilated, possibly as a result of stress, exhaustion, or food intolerance.

## HEADACHES

| AILMENT | SYMPTOMS | CAUSE & ONSET |
|---|---|---|
| **VIOLENT HEADACHE THAT COMES ON SUDDENLY** | ❑ Severe pain that comes on suddenly ❑ Brain feels too big for the head, and there is a sensation of a tight band or cap around the head ❑ Severe anxiety with a fear of dying, even to the point of predicting the time of death. | • *Exposure to cold winds or drafts*<br>• *Shock or fright* |
| **THROBBING HEADACHE FROM HEAT** | ❑ Splitting, throbbing, drumming headache ❑ Face becomes bright red and the pupils become enlarged, creating a staring appearance ❑ Headache may be associated with delirium if very severe ❑ Often worse on the right side. | • *Heat, either from a fever or from exposure to the hot sun*<br>• *Head getting cold, wet, or overheated* |
| **SPLITTING, CRUSHING HEADACHE** | ❑ Sharp, stabbing pain that results from even the slightest eye movement ❑ No desire to talk to anyone ❑ Head feels as if it is about to break into pieces. | • *Stress or worry, especially about work*<br>• *Exposure to cold, dry winds*<br>• *Rheumatism in the neck* |
| **HEADACHE CAUSED BY EMOTIONAL STRESS** | ❑ Pain is very severe, as if a nail is being forced through the side of the head ❑ Sensation of a tight band across the forehead. | • *Brought on by emotional stress, such as bereavement or a breakup with a loved one* |

Migraine is a very common complaint affecting one in ten people, with three times as many women sufferers as men. In women, there may be a hormonal connection. Migraines are often worse around menstruation and can be triggered by oral contraceptives. Menopause can also aggravate migraines in women who are susceptible.

## PRECAUTIONS

If the headache follows a head injury or is of sudden onset with nausea, vomiting, drowsiness, and intolerance of light, call an ambulance and give *Arnica* 30c every 15 minutes until help arrives.

If the headache is severe and associated with a fever of more than 100° F (38° C) and intolerance of light or if there is pain behind one eye with blurred vision, call a doctor within 2 hours.

If the headache has lasted more than a few days, is worse in the mornings and accompanied by nausea and vomiting, call a doctor within 12 hours.

## SELF-HELP TREATMENTS

**Headaches & Migraines** *Avoiding stress, fatigue, and physical tension and learning to relax can help prevent and reduce the frequency of headaches and migraines. For headaches, take potassium supplements and vitamin B₃ (see pp. 225–6) and avoid vitamin A supplements.*

*Another means of preventing migraines is to avoid foods and drinks that are known to trigger them (see p. 229). Eliminate these one at a time for about 4 weeks and then gradually reintroduce them to see if any trigger a migraine. Avoid all food additives. If the migraine is worse around menstruation, avoid salty foods, eat protein-rich or complex carbohydrate snacks, rather than large meals (see p. 229), and take 30 minutes outdoor exercise every day.*

*Migraine sufferers should also stop smoking and taking oral contraceptives, and avoid wearing perfumes and using perfumed products. Take evening primrose oil and vitamins B₆, C, and E (see pp. 225–6), and add fresh ginger to cooking. If a migraine is coming on, splash the face with cold water for a few minutes, lie down in a darkened, quiet room, and try to sleep. If the migraine does not respond to this treatment, apply hot compresses to the forehead.*

| YOU FEEL BETTER | YOU FEEL WORSE | REMEDY & DOSAGE |
|---|---|---|
| ◆ From fresh, warm air | ◆ In intensely hot weather<br>◆ From exposure to dry, cold, windy weather<br>◆ Near tobacco smoke | **Aconite – see p. 82**<br>*Take 30c every 10–15 minutes for up to 10 doses.*  |
| ◆ Standing or sitting upright<br>◆ With warmth | ◆ At the slightest knock or jar<br>◆ With movement or noise<br>◆ Lying down<br>◆ In bright light or the sun<br>◆ At night | **Belladonna – see p. 86**<br>*Take 30c every 10–15 minutes for up to 10 doses.* 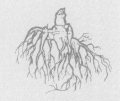 |
| ◆ From firm, cool pressure applied to the head | ◆ From excitement or noise<br>◆ From touch or movement<br>◆ From eating or in bright light | **Bryonia – see p. 88**<br>*Take 30c every 10–15 minutes for up to 10 doses.* 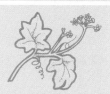 |
| ◆ From eating<br>◆ After urinating<br>◆ Walking or resting<br>◆ Lying on the painful side<br>◆ With heat and firm pressure | ◆ From fresh air and cold<br>◆ From drinking coffee or alcohol<br>◆ Near tobacco smoke<br>◆ Around strong smells | **Ignatia – see pp. 58–9**<br>*Take 30c every 10–15 minutes for up to 10 doses.*  |

**HEADACHES** *continued*

## HEADACHES *continued*

| AILMENT | SYMPTOMS | CAUSE & ONSET |
|---|---|---|
| **HEADACHE FROM MUSCULAR TENSION IN THE NECK** | ❑ Headache at the top of the head or spreading to or from the neck ❑ A feeling of pressure at the top of the head or a full sensation as if it might open up ❑ Eye pain ❑ Neck stiffness, spreading across the shoulders ❑ Neck spasms. | • *Spasm in the neck and back muscles* <br> • *Emotional stress, particularly in women* <br> • *Back injury* <br> • *Eyestrain* |
| **HEADACHE FROM A HANGOVER, WITH NAUSEA** | ❑ Headache with a sensation of a great weight bearing down on the head ❑ Extreme irritability and a tendency to be hypercritical ❑ Dizziness. | • *Drinking too much alcohol or coffee* |

## MIGRAINES

| AILMENT | SYMPTOMS | CAUSE & ONSET |
|---|---|---|
| **MIGRAINE THAT IS WORSE ON THE LEFT SIDE** | ❑ Headache accompanied by severe nausea and vomiting ❑ Pain may extend to the face, mouth, teeth, or root of the tongue ❑ Vomiting does not relieve the headache ❑ Tongue feels clean and not thickly coated, despite constant nausea. | • *Stress* <br> • *Indigestible foods* |
| **BLINDING, THROBBING MIGRAINE** | ❑ Often begins with numbness and tingling in the lips and tongue ❑ Pain is severe and pulsating ❑ Head feels as if there is too much blood in it. | • *Brought on by the stress of suppressing emotions* <br> • *Grief* <br> • *Hormonal changes caused by PMS or menopause* |
| **MIGRAINE ACCOMPANIED BY TEARFULNESS** | ❑ Often associated with moodiness and changeable emotions ❑ Head feels as if it is about to burst ❑ The slightest stress causes crying. | • *Hormonal changes, particularly in women suffering from PMS* <br> • *Emotional stress* <br> • *Eating rich, fatty foods* |
| **MIGRAINE THAT SETTLES OVER THE RIGHT EYE** | ❑ Headache usually starts in the morning at the back of the head and gradually spreads upward to the forehead above the right eye ❑ Veins in the temple feel distended ❑ Pain is sharp and sudden and may radiate to the right shoulder. | • *Hormonal changes, particularly during menopause* |
| **MIGRAINE WITH A STRONG DESIRE TO COVER THE HEAD** | ❑ Pain starts in the back of the head and then shifts upward, settling over one eye ❑ Worse around midday ❑ There may be head sweats, often on the right side ❑ Pain relieved by pressure and urinating. | • *Stress* <br> • *Exhaustion* |

| YOU FEEL BETTER | YOU FEEL WORSE | REMEDY & DOSAGE |
|---|---|---|
| ◆ With warmth<br>◆ From eating | ◆ During menstruation<br>◆ In a draft<br>◆ If cold | **Cimic. – see p. 93**<br>*Take 6c every hour for up to 6 doses.* 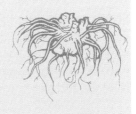 |
| ◆ With warmth<br>◆ With sleep<br>◆ From firm pressure applied to the affected part<br>◆ From washing the hair | ◆ In cold, windy weather<br>◆ Around noise<br>◆ From more alcohol<br>◆ If touched<br>◆ Between 3 a.m. and 4 a.m. | **Nux vomica – see pp. 74–5**<br>*Take 6c every hour for up to 6 doses.*  |
| ◆ With rest<br>◆ From pressure applied to the affected part<br>◆ With the eyes closed | ◆ From rich foods<br>◆ From lemon peel, ices, raisins, and salads<br>◆ With movement<br>◆ From vomiting or coughing | **Ipecac. – see p. 91**<br>*Take 6c every 15 minutes for up to 10 doses.* 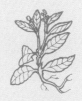 |
| ◆ From fresh air<br>◆ From fasting<br>◆ Sleeping on a firm bed<br>◆ From cold compresses applied to the affected part | ◆ From mental fatigue<br>◆ From physical exertion<br>◆ From talking, noise or music<br>◆ With warmth<br>◆ In bright light or hot sun<br>◆ From too much sympathy<br>◆ In sea air or stormy weather | **Nux vomica – see pp. 74–5**<br>*Take 6c every hour for up to 6 doses.*  |
| ◆ From firm pressure, cold compresses, and cold drinks<br>◆ From crying and sympathy<br>◆ Raising the hands above the head<br>◆ From gentle exercise<br>◆ From fresh air | ◆ In the sun and heat<br>◆ From extremes of temperature<br>◆ From rich, fatty foods<br>◆ From early evening onward | **Pulsatilla – see pp. 68–9**<br>*At the first sign of an attack, take 6c every 15 minutes for up to 10 doses.*  |
| ◆ From acidic drinks or foods<br>◆ With sleep<br>◆ Lying in darkness | ◆ From eating candy<br>◆ If touched<br>◆ In the sun | **Sanguinaria – see p. 144**<br>*At the first sign of an attack, take 6c every 15 minutes for up to 10 doses.* 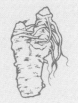 |
| ◆ From wrapping the head warmly<br>◆ After urinating<br>◆ In warm, wet weather | ◆ Lying on the left side<br>◆ After getting undressed<br>◆ From using antiperspirants<br>◆ In cold, windy weather | **Silica – see pp. 72–3**<br>*At the first sign of an attack, take 6c every 15 minutes for up to 10 doses.* 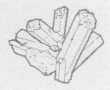 |

# TEETH, MOUTH & GUMS

Problems with the teeth, mouth, and gums are very common but can be prevented by good oral hygiene, regular checkups, and eating fibrous, chewy, nonsugary foods. Soft, acidic, refined, and sweet foods cause tooth decay.

**TOOTHACHE** is often a sign of tooth decay and requires a visit to the dentist. It can also be a symptom of infection such as an abscess, gum disease, or sinus congestion.

**INFLAMED GUMS (GINGIVITIS)** is caused by a buildup of plaque on the teeth that occurs because of poor brushing. The gums bleed and become darker, swollen, and infected. Less often it may be due to a vitamin deficiency, a serious

blood disorder, a drug side effect, or a weakened immune system caused by stress or grief.

**MOUTH ULCERS** occur because of careless brushing, accidentally biting the side of the mouth, or eating very hot food. They may also result from stress, an allergy, or being run-down, and can be aggravated by acidic or spicy foods.

**COLD SORES** are caused by a viral infection, which can be triggered by being run-down, or exposure to hot sun or cold, windy weather.

**BAD BREATH (HALITOSIS)** can be due to tooth decay, inflamed gums, indigestion, tonsillitis, diabetes, fasting, or smoking.

## TOOTHACHE

| AILMENT | SYMPTOMS | CAUSE & ONSET |
|---|---|---|
| **TOOTHACHE WITH SEVERE SHOOTING PAIN** | ❏ Overreaction to the pain ❏ Thrashing around in agony ❏ Pain makes it difficult to sleep at night ❏ Inability to relax ❏ Mind is hyperactive. | • *Tooth decay* |
| **TOOTHACHE WITH UNBEARABLE PAIN** | ❏ Irritability ❏ Easily angered ❏ A desire to be left alone and not be troubled by anything. | • *Tooth decay* |
| **TOOTHACHE WITH THROBBING PAIN** | ❏ Gums and cheeks are swollen, painful, and hot to the touch ❏ Pain may shoot downward from the ear ❏ Pain gradually increases in severity to an excruciating level and then subsides. | • *Infection* |

## GINGIVITIS (INFLAMED GUMS)

| | | |
|---|---|---|
| **BLEEDING GUMS WITH BAD BREATH** | ❏ Gums are tender, spongy, and bleed easily ❏ Excessive saliva that dribbles onto the pillow during sleep ❏ Teeth may feel loose. | • *Poor oral hygiene* <br> • *Weakened immune system due to stress* <br> • *Gum disease* |
| **SWOLLEN, BLEEDING GUMS WITH ULCERS** | ❏ A taste of pus in the mouth ❏ Teeth are very sensitive to heat and cold ❏ Possible mouth ulcers and cold sores ❏ A desire to be left alone. | • *Weakened immune system due to emotional stress or grief* |

**FEAR OF DENTISTS** and dental treatment is very common. Homeopathy can help steady the nerves and make waiting more bearable.

**DISCOMFORT AFTER DENTAL TREATMENT** is usually caused by injury or bruising around the tooth. Pain may occur after an anesthestic has worn off. If it persists there may be an infection.

## PRECAUTIONS

**Toothache** If there is fever and swelling of the gums or face, or a tooth feels loose, see a dentist within 12 hours. If a tooth is sensitive to food and drink that is hot, cold, or sweet, or if there is pain on biting, see a dentist within 48 hours.

**Dental treatment** If pain persists after an anesthetic has worn off, see a dentist.

## SELF-HELP TREATMENTS

**Toothache** *Rub oil of cloves on the affected tooth and surrounding gums, except when taking a homeopathic remedy, which may be antidoted by the oil.*

**Inflamed gums** *Use calendula and hypericum solution as a mouthwash (see p. 227).*

**Mouth ulcers** *Avoid spicy, sweet, and acidic foods (see p. 229). Rinse the mouth with warm salt solution several times a day. Take vitamin B complex (see p. 226).*

**Cold sores** *Take bioflavonoids, lysine, vitamin C, and zinc (see pp. 224–6). Avoid foods that contain arginine (see p. 229).*

**Bad breath** *Stop smoking. Avoid spicy foods and alcohol.*

| YOU FEEL BETTER | YOU FEEL WORSE | REMEDY & DOSAGE | |
|---|---|---|---|
| ◆ From ice-cold water in mouth | ◆ With heat<br>◆ From eating hot food | **Coffea – see p. 125**<br>*Take 6c every 5 minutes for up to 10 doses.* | 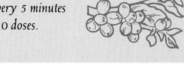 |
| ◆ From sympathy | ◆ At night<br>◆ If angry<br>◆ From warm food and drinks<br>◆ From cold air | **Chamomilla – see pp. 134–5**<br>*Take 6c every 5 minutes for up to 10 doses.* | 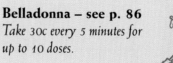 |
| ◆ From food, but eating is painful | ◆ If touched<br>◆ From eating<br>◆ At night<br>◆ From fresh air | **Belladonna – see p. 86**<br>*Take 30c every 5 minutes for up to 10 doses.* | 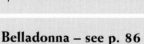 |
| ◆ With rest<br>◆ If warmly dressed | ◆ From extremes of temperature<br>◆ From sweating at night | **Merc. sol. – see pp. 62–3**<br>*Take 6c every 4 hours for up to 3 days.* |  |
| ◆ From fresh air<br>◆ From fasting | ◆ From mental and physical exertion<br>◆ From warmth and hot sun<br>◆ With noise or jarring | **Natrum mur. – see pp. 64–5**<br>*Take 6c every 4 hours for up to 3 days.* | 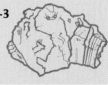 |

# MOUTH ULCERS

| AILMENT | SYMPTOMS | CAUSE & ONSET |
|---|---|---|
| BURNING MOUTH ULCERS | ❏ Mouth feels dry ❏ Smarting pain ❏ Restlessness and anxiety. | • *Stress and worry*<br>• *Being run-down* |

# COLD SORES

| AILMENT | SYMPTOMS | CAUSE & ONSET |
|---|---|---|
| COLD SORES ON THE LIPS AND AROUND THE MOUTH | ❏ Mouth feels very dry ❏ Lips are swollen and burning with pearllike blisters on the cold sores ❏ Deep, painful crack in the middle of the lower lip ❏ Mental or physical exertion aggravates the discomfort ❏ Depression ❏ A desire to be left alone. | • *Infection*<br>• *Emotional stress*<br>• *Grief* |

# BAD BREATH (HALITOSIS)

| AILMENT | SYMPTOMS | CAUSE & ONSET |
|---|---|---|
| BAD BREATH ASSOCIATED WITH TOOTH DECAY AND INFLAMED GUMS | ❏ Breath and sweat smell offensive ❏ Excessive saliva that dribbles onto the pillow during sleep ❏ Tongue is yellow and thickly coated. | • *Tooth decay*<br>• *Tonsillitis*<br>• *Sinus congestion*<br>• *Inflamed gums* |

# FEAR OF DENTISTS

| AILMENT | SYMPTOMS | CAUSE & ONSET |
|---|---|---|
| ACUTE PANIC | ❏ Intense feelings of anxiety and panic that may be severe enough to fear death as a result of impending dental treatment. | • *Sudden onset of fear* |
| FEAR WITH TREMBLING | ❏ Extreme apprehension that causes the whole body to tremble ❏ Legs feel wobbly and weak, as if they will not support the body. | • *Gradual onset of fear* |

# DISCOMFORT AFTER DENTAL TREATMENT

| AILMENT | SYMPTOMS | CAUSE & ONSET |
|---|---|---|
| IMMEDIATE DISCOMFORT | ❏ Discomfort immediately after any type of dental treatment, especially when there has been a lot of trauma and bruising. | • *Bruising or blood loss during dental treatment* |
| PERSISTENT PAIN | ❏ Pain continues after initial discomfort or returns once the anesthetic has worn off. | • *Bruising of a nerve caused by dental treatment* |

| YOU FEEL BETTER | YOU FEEL WORSE | REMEDY & DOSAGE |
|---|---|---|
| ◆ From a warm mouthwash<br>◆ From warm compresses applied to the face | ◆ From cold foods and drinks<br>◆ In cold, dry, windy weather<br>◆ Between midnight and 2 a.m. | **Arsen. alb. – see pp. 52–3**<br>*Take 6c 4 times a day for up to 5 days.*  |
| ◆ From fresh air<br>◆ From fasting | ◆ Around 10 a.m.<br>◆ In cold, stormy weather<br>◆ In sea air, hot sun, and a draft<br>◆ With warmth<br>◆ Near music or noise<br>◆ From jarring or talking | **Natrum mur. – see pp. 64–5**<br>*Take 6c 4 times a day for up to 5 days.*  |
| ◆ With rest<br>◆ From dressing warmly | ◆ From cold and extremes of temperature<br>◆ From sweating at night | **Merc. sol. – see pp. 62–3**<br>*Take 6c 3 times a day for up to 7 days.* 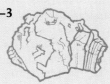 |
| ◆ From fresh air | • Thinking about visiting the dentist<br>• With warmth | **Aconite – see p. 82**<br>*Take 30c every hour as necessary.*  |
| ◆ From fresh air<br>◆ After urinating<br>◆ From exercise<br>◆ From drinking alcohol<br>◆ Bending forward | ◆ The more you think about visiting the dentist<br>◆ With heat<br>◆ Early in the morning | **Gelsemium – see p. 99**<br>*Take 30c every hour as necessary.* 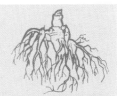 |
| ◆ With movement<br>◆ Lying down with the head lower than the feet | ◆ With heat<br>◆ From pressure applied to the affected part | **Arnica – see p. 85**<br>*Take 30c every hour for up to 10 doses.*  |
| ◆ Tilting the head back | ◆ In cold or damp weather<br>◆ In warm, stuffy rooms<br>◆ From touch | **Hypericum – see p. 102**<br>*Take 6c every 30 minutes for up to 10 doses and then 4 times a day for up to 5 days.*  |

# EAR, EYE & NOSE AILMENTS

The ears, eyes, and nose are continually assaulted by dust particles, spores, chemicals, viruses, bacteria, smoke, and pollution, all of which can cause problems. Drafts, extremes of temperature, getting the head wet, emotional and physical stress, and fatigue all aggravate complaints in these organs by weakening the immune system's ability to fight infection.

**EARACHE** can be due to a buildup of wax or an infection in the outer, middle, or inner ear, for example, after a cold. Exposure to temperature extremes may make it more difficult for the body's own healing powers to fight infection.

**EYESTRAIN** can be caused by overwork or working in poor light. Stress, especially after an emotional upset or resulting from grief, can weaken the eye muscles and cause strain.

**CONJUNCTIVITIS**, or swelling of the eyelid lining, is caused by an infection or allergy.

**STIES** are small, pus-filled boils that form at the base of the eyelashes. They are caused primarily by infection and can be aggravated by fatigue.

**HAY FEVER**, or allergic rhinitis is a seasonal allergic reaction to air-borne irritants – usually grass, tree, or flower pollens. If it continues throughout the year, it is most often due to house dust or animal fur.

**PHLEGM** is a discharge of runny or sticky mucus, which may block the nose, causing pain. It can be caused by an infection or allergy. Pollution irritates the mucous membranes causing increased mucus in an attempt to lubricate the membranes and remove the irritation; vigorous

## EARACHE

| AILMENT | SYMPTOMS | CAUSE & ONSET |
|---|---|---|
| EARACHE WITH SHARP PAIN | ❑ Acute pain ❑ Affected ear is very sensitive to touch ❑ Irritability. | • *Exposure to cold air and drafts* |
| THROBBING EARACHE WITH REDNESS | ❑ Affected ear is bright red ❑ Throbbing pain ❑ High fever, and dry mouth and throat are possible ❑ Eyes may be wide and staring. | • *Infection* <br> • *Head getting chilled, such as after having the hair washed* |

## EYESTRAIN

| AILMENT | SYMPTOMS | CAUSE & ONSET |
|---|---|---|
| EYES ACHE ON MOVEMENT | ❑ Dull, aching pain in the eyes on looking up, down, or sideways ❑ A dislike of sympathy and consolation. | • *Too much studying or reading* <br> • *Working in poor light* |
| BURNING EYES | ❑ Eyes burn and feel strained after prolonged studying or reading ❑ Eyes are red and feel hot ❑ Possible headache. | • *Too much studying or reading* <br> • *Working in poor light* |

exercise makes the mucous membranes produce more mucus.

**SINUS CONGESTION (SINUSITIS)** occurs if the sinuses (the air-filled cavities in the bones around the nose) become irritated or inflamed. They may fill up with fluid, which creates pressure and causes pain. This may be caused by pollution, tobacco smoke, or a viral infection.

### PRECAUTIONS

**Earache** All earaches, especially in children, should be referred promptly to a doctor.

**Conjunctivitis** If there is no improvement within 24 hours, see a doctor.

**Sties** If there is no improvement within 7 days, see a doctor.

**Sinus congestion** If pains are very severe, see a doctor within 12 hours.

### SELF-HELP TREATMENTS

**Conjunctivitis** *Bathe the eyes with an eyewash made from euphrasia tincture (see p. 227). Rest the eyes.*

**Sties** *Avoid touching or rubbing the eyes, especially with dirty hands. Do not squeeze sties. Rest the eyes.*

**Hay fever or allergic rhinitis** *Eat lots of fresh, raw fruits and vegetables. Take magnesium, vitamin C, and combination H tissue salts (see pp. 225–7).*

**Phlegm** *Take iron, vitamins B complex and C, zinc, and combination Q tissue salts (see pp. 225–7). Do not eat any dairy products for two weeks and note any changes. Drink plenty of fluids.*

**Sinus congestion** *Humidify all rooms and try a steam inhalation. Blow the nose very gently, one nostril at a time. Take iron, vitamins B complex and C, zinc, and combination Q tissue salts (see pp. 225–7), and drink plenty of fluids. Stop smoking and avoid decongestants.*

| YOU FEEL BETTER | YOU FEEL WORSE | REMEDY & DOSAGE |
|---|---|---|
| ◆ With warmth<br>◆ From warm compresses applied to the forehead<br>◆ From wrapping the head warmly | ◆ In cold air and in a draft<br>◆ From getting cold on undressing<br>◆ From touching the affected ear<br>◆ Lying on the affected side | **Hepar sulf. – see p. 101** *Provided the pain is not associated with fever or discharge, take 6c every 30 minutes until you see a doctor.*  |
| ◆ Standing or sitting upright<br>◆ From cold compresses applied to the forehead | ◆ From jarring, motion, noise, light, and pressure<br>◆ Lying on the right side<br>◆ At night | **Belladonna – see p. 86** *Take 30c every 30 minutes until you see a doctor.* |
| ◆ From fresh air<br>◆ From fasting<br>◆ From cold compresses applied to the affected eye | ◆ In cold, stormy weather, and by the sea<br>◆ From exertion<br>◆ In a draft and hot sun<br>◆ From emotional stress or grief | **Natrum mur. – see pp. 64–5** *Take 6c 4 times a day for up to 7 days.* |
| ◆ With movement | ◆ In cold, damp weather<br>◆ From rest or lying down<br>◆ From drinking alcohol | **Ruta grav. – see p. 109** *Take 6c 4 times a day for up to 7 days.*  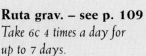 |

## CONJUNCTIVITIS (PINK EYE)

| AILMENT | SYMPTOMS | CAUSE & ONSET |
|---|---|---|
| SWOLLEN EYELIDS WITH A BURNING DISCHARGE | ❑ Eyes water continuously, which irritates the skin under the eyes ❑ Eyelids are swollen and burning with a need to blink frequently ❑ Little blisters may form inside the eyelid ❑ Nasal discharge is bland. | • *Allergy*<br>• *Infection* |

## STIES

| AILMENT | SYMPTOMS | CAUSE & ONSET |
|---|---|---|
| SWOLLEN EYES WITH ITCHY EYELIDS | ❑ Eyes are red and inflamed with itchy eyelids ❑ Small boil on the eyelid develops a head of pus ❑ Depression and self-pity may accompany the physical symptoms. | • *Infection* |
| SWOLLEN, RED, PAINFUL EYES | ❑ Starts as a small boil and then develops a head of pus. | • *Infection*<br>• *Curiously, the sties may occur when feeling deeply resentful of, and angry with, a loved one* |

## HAY FEVER (OR ALLERGIC RHINITIS)

| AILMENT | SYMPTOMS | CAUSE & ONSET |
|---|---|---|
| HAY FEVER WITH A BURNING NASAL DISCHARGE | ❑ Streaming, burning nasal discharge that tends to start in the left nostril and moves to the right, making the upper lip sore ❑ Pain in the forehead ❑ Larynx feels as if there are hooks sticking into it ❑ Eyes stream with a bland discharge. | • *Allergy* |
| HAY FEVER WITH A CONSTANT DESIRE TO SNEEZE | ❑ Thick, honey-colored nasal discharge comes on after three or four days of continuous, violent sneezing, which brings no relief ❑ Nostrils are sore, red, and painful ❑ Throat burns and there is an irritating cough ❑ Anxiety and worry. | • *Allergy* |
| HAY FEVER IN WHICH THE EYES ARE MAINLY AFFECTED | ❑ Eyes are swollen and sensitive to bright light ❑ Thick burning discharge irritates the skin under the eyes ❑ Discharge from the nose is bland ❑ Mucus drips down the back of the throat. | • *Allergy* |
| HAY FEVER WITH A SORE THROAT | ❑ A sore throat that often starts on the left-hand side ❑ Swallowing is very painful ❑ Throat is dry and it feels as if there is a lump in it that makes it necessary to swallow constantly ❑ Eyelids are red and swollen ❑ Eyes water and there is violent sneezing ❑ The head aches as if shrinking in size. | • *Allergy* |

| YOU FEEL BETTER | YOU FEEL WORSE | REMEDY & DOSAGE |
|---|---|---|
| ♦ From closing the eyes<br>♦ From drinking coffee | ♦ In the evening<br>♦ From being indoors<br>♦ With warmth and light<br>♦ In warm, windy weather | **Euphrasia – see p. 97**<br>*Take 6c every hour for up to 10 doses.*  |
| ♦ With heat | ♦ No specific factors | **Pulsatilla – see pp. 68–9**<br>*Take 6c every hour for up to 10 doses.*  |
| ♦ With heat | ♦ No specific factors | **Staphysagria – see p. 127**<br>*Take 6c every hour for up to 10 doses.*  |
| ♦ In cool rooms<br>♦ From fresh air | ♦ In warm rooms<br>♦ In cold or damp weather<br>♦ From warm foods and drinks | **Allium – see p. 83**<br>*Take 6c as required for up to 10 doses.* 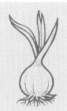 |
| ♦ No specific factors | ♦ From sneezing<br>♦ With warmth | **Arsen. iod. – see p. 117**<br>*Take 6c as required for up to 10 doses.* 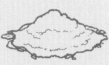 |
| ♦ Lying down in a darkened room<br>♦ From drinking coffee | ♦ With warmth<br>♦ In warm, windy weather<br>♦ In bright light<br>♦ From being indoors<br>♦ In the evening | **Euphrasia – see p. 97**<br>*Take 6c as required for up to 10 doses.*  |
| ♦ With warmth<br>♦ From eating<br>♦ From warm drinks<br>♦ If warmly dressed | ♦ From cold<br>♦ From cold drinks | **Sabadilla – see p. 143**<br>*Take 6c as required for up to 10 doses.*  |

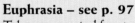

# PHLEGM

| AILMENT | SYMPTOMS | CAUSE & ONSET |
| --- | --- | --- |
| THICK WHITE MUCUS | ❑ Mucus that occurs in the second stage of a cold, after the inflammation has gone down ❑ Mucus is discharged through the nose or down the back of the throat. | • *Infection*<br>• *Allergy* |
| MUCUS LIKE THE WHITE OF A RAW EGG | ❑ Excessive, fluid, transparent mucus that may be so profuse that it is necessary to put a handkerchief under the nose ❑ Loss of smell and taste. | • *Infection*<br>• *Allergy* |
| PHLEGM WITH A CONSTANTLY RUNNY NOSE | ❑ Nose runs constantly with a need to blow it all the time ❑ Nasal discharge is yellow or green, and thin and burning ❑ Thick mucus drips down the back of the throat ❑ Small ulcers on the septum (the bone that separates the nostrils) are possible. | • *Infection* |
| PHLEGM WITH EXTREME SENSITIVITY TO STRONG SMELLS | ❑ Crusts and cracks inside the nose make it painful to blow ❑ Possible nosebleeds ❑ An acute sense of smell may make even the scent of flowers unbearable ❑ Eczema may accompany the symptoms ❑ The face feels as if it is covered by a cobweb. | • *Vigorous physical exercise*<br>• *Pollution* |

# SINUS CONGESTION (SINUSITIS)

| | | |
| --- | --- | --- |
| SINUS CONGESTION WITH STRINGY MUCUS | ❑ Stringy, stretchy mucus that is greenish yellow ❑ A feeling of fullness and blockage on either side of the nose ❑ Mucus drips down the back of the throat ❑ Violent sneezing ❑ Loss of smell. | • *Infection* |
| SINUS CONGESTION ACCOMPANIED BY TEARFULNESS | ❑ Pain above the eyes or in the right cheekbone with nerve pains in the right side of the face ❑ Yellow mucus ❑ Nose is stuffed up ❑ A tearful and self-pitying attitude. | • *Infection* |
| SINUS CONGESTION WITH FACIAL TENDERNESS | ❑ Facial bones are very tender, even to the slightest touch ❑ Excessive yellow mucus, with sneezing ❑ Irritability ❑ Subject to chills. | • *Infection*<br>• *Exposure to cold, dry, windy weather* |

| YOU FEEL BETTER | YOU FEEL WORSE | REMEDY & DOSAGE |
|---|---|---|
| ◆ From cold drinks<br>◆ With massage | ◆ From fresh air<br>◆ From cold and drafts<br>◆ From eating fatty foods<br>◆ During menstruation | **Kali mur. – see p. 132**<br>*Take 6c 4 times a day for up to 14 days.* 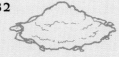 |
| ◆ With rest<br>◆ From fresh air<br>◆ From sweating<br>◆ From pressure<br>◆ From fasting | ◆ From sun and heat<br>◆ Before menstruation<br>◆ From damp air<br>◆ From exertion<br>◆ From sympathy<br>◆ From too much salt | **Natrum mur. – see pp. 64–5**<br>*Take 6c 4 times a day for up to 14 days.* 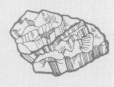 |
| ◆ No specific factors | ◆ No specific factors | **Hydrastis – see p. 130**<br>*Take 6c 4 times a day for up to 14 days.* 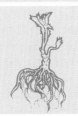 |
| ◆ With sleep | ◆ From eating cold or sweet foods, or seafood | **Graphites – see pp. 56–7**<br>*Take 6c 4 times a day for up to 14 days.* 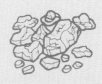 |
| ◆ From hot compresses applied to the sinuses | ◆ From drinking beer<br>◆ In the morning<br>◆ In hot weather<br>◆ From getting cold on undressing | **Kali bich. – see p. 103**<br>*Take 6c every 2 hours for up to 2 days.*  |
| ◆ From crying and sympathy<br>◆ Raising the hands above the head<br>◆ From gentle exercise<br>◆ From fresh air<br>◆ From cold drinks and cold compresses | ◆ In stuffy rooms<br>◆ From sun, heat, and extremes of temperature<br>◆ From rich, fatty foods<br>◆ Lying on the painful side<br>◆ In the evening and at night | **Pulsatilla – see pp. 68–9**<br>*Take 6c every 2 hours for up to 2 days.* |
| ◆ Sitting in warm surroundings<br>◆ From wrapping the head warmly | ◆ In a draft<br>◆ If touched<br>◆ From getting cold on undressing | **Hepar sulf. – see p. 101**<br>*Take 6c every 2 hours for up to 2 days.* 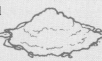 |

# COLDS, COUGHS & FLU

Colds, coughs, and flu occur when the immune system is weakened, making the body more susceptible to infections. Homeopathy emphasizes treating the underlying imbalance in the immune system rather than simply fighting the infection, although both approaches are sometimes needed.

Contributory causes to a weakened immune system include: too much food and alcohol or a poor diet; exposure to dry, cold winds; becoming chilled after getting the head wet; overwork and not enough rest; emotional stress, especially after a shock or scare; anxiety or embarrassment about financial matters or a future event. Infections may be brought on by anything that saps the vital energy (see pp. 18–19), and occasionally, very hot weather.

**COLDS** are caused by a viral infection and affect the respiratory system. Early symptoms include a mild sore throat, a watery nasal discharge, and sneezing. As the body fights the infection, the nasal discharge becomes thicker and possibly yellow. Colds are usually self-limiting, but a neglected cold can turn into a more serious complaint, such as a chest infection, or spread to the ears, sinuses, throat, or larynx.

**COUGHS** are dry or productive (bringing up mucus). They are usually caused by an irritation of the lining of the air passages, such as mucus dripping down the throat during a cold, smoking, or by pollen in hay fever sufferers. To get rid of the irritation, the lungs build up a pressure of air, which is suddenly expelled.

## COLDS

| AILMENT | SYMPTOMS | CAUSE & ONSET |
|---|---|---|
| COLD THAT COMES ON SLOWLY | ❏ Mouth feels hot ❏ Throat is red and swollen ❏ Mild fever is possible ❏ Nosebleeds are possible. | • *Infection* • *Overheating without perspiring* |
| COLD WITH IRRITABILITY | ❏ Tendency to be overly critical of others ❏ Subject to chills ❏ A runny nose during the day and a blocked nose at night ❏ Watery eyes ❏ Sneezing ❏ Headache ❏ Sore throat. | • *Infection* • *Emotional stress due to overwork, lack of sleep, or from something that has caused anger* |
| EARLY STAGES OF A COLD WITH SNEEZING | ❏ Cold starts with violent sneezing and a thin mucus discharge, like the white of a raw egg ❏ Nose may also be blocked and cold sores may develop ❏ A desire to be left alone ❏ A dislike of sympathy. | • *Infection* • *Emotional stress* |
| COLD WITH YELLOW MUCUS | ❏ Nose is blocked at night but runny during the day ❏ Mucus is bland and yellow ❏ Lack of thirst and a loss of smell ❏ Nosebleeds may occur ❏ Headache above the eyes may develop. | • *Infection* |

**FLU (INFLUENZA)** is caused by a viral infection. Symptoms include a fever, muscle aches and pains, a headache, a sore throat, and a cough. Children, the elderly, smokers, and diabetics are likely to be most seriously affected.

## PRECAUTIONS

**Colds** If a cold becomes complicated by pain in the throat, larynx, chest, sinuses, or ears, see also: Sore throats pp. 176–7; Tonsillitis and Laryngitis pp. 178–9; Coughs pp. 174–5; Sinus congestion pp. 170–1; Earache pp. 166–7.

**Cough** If it is accompanied by a high fever, and/or difficulty in breathing or severe chest pain, see a doctor. If there is no improvement within 1–2 days after a sudden onset of coughing from inhaling dust or fumes, see a doctor.

**Flu** If it is accompanied by a fever that does not clear within 4 days, see a doctor.

## SELF-HELP TREATMENTS

**Colds & flu** *Ensure that you get plenty of rest and drink lots of fluids, especially hot water mixed with fresh lemon juice and a little honey. Eat plenty of fresh fruit and vegetables. Take vitamins A and C, zinc, and combination Q tissue salts (see pp. 226–7). It is important to get some fresh air.*

**Coughs** *Humidify the air in all rooms, do not smoke, and avoid dusty or smoky areas. Exposure to cold, damp weather may aggravate symptoms. Get lots of rest and avoid strenuous physical exertion. Drink plenty of fluids, especially hot water with fresh lemon juice and a little honey. If you are coughing up a lot of phlegm, avoid dairy products and starchy foods such as bread and potatoes, which may increase the flow of mucus. Homeopathic cough mixtures and herbal cough mixtures are available over the counter. These are preferable to orthodox cough syrups, which may contain drugs that cause drowsiness.*

| YOU FEEL BETTER | YOU FEEL WORSE | REMEDY & DOSAGE |
|---|---|---|
| ◆ From cold compresses applied to the forehead<br>◆ From gentle exercise | ◆ From jarring and touch<br>◆ Lying on the right side<br>◆ From fresh air<br>◆ In the sun<br>◆ Between 4 a.m. and 6 a.m. | **Ferrum phos. – see p. 98**<br>*Take 6c every 2 hours for up to 4 doses.* 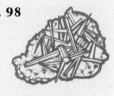 |
| ◆ With warmth<br>◆ With sleep<br>◆ From firm pressure<br>◆ From washing and compresses<br>◆ In the evening | ◆ In cold, dry, windy weather<br>◆ In public places<br>◆ Between 3 a.m. and 4 a.m.<br>◆ From overindulging in spicy foods and stimulants, such as coffee | **Nux vomica – see pp. 74–5**<br>*Take 6c every 2 hours for up to 4 doses.*  |
| ◆ From fresh air<br>◆ From fasting<br>◆ From applying cold compresses to the sinuses | ◆ Around 10 a.m.<br>◆ In cold, stormy weather<br>◆ From mental and physical exertion<br>◆ In a draft, sea air, or hot sun<br>◆ Near noise, talking, and music | **Natrum mur. – see pp. 64–5**<br>*Take 6c every 2 hours for up to 4 doses.* 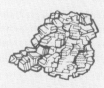 |
| ◆ Raising the hands above the head<br>◆ From exercise and fresh air<br>◆ From cold drinks and cold compresses<br>◆ From crying and sympathy | ◆ In the sun<br>◆ With heat<br>◆ From rich, fatty foods<br>◆ In the evening and at night | **Pulsatilla – see pp. 68–9**<br>*Take 6c every 2 hours for up to 4 doses.*  |

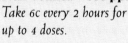

## COUGHS

| AILMENT | SYMPTOMS | CAUSE & ONSET |
|---|---|---|
| DRY, IRRITATING COUGH THAT COMES ON SUDDENLY | ❑ Dry, hollow-sounding, croaking cough ❑ Great thirst ❑ A rapid rise in temperature is common ❑ Feelings of extreme anxiety to the point of fearing death ❑ Especially sensitive to smoke. | • A cold or flu<br>• Fright<br>• Exposure to dry, cold wind or intensely hot weather<br>• Pollen |
| CHEST PAIN FROM COUGHING | ❑ Splitting headache, aggravated by the slightest cough ❑ Extreme thirst, usually for warm drinks, but at infrequent intervals ❑ Whole body feels dried out ❑ A fever may accompany the cough. | • A cold or flu<br>• Stress and worry, particularly about financial or business matters |
| COUGH WITH THICK, GREEN MUCUS | ❑ Thick, green, bitter-tasting mucus is coughed up, leaving a bad taste in the mouth ❑ Poor appetite ❑ Tongue is coated white ❑ A green, bland discharge from the nose may occur ❑ Little or no thirst. | • A cold or flu<br>• Chest infection<br>• Pollen |

## FLU (INFLUENZA)

| AILMENT | SYMPTOMS | CAUSE & ONSET |
|---|---|---|
| FLU WITH RESTLESSNESS | ❑ High fever that comes on abruptly ❑ Sore throat ❑ Feelings of great apprehension and fear often accompany the physical symptoms. | • Infection<br>• Exposure to dry, cold, windy or very hot weather<br>• Emotional shock or fright |
| FLU WITH A HIGH FEVER | ❑ High fever that comes on suddenly ❑ Face is flushed and bright red ❑ Sore throat ❑ Eyes are wide and staring ❑ Possible confusion and delirium. | • Infection<br>• Head getting cold, wet, or overheated |
| FLU WITH CHILLS AND WEAKNESS | ❑ Lack of thirst despite fever ❑ Sore throat ❑ Chills up and down the spine ❑ Splitting headache, which is better after urinating ❑ Fatigue ❑ Legs feel weak and shaky ❑ Strong bone pain ❑ Feeling apprehensive and stressed about a forthcoming event or task. | • Infection<br>• Worry about a forthcoming event, such as public speaking |
| FLU WITH A SEVERE, THROBBING HEADACHE | ❑ Violent headache that is made worse by coughing, or by moving the eyes slightly ❑ Dehydration with a need to drink lots of fluids at infrequent intervals ❑ Irritability ❑ A desire to be at home. | • Infection<br>• Stress and worry about financial problems |

| YOU FEEL BETTER | YOU FEEL WORSE | REMEDY & DOSAGE |
|---|---|---|
| ◆ From fresh air | ◆ In warm rooms<br>◆ Near tobacco smoke<br>◆ In the evening and at night | **Aconite – see p. 82**<br>*Take 30c every 4 hours<br>for up to 10 doses.* 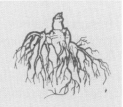 |
| ◆ In cool surroundings<br>◆ From firm, cool pressure<br>applied to the head<br>and chest | ◆ With movement<br>◆ In bright light<br>◆ Near noises, if touched<br>◆ In the morning and around<br>9 p.m. and 3 a.m. | **Bryonia – see p. 88**<br>*Take 30c every 4 hours<br>for up to 10 doses.* 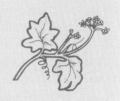 |
| ◆ From fresh air | ◆ In the evening<br>◆ In warm, stuffy rooms | **Pulsatilla – see pp. 68–9**<br>*Take 30c every 4 hours<br>for up to 10 doses.*  |
| ◆ From fresh air | ◆ In warm rooms<br>◆ Lying on the affected side<br>◆ In the evening or at night<br>◆ Near tobacco smoke<br>◆ Near music | **Aconite – see p. 82**<br>*Take 30c every 2 hours<br>for up to 10 doses.* 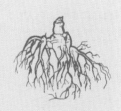 |
| ◆ Standing<br>◆ Sitting upright<br>◆ In warm rooms | ◆ With jarring, movement,<br>noise, and light<br>◆ In hot sun<br>◆ Lying down<br>◆ On the right side<br>◆ At night | **Belladonna – see p. 86**<br>*Take 30c every 2 hours<br>for up to 10 doses.*  |
| ◆ From fresh air<br>◆ With movement<br>◆ After urinating<br>◆ From drinking alcohol<br>◆ Bending forward | ◆ Early in the morning and<br>last thing at night<br>◆ In the sun or in fog<br>◆ Before a thunderstorm<br>◆ From humidity<br>◆ Near tobacco smoke | **Gelsemium – see p. 99**<br>*Take 6c every 2 hours<br>for up to 10 doses.* 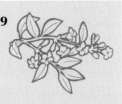 |
| ◆ In cool surroundings<br>◆ From firm pressure<br>applied to the head<br>◆ With sleep | ◆ With excitement, noise, touch,<br>movement, and bright light<br>◆ From eating<br>◆ Around 3 a.m. and 9 p.m.<br>◆ From coughing | **Bryonia – see p. 88**<br>*Take 30c every 2 hours<br>for up to 10 doses.* 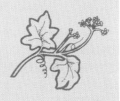 |

# THROAT COMPLAINTS

Throat complaints range from mild sore throats to more severe ailments such as tonsillitis and laryngitis. All these disorders make breathing and swallowing difficult to a greater or lesser extent. Throat infections may affect the whole throat or cause acute discomfort in specific areas. Characteristic symptoms include the following: a dry mouth and throat, inflammation of the throat and tonsils causing a constricted sensation with pain on swallowing, hoarseness, foul-tasting saliva, bad breath, fatigue, and feeling flushed, feverish, or irritable.

There are numerous types of infection but usually the offending microbes are viruses that cause colds, flu, and glandular fever. Some infections can be due to a bacterium, as in "strep throat," or a fungus, as in thrush. Heavy smoking and drinking, exposure to cold or damp winds, vocal exertion, food allergy, or a general vitamin deficiency can cause or exacerbate inflammation and infection. A throat complaint may also occur as a result of being generally run-down due to lack of sleep, overexertion, cooling down too quickly after sweating, becoming chilled after getting the head wet, and emotional or physical stress, such as a shock or scare. Recurrent sore throats indicate a weakened immune system, and constitutional treatment by a homeopath is recommended (see pp. 24–5).

**SORE THROAT** describes any inflammation or infection of the larynx, tonsils, adenoids, pharynx, and vocal cords.

**TONSILLITIS** is an inflammation due to infection of the tonsils, which are located in the back of the mouth at the top of the throat. Occasionally, the lymph glands may become enlarged and cause the neck or face to swell.

## SORE THROATS

| AILMENT | SYMPTOMS | CAUSE & ONSET |
|---|---|---|
| **ACUTE, PAINFUL SORE THROAT** | ❑ Sudden onset of the sore throat and its severity cause extreme anxiety, even to the point of fear of death ❑ Skin is dry and hot ❑ Great thirst ❑ Swollen tonsils ❑ Throat looks red and feels dry, rough, constricted, burning, and tingly ❑ A hoarse voice may accompany the sore throat. | • *Exposure to cold winds*<br>• *A severe fright* |
| **RAW, BURNING SORE THROAT** | ❑ Acute sore throat with thick saliva and a hoarse voice ❑ Cold sores possible around the mouth ❑ Possible hives (urticaria) ❑ Thirst for cold drinks ❑ May be associated with mucus dripping down the throat from the nose, lumbago, or an earache. | • *Exposure to cold, damp weather*<br>• *Cooling down rapidly after sweating* |
| **PAIN EXTENDS TO THE NECK AND EARS** | ❑ Bad taste in the mouth ❑ Swallowing hurts and drinking is difficult ❑ Alternately hot and cold due to a fever ❑ Heavy, exhausted, weak, and shaky, with dullness and drowsiness ❑ The head is heavy and feels as if there is a tight band around it. | • *Viral infection, especially in the summer* |
| **BACK OF THE THROAT IS BRIGHT RED AND SEVERELY SWOLLEN** | ❑ Burning and stinging pains ❑ Back of the throat is red, shiny, and swollen ❑ Depression and irritability. | • *Allergy* |

**LARYNGITIS**, which results in hoarseness or voice loss, is caused by an inflammation of the larynx due to an allergy or infection. It may also be caused by overuse of the voice, continued coughing to bring up phlegm, vomiting, heavy smoking or drinking, inhaling toxic fumes, or continually breathing through the mouth rather than the nose. If the larynx is a weak spot, then any scare or emotional shock may cause inflammation. Laryngitis is an occupational hazard of teachers, singers, and market traders.

## PRECAUTIONS

**Sore throats** If inflammation is accompanied by a high fever, see a doctor within 12 hours for children and within 48 hours for adults.

**Tonsillitis** If infection is accompanied by a high fever, see a doctor within 12 hours.

**Laryngitis** If there is no improvement within 7–10 days, or hoarseness or voice loss persist, see a doctor.

## SELF-HELP TREATMENTS

**Sore throats** *Take garlic, vitamin C, and zinc (see pp. 225–6). Gargle with calendula and hypericum solution (5 drops mother tincture of each in half a pint [300 ml] of boiled, cooled water every 4 hours). Drink plenty of fluids.*

**Tonsillitis** *Rest in bed for several days and drink plenty of fluids. Take iron, vitamins B complex and C, and zinc (see pp. 225–6).*

**Laryngitis** *Do not smoke or drink alcohol, and avoid hot, smoky rooms. Rest the voice and increase your fluid intake. Take iron, vitamins B complex and C, and zinc (see pp. 225–6). Gargle with calendula and hypericum solution (5 drops mother tincture of each in half a pint [300 ml] of boiled, cooled water every 4 hours). If you are a singer and your voice is persistently troublesome, it may be that your voice needs retraining. Seek professional help from a singing teacher. Recurrent laryngitis can also be due to poor posture; the Alexander technique, a special method of adjusting body posture, may be helpful.*

| YOU FEEL BETTER | YOU FEEL WORSE | REMEDY & DOSAGE |
|---|---|---|
| • From fresh air | • In warm rooms<br>• Near tobacco smoke<br>• Near music<br>• In the evening and at night | **Aconite – see p. 82** *Take 30c every 2 hours for up to 10 doses.* 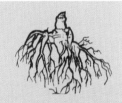 |
| • With movement<br>• With warmth | • At night<br>• In damp or cold weather<br>• With rest | **Dulcamara – see p. 145** *Take 6c every 2 hours for up to 10 doses.*  |
| • From fresh air<br>• From exercise<br>• From stimulants<br>• With local heat<br>• Bending forward | • Early in the morning and last thing at night<br>• In the sun, fog, and damp<br>• Before a thunderstorm<br>• From emotional stress or worry | **Gelsemium – see p. 99** *Take 6c every 2 hours for up to 10 doses.*  |
| • From fresh air<br>• From cold compresses applied to the throat<br>• From loosening the clothes | • With sleep<br>• From touch, pressure, and heat<br>• In stuffy rooms<br>• In the late afternoon | **Apis – see p. 84** *Take 30c every 2 hours for up to 10 doses.* 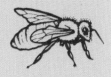 |

## TONSILLITIS

| AILMENT | SYMPTOMS | CAUSE & ONSET |
|---|---|---|
| **TONSILLITIS WITH BURNING PAIN THAT SHOOTS INTO THE HEAD** | ❑ Throat is very sore and tender ❑ Spasms of pain on moving ❑ Often the right tonsil is the most affected ❑ Neck is tender and stiff ❑ Face is red ❑ Pupils are dilated ❑ Tongue has a strawberrylike appearance ❑ High fever. | • *Infection* <br> • *Head getting chilled, for example after washing the hair* |
| **TONSILLITIS WITH STABBING PAIN IN THE THROAT** | ❑ Pain in the throat that feels as if a fish bone is stuck in it ❑ Bad breath may accompany hoarseness or voice loss ❑ Yellow pus may be coughed up ❑ Neck glands are often swollen ❑ Possible pain in the ear on swallowing ❑ Chills and shivering ❑ Emotional sensitivity and unreasonableness. | • *Infection* |
| **TONSILLITIS WITH BAD BREATH** | ❑ Throat is dark red, sore, and swollen ❑ Saliva burns on swallowing ❑ Tongue may feel swollen and appear yellow-coated with teeth imprints on it ❑ Possible tendency to dribble excess saliva during sleep ❑ Swallowing hurts. | • *Infection* |

## LARYNGITIS

| AILMENT | SYMPTOMS | CAUSE & ONSET |
|---|---|---|
| **LARYNGITIS WITH A HIGH FEVER** | ❑ Hoarseness and loss of voice ❑ Sudden onset of laryngitis causes anxiety, even to the point of fear of death ❑ Restlessness ❑ May be associated with an acute onset of croup in children. | • *Exposure to cold, dry, windy weather* <br> • *Emotional shock* |
| **LARYNGITIS WITH A DRY, TICKLY COUGH** | ❑ Throat feels dry and sore ❑ Talking is painful because of hoarseness or total loss of voice ❑ Thirst for ice-cold drinks, which are vomited up as soon as they become warm in the stomach ❑ A strong desire for company and sympathy. | • *Changes in temperature* |
| **DRY, RAW THROAT WITH VIOLENT COUGH** | ❑ Cough is due to mucus dripping down the back of the throat, which is so copious it makes speaking difficult ❑ Cough can be violent enough to cause accidental leakage of urine ❑ Often associated with depression and extreme sensitivity to the suffering of others ❑ Drinking cold water may stop a cough from developing ❑ Occasionally, the loss of voice with laryngitis may be quite painless. | • *Exposure to cold, dry, windy weather* <br> • *After grief or a scare* |
| **LOSS OF VOICE FROM TOO MUCH SINGING OR SHOUTING** | ❑ Tickly larynx ❑ Voice is weak, trembles, and tends to break ❑ Hoarseness. | • *Overuse of the voice from too much singing or shouting* |

| YOU FEEL BETTER | YOU FEEL WORSE | REMEDY & DOSAGE |
|---|---|---|
| ◆ Standing<br>◆ Sitting upright<br>◆ With warmth | ◆ With the slightest jar or movement<br>◆ From light or noise<br>◆ If the throat is touched<br>◆ At night | **Belladonna – see p. 86**<br>*Take 30c every 2 hours for up to 10 doses.*  |
| ◆ From eating<br>◆ With warmth<br>◆ From wrapping up the neck warmly | ◆ In cold air and a draft<br>◆ From getting cold on undressing<br>◆ If the throat is touched<br>◆ Lying on the affected side | **Hepar sulf. – see p. 101**<br>*Take 6c every 2 hours for up to 10 doses.* 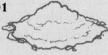 |
| ◆ With rest<br>◆ From dressing warmly | ◆ From extremes of temperature<br>◆ From sweating<br>◆ At night<br>◆ Lying on the right side | **Merc. sol. – see pp. 62–3**<br>*Take 6c every 2 hours for up to 10 doses.* 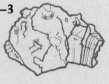 |
| ◆ From fresh air | ◆ In warm rooms<br>◆ Near tobacco smoke<br>◆ Near music<br>◆ In the evening and at night | **Aconite – see p. 82**<br>*Take 30c 4 times a day for up to 7 days.* 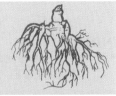 |
| ◆ With sleep<br>◆ With massage<br>◆ From fresh air<br>◆ From drinking | ◆ From talking and laughing<br>◆ From hot food and drinks<br>◆ Lying on the left or painful side<br>◆ Between sunset and midnight | **Phos. – see pp. 66–7**<br>*Take 6c 4 times a day for up to 7 days.*  |
| ◆ In warm, humid weather | ◆ From sweet foods<br>◆ From coffee | **Causticum – see p. 123**<br>*Take 6c 4 times a day for up to 7 days.*  |
| ◆ From fresh air | ◆ If touched<br>◆ Around noon | **Argent. nit. – see pp. 50–1**<br>*Take 6c 4 times a day for up to 6 days.* 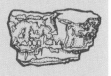 |

# DIGESTIVE DISORDERS

Digestion is a complex process involving not only the intestines but also the liver, gallbladder, and pancreas. Irregular eating habits, a poor diet, stress, anxiety, and a sedentary lifestyle all aggravate digestive complaints, which are extremely common. In order to help the digestive system perform properly, it is vital to eat a good variety of fresh, unprocessed, low-fat, high-fiber foods. Eat slowly in calm, relaxed surroundings and get regular exercise to help speed up digestion.

**INDIGESTION** is a blanket term that describes various symptoms, such as heartburn, stomachache, nausea, and excessive flatulence and burping, which are brought on by eating. Very rich, fatty, or spicy foods, eating too much too quickly, and swallowing air also cause indigestion. Smokers and those who are constipated or overweight are more susceptible to indigestion, which is also common in pregnancy, when discomfort after eating increases as the uterus enlarges and presses against the stomach. Nervous indigestion is caused by stress.

**NAUSEA & VOMITING** may be due to an infection such as stomach flu, a migraine, stress, overindulgence in food or alcohol, a hiatus hernia, contaminated food or water, gallbladder or liver disorders, hormone changes associated with pregnancy and menstruation, or problems with the inner ear and associated dizziness.

**STOMACH FLU (GASTROENTERITIS)** is an inflammation of the digestive tract that may lead to sudden, violent upsets. It is usually due to a viral infection caused by contaminated food or water. It may also be due to an allergic reaction, sudden changes in the diet, anger, or indignation, or it may be a drug side effect.

**DIARRHEA** is a symptom of stomach flu or irritable bowel syndrome, which is a combination of intermittent cramplike pains in the abdomen and irregular bowel habits. Diarrhea can also be a symptom of more serious forms of bowel disease, and it may be a side effect of certain drugs. It is also associated with food allergy, food intolerance, stress, and anxiety.

## INDIGESTION

| AILMENT | SYMPTOMS | CAUSE & ONSET |
|---|---|---|
| **INDIGESTION WITH EXCESSIVE FLATULENCE** | ❑ Digestion seems slower than usual and eating even plain food causes pain ❑ Possible burning sensation in the stomach that radiates through to the back ❑ Headache ❑ A craving for salty, acidic, or sweet foods, and coffee ❑ An aversion to meat and milk. | • *Overeating* <br> • *Eating rich, fatty foods* <br> • *Eating too late in the evening* |
| **INDIGESTION WITH PAINFUL RETCHING** | ❑ Overwrought from stress and lack of sleep ❑ Irritability ❑ Critical of others ❑ Heartburn 30 minutes after eating, with a putrid taste in the mouth ❑ A craving for alcohol and fatty, sour, or spicy foods, even though they upset the digestion. | • *Mental and physical exhaustion due to stress* |
| **INDIGESTION WITH NAUSEA AND VOMITING** | ❑ Indigestion begins two hours after eating, especially in the evening ❑ Sense of pressure under the breastbone ❑ Pounding heart ❑ Bad taste in the mouth ❑ There may be a headache around the eyes ❑ Depression, tearfulness, and self-pitying attitude. | • *Eating rich, fatty foods* <br> • *Emotional stress* <br> • *Hormonal changes associated with menstruation or pregnancy* |

**BLOATING & FLATULENCE** can be caused by constipation, premenstrual tension, swallowing air, food intolerance, or nervous apprehension.

**CONSTIPATION** is most often caused by a diet that is too low in fiber, although emotional tension, poor bowel habits, sluggish bowels, and a sedentary lifestyle may also contribute.

**HEMORRHOIDS (PILES)** are inflamed veins in the lining of the anus usually due to constipation, pregnancy, childbirth, persistent coughing, standing for long periods, overuse of laxatives, or sitting on cold, hard surfaces for a long time.

## PRECAUTIONS

If there is severe abdominal pain with or without vomiting, vomited blood, or an associated fever, call an ambulance.

If vomiting or diarrhea persist for more than 48 hours, there is blood in the stools or an associated fever, see a doctor within 2 hours.

If there is bleeding from the anus, see a doctor within 12 hours. For persistent constipation or a prolonged change in bowel habits, see a doctor.

## SELF-HELP TREATMENTS

**Indigestion** *Relax for 15 minutes before eating and avoid eating late at night. Reduce coffee, tea, and alcohol consumption, and stop smoking. If there is associated flatulence, avoid the foods listed on p. 229.*

**Nausea & vomiting** *Drink small amounts of fluids frequently. Avoid solid foods for a few days. Stop smoking.*

**Stomach flu** *Rest and drink plenty of fluids. Drink only fluids until the stomach settles down.*

**Diarrhea** *Drink plenty of boiled, cooled water mixed with a little honey or water in which rice or barley has been cooked. If you have recently been on antibiotics, take acidophilus, folic acid, and vitamin B complex (see pp. 224–6). Avoid vitamin D supplements.*

**Bloating & flatulence** *For foods to avoid, see p. 229.*

**Constipation** *Take magnesium and vitamin C (see pp. 225–6) and eat plenty of raw vegetables.*

**Hemorrhoids** *Try the liver diet (see p. 229) and apply peony ointment or use hamamelis suppositories (see p. 227).*

| YOU FEEL BETTER | YOU FEEL WORSE | REMEDY & DOSAGE |
|---|---|---|
| • From cold, fresh air<br>• After burping | • In warm, wet weather<br>• In the evening<br>• Lying down | **Carbo veg. – see p. 90** *Take 30c every 10–15 minutes for up to 7 doses.* 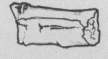 |
| • With warmth and sleep<br>• From firm pressure applied to the stomach<br>• In the evening<br>• When left alone | • In cold, windy weather<br>• Around noise<br>• If touched<br>• From fatty, sour, or spicy foods and alcohol | **Nux vomica – see pp. 74–5** *Take 6c every 10–15 minutes for up to 7 doses.*  |
| • From crying<br>• Raising the hands above the head<br>• From gentle exercise<br>• From fresh air<br>• From cold drinks | • In hot, stuffy rooms<br>• In the evening<br>• At night | **Pulsatilla – see pp. 68–9** *Take 6c every 10–15 minutes for up to 7 doses.* 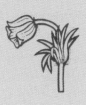 |

# NAUSEA & VOMITING

| AILMENT | SYMPTOMS | CAUSE & ONSET |
|---------|----------|---------------|
| CONSTANT NAUSEA | ❑ Nausea that is constant and not relieved by vomiting ❑ Headache, perspiration, and diarrhea may accompany the headache ❑ Spasmodic pain in the abdomen ❑ Copious saliva ❑ Vomiting of green mucus may occur. | • *Stress due to embarrassment* |
| VOMITING WITH GREAT THIRST | ❑ Great thirst for ice-cold drinks, which are vomited once they warm up in the stomach ❑ Burning pain in the pit of the stomach with retching and vomiting ❑ Associated anxiety and fearfulness. | • *Nervous tension*<br>• *Liver disorders* |
| NAUSEA AND VOMITING WITH TEARFULNESS | ❑ Tearfulness, depression, and a desire for sympathy ❑ Nausea may be associated with mucus dripping down the back of the throat. | • *Emotional stress*<br>• *Hormonal changes associated with pregnancy or menstruation*<br>• *Gallbladder disease*<br>• *Migraine* |

# STOMACH FLU (GASTROENTERITIS)

| AILMENT | SYMPTOMS | CAUSE & ONSET |
|---------|----------|---------------|
| VOMITING AND DIARRHEA AT THE SAME TIME | ❑ Chilliness, restlessness, and anxiety ❑ Thirst for small, frequent sips of water ❑ Preference for cold drinks, but these are often vomited ❑ Burning pain in the abdomen with diarrhea that causes soreness in the anus and stinging pain in the rectum. | • *Viral infection from eating or drinking contaminated food and water, especially when traveling*<br>• *Eating too much ripe fruit or ice-cold food*<br>• *Drinking too much alcohol* |
| STOMACH FLU WITH SEVERE CRAMPING PAINS | ❑ Colicky pains that are better when bending double ❑ Possible diarrhea ❑ Pain is relieved by passing gas ❑ Irritability and extreme sensitivity. | • *Viral infection*<br>• *Anger and indignation* |
| STOMACH FLU WITH DIFFERENT TYPES OF STOOLS | ❑ Rumbling, gurgly stomach ❑ A feeling of pressure under the breastbone after meals ❑ No two stools are alike in texture or color ❑ Possible vomiting ❑ Depression and self-pitying attitude. | • *Viral infection*<br>• *Too much rich, fatty food*<br>• *Stress* |

# DIARRHEA

| AILMENT | SYMPTOMS | CAUSE & ONSET |
|---------|----------|---------------|
| DIARRHEA FROM FOOD INTOLERANCE | ❑ Uncertainty as to whether gas or a stool will be passed ❑ Tip of the tongue appears red ❑ Urination is painful ❑ Stools are yellowish green, and there is a lot of flatulence. | • *Food intolerance*<br>• *An angry outburst*<br>• *Catching a summer chill* |

| YOU FEEL BETTER | YOU FEEL WORSE | REMEDY & DOSAGE |
|---|---|---|
| ◆ No specific factors | ◆ In a car, or looking at moving objects<br>◆ With movement<br>◆ Lying down | **Ipecac. – see p. 91**<br>*If severe, take 6c every 15 minutes for up to 10 doses. If less severe, take 6c every hour for up to 10 doses.*  |
| ◆ With sleep<br>◆ With massage and relaxation<br>◆ Lying on the right side | ◆ From physical or mental exertion<br>◆ From hot meals and drinks<br>◆ Between sunset and midnight<br>◆ Putting the hands in cold water | **Phos. – see pp. 66–7**<br>*If severe, take 6c every 15 minutes for up to 10 doses. If less severe, take 6c every hour for up to 10 doses.*  |
| ◆ From crying and sympathy<br>◆ From gentle exercise<br>◆ From fresh air<br>◆ From cold drinks<br>◆ Raising the hands above the head | ◆ From rich, fatty foods<br>◆ In warm, stuffy rooms<br>◆ In the sun<br>◆ In the evening and at night | **Pulsatilla – see pp. 68–9**<br>*If severe, take 6c every 15 minutes for up to 10 doses. If less severe, take 6c every hour for up to 10 doses.*  |
| ◆ With warmth<br>◆ From hot drinks | ◆ From the sight or smell of food<br>◆ Between midnight and 2 a.m.<br>◆ From cold drinks | **Arsen. alb. – see pp. 52–3**<br>*Take 6c every hour for up to 10 doses.*  |
| ◆ Lying sideways with the knees tucked up under the chin<br>◆ With warmth and sleep<br>◆ From coffee | ◆ From eating or drinking<br>◆ In cold, damp weather<br>◆ Around 4 p.m. | **Colocynthis – see p. 94**<br>*Take 6c every hour for up to 10 doses.*  |
| ◆ From crying and sympathy<br>◆ From fresh air<br>◆ From cold drinks | ◆ In hot, stuffy rooms<br>◆ In the evening and at night<br>◆ From rich, fatty foods | **Pulsatilla – see pp. 68–9**<br>*Take 6c every hour for up to 10 doses.*  |
| ◆ From cold<br>◆ From fresh air<br>◆ From fasting | ◆ In hot weather<br>◆ From eating or drinking<br>◆ Early in the morning | **Aloe – see p. 115**<br>*Take 6c every hour for up to 10 doses.*  |

**DIARRHEA** *continued*

## DIARRHEA *continued*

| AILMENT | SYMPTOMS | CAUSE & ONSET |
|---|---|---|
| **DIARRHEA FROM NERVOUS EXCITEMENT** | ❑ Diarrhea accompanied by severe flatulence ❑ Stools may be greenish ❑ Craving for salty, sweet, and cold foods ❑ Flatulence is not relieved by burping. | • *Nervous anxiety or fear, such as before an exam or performance* |
| **DIARRHEA WITH IRRITATION OF SKIN AROUND THE ANUS** | ❑ Urgent need to pass a stool first thing in the morning, characteristically causing early rising from bed at around 5 a.m. ❑ Possible hemorrhoids. | • *Eating foods that upset the stomach, especially fatty, salty, sweet, or spicy foods* |

## BLOATING & FLATULENCE

| AILMENT | SYMPTOMS | CAUSE & ONSET |
|---|---|---|
| **BLOATING AFTER EATING ONLY SMALL AMOUNTS OF FOOD** | ❑ Constipation makes it impossible to pass stools without straining ❑ Discomfort is often felt on the right-hand side of the abdomen and is not relieved by passing gas. | • *Nervous apprehension* |
| **BLOATING AND FLATULENCE RELIEVED BY BURPING** | ❑ Burning sensation in the stomach with much flatulence no matter what kind of food is eaten ❑ A craving for salty, acidic, and sweet foods, and coffee ❑ An aversion to meat and milk. | • *Overeating* • *Eating rich, fatty foods* • *Eating too late in the evening* |

## CONSTIPATION

| AILMENT | SYMPTOMS | CAUSE & ONSET |
|---|---|---|
| **CONSTIPATION WITH SOFT STOOLS THAT ARE DIFFICULT TO PASS** | ❑ Lack of desire to move the bowels until the rectum is completely full ❑ Stools are soft and clayey or covered with mucus ❑ Sensation as if stools are trapped in the top left-hand side of the abdomen ❑ An associated sense of confusion and apprehension ❑ A craving for fruits, vegetables, and indigestible foods ❑ An aversion to meat and beer. | • *Sluggish bowels, often due to a low-fiber diet* |
| **CONSTIPATION WITH STRONG URGE TO PASS STOOLS** | ❑ Despite great urgency to pass stools, few or none are passed ❑ Associated feelings of anger and irritability ❑ Extreme sensitivity to noise, touch, and pressure. | • *Cramping and spasm in the anus* • *Chronic use of laxatives* • *Sedentary lifestyle* |

## HEMORRHOIDS (PILES)

| AILMENT | SYMPTOMS | CAUSE & ONSET |
|---|---|---|
| **HEMORRHOIDS WITH BURNING AND SORENESS** | ❑ A bruised, sore feeling in the anus; the hemorrhoids may bleed ❑ Hemorrhoids feel strained and rigid. | • *Inflamed veins* |

| YOU FEEL BETTER | YOU FEEL WORSE | REMEDY & DOSAGE |
|---|---|---|
| ◆ From fresh air<br>◆ From cold | ◆ With warmth<br>◆ From sweet foods<br>◆ At night | **Argent. nit. – see pp. 50–1**<br>*Take 6c every 30 minutes for up to 10 doses.* 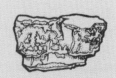 |
| ◆ From fresh air<br>◆ Lying on the right side | ◆ From eating irregular meals<br>◆ Between 11 a.m. and 11 p.m.<br>◆ With warmth | **Sulfur – see pp. 76–7**<br>*Take 6c every 30 minutes for up to 10 doses.* 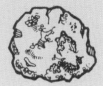 |
| ◆ In cool surroundings<br>◆ From hot meals or drinks<br>◆ After midnight | ◆ In stuffy rooms<br>◆ Wearing tight clothing<br>◆ From overeating<br>◆ Between 4 p.m. and 8 p.m. | **Lycopodium – see pp. 60–1**<br>*Take 6c every 30 minutes for up to 10 doses.*  |
| ◆ From cold<br>◆ From fresh air<br>◆ After burping | ◆ In the evening<br>◆ Lying down | **Carbo veg. – see p. 90**<br>*Take 6c every 30 minutes for up to 10 doses.*  |
| ◆ With warmth<br>◆ From warm food and drink | ◆ From cold air<br>◆ Early in the morning<br>◆ From eating starchy foods, vinegar, salt, pepper, and from drinking wine | **Alumina – see p. 115**<br>*Take 6c every 2 hours for up to 10 doses.*  |
| ◆ With heat<br>◆ After a nap<br>◆ In the evening | ◆ Early in the morning<br>◆ From cold<br>◆ From coffee and alcohol<br>◆ With too much mental stimulation | **Nux vomica – see pp. 74–5**<br>*Take 6c every 2 hours for up to 10 doses.*  |
| ◆ No specific factors | ◆ With warmth<br>◆ In warm, humid weather<br>◆ With pressure and movement | **Hamamelis – see p. 100**<br>*Take 6c 4 times a day for up to 5 days.*  |

# SKIN & HAIR

Homeopaths view skin complaints as a reflection of overall health, rather than just a local condition. Any general upset in the body, whether due to stress or poor nutrition, can manifest itself as a skin problem. Other causes include allergy and infection. Lack of exercise, constipation, sugar and refined carbohydrates, spices, caffeine, alcohol, and cosmetics are the main aggravating factors.

ECZEMA is a skin inflammation that causes itching and redness. If scratched, the skin may blister and bleed. Eczema may be due to an underlying allergy to plants, metals, detergents, and chemical irritants. It may also be hereditary. Emotional stress, menstruation, or a poor diet can aggravate any of these causes.

ACNE is a common skin condition in teenagers. It is caused mainly by high hormone levels associated with puberty. These increase the production of sebum (an oily secretion made by the skin), which leads to clogged pores. Pores may become inflamed and infected, causing pimples, which should not be picked or squeezed. Stress may make them worse.

HIVES (URTICARIA) is a rash with very itchy raised red patches on the skin, often with paler areas in the center. It is usually due to an allergy to certain plants, foods, drugs, or insect bites. It is also caused by extreme emotional stress, particularly after the death of a loved one. In some people who have very sensitive skin, hives can be brought on by extremes of temperature or light touch.

BOILS are caused by infected hair follicles, resulting in inflamed and pus-filled areas on the skin. Illness, fatigue, or being run-down can weaken the body's immune system and cause boils to form. Boils should not be squeezed.

## ECZEMA

| AILMENT | SYMPTOMS | CAUSE & ONSET |
|---|---|---|
| MOIST ECZEMA WITH HONEYLIKE DISCHARGE | ❑ Rough, dry, or cracked skin ❑ The palms of the hands and behind the ears are especially affected ❑ The face may feel as if there is a cobweb over it ❑ A tendency for the eczematous skin to turn septic. | • *Allergy* <br> • *Inherited tendency* |
| DRY ECZEMA | ❑ Skin is dry, rough, red, and itchy ❑ Eczema may be associated with diarrhea and a tendency to eat fatty, salty, sweet, or spicy foods, and to drink alcohol. | • *Allergy* <br> • *Inherited tendency* |
| MOIST ECZEMA WITH SKIN THAT CRACKS EASILY | ❑ Skin is very sensitive, rough, and broken ❑ The slightest scratch can cause the skin to become pus-filled, with cracking and bleeding ❑ Crusts may be greenish, with burning and itching. | • *Allergy* <br> • *Chronic stress* <br> • *Aftereffects of a scare or shock* |

## ACNE

| AILMENT | SYMPTOMS | CAUSE & ONSET |
|---|---|---|
| ITCHY PIMPLES ON THE FACE, CHEST, AND SHOULDERS | ❑ Blackheads ❑ Pustules with a depressed center ❑ Acne may be associated with increased sexual urges. | • *Hormonal changes, sometimes associated with puberty* |

**WARTS** are caused by a viral infection in the skin but may be precipitated by stress. To prevent the virus from spreading, the body "walls" it off, resulting in these common raised growths.

**HAIR LOSS** and graying are common in men and women as they get older. Hair loss can also be caused by a fever, childbirth, shock, stress, or an excess or lack of vitamin A and selenium. Baldness is hereditary and occurs mainly in men.

## PRECAUTIONS

**Hives** If the throat swells suddenly and acutely, call an ambulance immediately. Take *Apis* 30c every minute until help arrives.

**Boils** If boils are recurrent, occur with a fever, or do not heal within a week of onset, or if redness spreads and there is severe pain, see a doctor.

**Warts** If warts change size or color, or if they itch or bleed, see a doctor.

**Hair loss** If there is unexplained, sudden hair loss, see a doctor.

## SELF-HELP TREATMENTS

**Eczema** *Avoid known irritants, dry the skin thoroughly after washing, and use calendula cream on affected areas. Rub evening primrose oil on affected areas (see p. 225). Take vitamins B complex and C, and zinc (see p. 226). Try the liver diet for a month (see p. 229).*

**Acne** *Take vitamins A, B complex, and C, and zinc (see p. 226). Avoid iodine (found in cough mixtures, seaweed, and salt). Try the liver diet (see p. 229).*

**Hives (urticaria)** *Place an ice pack on affected areas or take a cold shower. Apply urtica ointment (see p. 227).*

**Boils** *Bathe the affected area with calendula and hypericum solution (see p. 227). Avoid handling food.*

**Warts** *To help kill warts, use thuja tincture (see p. 227).*

**Hair loss** *Avoid harsh hair treatments. Take iron, vitamins B complex and C, and zinc (see pp. 225–6). Make sure that your intake of vitamin A and selenium is neither excessive nor deficient (see p. 225).*

| YOU FEEL BETTER | YOU FEEL WORSE | REMEDY & DOSAGE |
|---|---|---|
| ◆ With sleep | ◆ From eating cold or sweet food, or seafood<br>◆ During menstruation | **Graphites – see pp. 56–7**<br>*Take 6c 4 times a day for up to 14 days.* 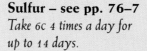 |
| ◆ From fresh air | ◆ From prolonged standing<br>◆ From washing<br>◆ If overheated<br>◆ Early in the morning | **Sulfur – see pp. 76–7**<br>*Take 6c 4 times a day for up to 14 days.* |
| ◆ From warm air<br>◆ In dry weather | ◆ In damp, wet weather<br>◆ In winter | **Petroleum – see p. 139**<br>*Take 6c 4 times a day for up to 14 days.* |
| ◆ From physical exercise or mental stimulation | ◆ During menstruation | **Kali brom. – see p. 131**<br>*Take 6c 4 times a day for up to 14 days.* 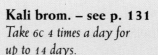 |

**ACNE** *continued*

## ACNE *continued*

| AILMENT | SYMPTOMS | CAUSE & ONSET |
|---|---|---|
| LARGE, PAINFUL, PUS-FILLED PIMPLES | ❑ Acne that is extremely painful when touched ❑ Blackheads that are worse on the forehead. | • *Hormonal changes associated with puberty* |
| PIMPLES ASSOCIATED WITH A HORMONAL IMBALANCE | ❑ Pimples worse at puberty just as menstruation begins, especially in girls who are overweight. | • *Puberty* • *Hormonal changes, often associated with delayed or scanty menstruation* |

## HIVES (URTICARIA)

| AILMENT | SYMPTOMS | CAUSE & ONSET |
|---|---|---|
| SWELLING, PARTICULARLY ON THE LIPS AND EYELIDS | ❑ Skin is red, swollen, and burning ❑ A tendency to be depressed, irritable, suspicious, and extremely sensitive ❑ In a few cases the throat may become swollen (see *Precautions*). | • *Allergy* • *Sudden onset* |
| HIVES WITH VIOLENT, ITCHY BLOTCHES | ❑ A burning sensation, like scorching, especially on the hands and fingers ❑ Itchy, red or pale, slightly raised blotches. | • *Touching stinging nettles or another irritant plant* • *Food allergy* • *Associated with rheumatism* |

## BOILS

| AILMENT | SYMPTOMS | CAUSE & ONSET |
|---|---|---|
| EARLY STAGES, WHEN A BOIL IS FORMING | ❑ Skin around affected area is hard, swollen, painful, dry, burning, throbbing, and red. | • *Infection* • *Sudden onset* |
| LATER STAGES, WHEN PUS HAS FORMED | ❑ Boil is sensitive to the slightest touch, and is on the point of bursting. | • *Infection* |

## WARTS

| AILMENT | SYMPTOMS | CAUSE & ONSET |
|---|---|---|
| SOFT, FLESHY, CAULIFLOWER-SHAPED WARTS | ❑ Warts that ooze or bleed easily, found on any part of the body but especially the back of the head. | • *Viral infection* • *Some immunizations* |

## HAIR LOSS

| AILMENT | SYMPTOMS | CAUSE & ONSET |
|---|---|---|
| PREMATURE BALDING OR GRAYING | ❑ Great hair loss ❑ Graying at a young age. | • *Childbirth* • *Premature aging* |

| YOU FEEL BETTER | YOU FEEL WORSE | REMEDY & DOSAGE |
|---|---|---|
| ◆ With warmth<br>◆ From a warm, damp compress placed over the face | ◆ From cold<br>◆ In a draft<br>◆ In the morning | **Hepar sulf. – see p. 101**<br>*Take 6c 3 times a day for up to 14 days.* 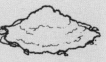 |
| ◆ From crying and sympathy<br>◆ From gentle exercise<br>◆ From fresh air<br>◆ From cold compresses | ◆ In hot, stuffy rooms<br>◆ From rich, fatty foods<br>◆ In the evening and at night | **Pulsatilla – see pp. 68–9**<br>*Take 6c 3 times a day for up to 14 days.*  |
| ◆ From fresh air<br>◆ From undressing<br>◆ After a cold bath | ◆ From heat and touch<br>◆ In late afternoon<br>◆ With sleep<br>◆ In stuffy rooms | **Apis – see p. 84**<br>*Take 30c every hour for up to 10 doses.* 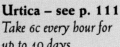 |
| ◆ Lying down | ◆ If touched<br>◆ In cold, damp air, water, and snow<br>◆ From scratching | **Urtica – see p. 111**<br>*Take 6c every hour for up to 10 days.*  |
| ◆ From pressure applied to the affected area<br>◆ At night<br>◆ With warmth | ◆ From cold compresses applied to the affected area | **Belladonna – see p. 86**<br>*Take 30c every hour for up to 10 doses.* 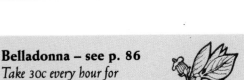 |
| ◆ With warmth<br>◆ From warm compresses applied to the affected area | ◆ In cold air and drafts | **Hepar sulf. – see p. 101**<br>*Take 6c every hour for up to 10 doses.* 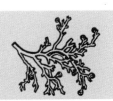 |
| ◆ No specific factors | ◆ No specific factors | **Thuja – see p. 110**<br>*Take 6c every 12 hours for up to 3 weeks.*  |
| ◆ From hot food and drink<br>◆ In cool surroundings | ◆ In stuffy rooms<br>◆ Between 4 p.m. and 8 p.m. | **Lycopodium – see pp. 60–1**<br>*Take 6c every 12 hours for up to 1 month.* 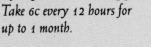 |

# EMOTIONAL PROBLEMS

Homeopathy has a lot to offer in the treatment of emotional problems. This is because it views them as only part of the whole picture, which also includes the spiritual, mental, and physical aspects of a person. Homeopaths diagnose what is happening to an individual on all levels.

**ANXIETY** or worry, is very common and is caused by stress, overwork, fear, or insecurity. In some people it manifests itself physically, for example, in a fast pulse rate, clammy skin, and appetite disturbances. Severe anxiety may cause chest pains that mimic a heart attack.

**BEREAVEMENT** has four stages: numbness and disbelief, denial that the person is dead, anger or guilt that not enough was done for the person, and, finally, depression that gradually fades. The grieving process takes a few years and may intensify on the anniversary of a loved one's death.

**FEAR** is a common emotion, but most people keep it under control. However, some fears, such as those resulting from shock, overwork or a scare, are more difficult to get over.

**IRRITABILITY & ANGER** are natural responses to events that seem threatening or frightening, and may be accompanied by symptoms such as a fast pulse, stomach flutters, and muscle tension. Too much food and alcohol, working too hard, and exhaustion also cause irritability and anger.

**SHOCK** is a reaction to a frightening or upsetting event, or can follow a serious injury. The rate of breathing increases and there is a churning sensation in the stomach.

**DEPRESSION** includes a wide range of feelings, from sadness to total despair. Where there is a specific cause, such as hormonal fluctuations

## ANXIETY

| AILMENT | SYMPTOMS | CAUSE & ONSET |
|---|---|---|
| **ANXIETY WITH A LACK OF CONFIDENCE** | ❑ Apprehension about performing in public ❑ Inability to sleep at night with continual reviewing of what happened during the day ❑ Appetite is disturbed ❑ A craving for sweet foods may accompany insomnia. | • *A forthcoming event or performance* • *More likely to occur in the very ambitious who have high standards* |
| **ANXIETY WITH RESTLESSNESS** | ❑ Chills ❑ Fatigue ❑ Appetite is disturbed ❑ A tendency to be fastidious and meticulously tidy ❑ Clammy skin ❑ Rapid pulse. | • *Deep insecurity* |
| **ANXIETY RELIEVED BY REASSURANCE** | ❑ Nervousness and edginess ❑ Sensitivity to the thoughts and feelings of others, but a desire be in the limelight ❑ Fear of many things, such as the dark, thunderstorms, being alone, or dying. | • *Overwork* |
| **ANXIETY WITH A FEAR OF INSANITY** | ❑ Forgetfulness, depression, and fear of making a fool of oneself ❑ Initial obsession with work, followed by a sense of defeat and complete failure ❑ A reluctance to answer questions ❑ A tendency to bore other people by repeatedly describing ailments. | • *Overwork* |

resulting in postpartum depression or after a
viral infection, it tends to disappear in time.
Sometimes there is no specific cause.

**INSOMNIA** is extremely common. It can happen
after a series of late nights, which can cause
severe exhaustion with disturbed sleep patterns,
difficulty getting to sleep, and frequent waking.
It is also caused by excess caffeine, food allergy,
alcohol, stress, anxiety, depression, or sleeping
in a stuffy bedroom.

## PRECAUTIONS

**Anxiety** If there is chest pain, call an ambulance.

**Shock** If it follows a injury and is accompanied
by nausea and vomiting, fainting, or clouding of
consciousness, call an ambulance.

**Depression** If it persists, see a doctor.

**Insomnia** If it does not improve within three
weeks, see a doctor.

## SELF-HELP TREATMENTS

**Anxiety** *Avoid anxiety-provoking situations and try
relaxation techniques. Take calcium, magnesium, and
vitamins B complex and C (see pp. 224–6). Avoid
drinking tea and coffee.*

**Irritability & anger** *Get more exercise. Take
bioflavonoids, calcium, magnesium, and vitamins
B complex and C (see pp. 224–6).*

**Depression** *Avoid excess copper, vitamin D, zinc, tea
and coffee (see pp. 224–6). Do not use oral contraceptives.
Increase your intake of bioflavonoids, biotin, calcium, folic
acid, magnesium, potassium, and vitamins B complex
and C (see pp. 224–6).*

**Insomnia** *Get more exercise and avoid eating late at night.
Stop working an hour before bedtime, drink herbal tea or a
hot milky drink, enjoy a warm bath, and read something
light. Sexual intercourse has a relaxing effect. Take biotin,
folic acid, vitamins B₁ and C, and zinc (see pp. 224–6).
Reduce vitamin A intake if taking supplements.*

| YOU FEEL BETTER | YOU FEEL WORSE | REMEDY & DOSAGE |
|---|---|---|
| • In cool surroundings<br>• From hot food and drinks<br>• After midnight<br>• With movement | • In stuffy rooms<br>• After overeating<br>• Between 4 p.m. and 8 p.m. | **Lycopodium – see pp. 60–1**<br>*Take 6c every 2 hours for up to 10 doses.*  |
| • With warmth<br>• From hot drinks<br>• Lying down with the head raised | • In cold, dry, windy weather<br>• Between midnight and 2 a.m.<br>• From cold food and drinks | **Arsen. alb. – see pp. 52–3**<br>*Take 6c every 2 hours for up to 10 doses.*  |
| • With sleep<br>• With massage<br>• From fresh air<br>• From reassurance | • From exercise<br>• From mental stimulation<br>• From hot food and drinks<br>• Before a thunderstorm | **Phos. – see pp. 66–7**<br>*Take 6c every 2 hours for up to 10 doses.* 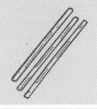 |
| • In the morning<br>• When slightly constipated | • In a draft<br>• In cool surroundings<br>• From exercise<br>• Between 2 a.m. and 3 a.m. | **Calc. carb. – see pp. 54–5**<br>*Take 6c every 2 hours for up to 10 doses.*  |

## BEREAVEMENT

| AILMENT | SYMPTOMS | CAUSE & ONSET |
| --- | --- | --- |
| SHOCK FOLLOWING BEREAVEMENT | ❑ A desire to be left alone ❑ A tendency to tell others to go away ❑ A dislike of being touched ❑ A tendency to insist you are all right. | • *Sudden death of a loved one* |
| BEREAVEMENT WITH RESTLESSNESS | ❑ Restless and a sense of being very hurried ❑ Tossing and turning when asleep ❑ Extreme fear of dying, even to the point of predicting the time of death. | • *Sudden onset of grief* |
| BEREAVEMENT WITH SUPPRESSION OF GRIEF | ❑ Inappropriate laughing, sighing, or crying, or even hysteria with rapid changes of mood because of an inability to express emotions ❑ Self-pitying attitude. | • *Slow onset of grief* |

## FEAR

| AILMENT | SYMPTOMS | CAUSE & ONSET |
| --- | --- | --- |
| MARKED FEAR OF DYING | ❑ Very strong fear of death, even to the point of predicting the time of death ❑ Fear of open spaces ❑ Restlessness and a sense of being hurried ❑ Tossing and turning when asleep. | • *Shock*<br>• *Sudden onset of fear* |
| FEAR WITH IMPULSIVE BEHAVIOR | ❑ Superstitious and anxious that something awful will happen at any moment ❑ Fear of crowds, heights, and being late ❑ Irrational fears ❑ Fear that a high building will fall down and crush you. | • *Fear of failure* |

## IRRITABILITY & ANGER

| AILMENT | SYMPTOMS | CAUSE & ONSET |
| --- | --- | --- |
| IRRITABILITY WITH AN OVERCRITICAL ATTITUDE | ❑ Slightest incident causes instant anger, which is over quickly but not before it has had a devastating effect ❑ Constantly finding fault with other people ❑ Very impatient, picky, and difficult to live with. | • *Overwork*<br>• *Too much food and alcohol*<br>• *Exhaustion* |
| ANGER WITH INSECURITY | ❑ Lack of self-confidence and deep feelings of cowardice, perhaps leading to angry outbursts at infrequent intervals ❑ Violent behavior is possible. | • *Fear of forthcoming events* |

## SHOCK

| AILMENT | SYMPTOMS | CAUSE & ONSET |
| --- | --- | --- |
| SHOCK WITH PHYSICAL AND EMOTIONAL NUMBNESS | ❑ Fear of going out ❑ Restlessness and a sense of being very hurried ❑ Tossing and turning while asleep ❑ Fear of dying, possibly to the point of predicting the hour of death. | • *Sudden onset* |

| YOU FEEL BETTER | YOU FEEL WORSE | REMEDY & DOSAGE |
|---|---|---|
| ◆ With movement<br>◆ Lying down with the head lower than the feet | ◆ With heat<br>◆ From light pressure | **Arnica – see p. 85**<br>*Take 30c every hour for up to 10 doses, then 4 times a day for up to 14 days.*  |
| ◆ From fresh air | ◆ In warm rooms<br>◆ Near tobacco smoke<br>◆ Near music<br>◆ In the evening and at night | **Aconite – see p. 82**<br>*Take 30c every hour for up to 10 doses.* 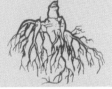 |
| ◆ From eating<br>◆ After urinating<br>◆ From walking<br>◆ With heat | ◆ From fresh air<br>◆ When warmly dressed<br>◆ From drinking coffee<br>◆ Near tobacco smoke | **Ignatia – see pp. 58–9**<br>*Take 6c every 2 hours for up to 10 doses then 3 times a day for up to 14 days.* 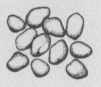 |
| ◆ From fresh air | ◆ In warm rooms<br>◆ Near tobacco smoke<br>◆ Near music<br>◆ In the evening and at night | **Aconite – see p. 82**<br>*Take 30c every 30 minutes for up to 10 doses.* 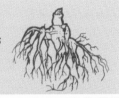 |
| ◆ From fresh air<br>◆ In cool surroundings | ◆ With warmth<br>◆ From eating sweet foods<br>◆ At night<br>◆ During menstruation | **Argent. nit. – see pp. 50–1**<br>*Take 6c every 30 minutes for up to 10 doses, then 4 times a day for up to 14 days.* 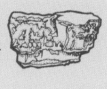 |
| ◆ With warmth<br>◆ With sleep<br>◆ From firm pressure<br>◆ In the evening | ◆ From being cold<br>◆ Near noise<br>◆ From spicy food and stimulants<br>◆ Between 3 a.m. and 4 a.m. | **Nux vomica – see pp. 74–5**<br>*Take 6c every 30 minutes for up to 10 doses.*  |
| ◆ From sympathy<br>◆ In cool surroundings<br>◆ From hot food and drinks<br>◆ After midnight | ◆ In stuffy rooms<br>◆ From wearing tight clothing<br>◆ After overeating<br>◆ Between 4 p.m. and 8 p.m. | **Lycopodium – see pp. 60–1**<br>*Take 6c every 30 minutes for up to 10 doses.* 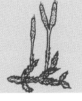 |
| ◆ From fresh air | ◆ In warm rooms<br>◆ Near tobacco smoke<br>◆ Near music<br>◆ In the evening and at night | **Aconite – see p. 82**<br>*Take 30c every 30 minutes for up to 10 doses.*<br>**SHOCK** *continued* 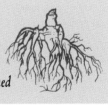 |

## SHOCK *continued*

| AILMENT | SYMPTOMS | CAUSE & ONSET |
|---|---|---|
| SHOCK AFTER A SCARE | ❑ Great apprehension develops before meeting new people, going to new places, or doing new things ❑ Examinations and new situations are considered dreadful ordeals ❑ Mental and physical weakness, with a sense of heaviness in the lower limbs ❑ Difficulty in getting the muscles to respond. | • *Emotional shock* • *Physical scare* |

## DEPRESSION

| AILMENT | SYMPTOMS | CAUSE & ONSET |
|---|---|---|
| DEPRESSION WITH WILDLY FLUCTUATING MOODS | ❑ Behavior is inappropriate – for example, suddenly bursting into tears or laughing for no reason ❑ Self-blame for everything that goes wrong ❑ A tendency to bottle up emotions ❑ Hysteria and sensitivity to noise, especially when studying. | • *Grief* |
| DEPRESSION WITH EXTREME TEARFULNESS | ❑ Self-pitying attitude ❑ A craving for comfort and reassurance ❑ Crying because of the slightest upset ❑ Great sympathy for people or animals that are suffering ❑ Lack of self-esteem and willpower. | • *Hormonal changes* |

## INSOMNIA

| AILMENT | SYMPTOMS | CAUSE & ONSET |
|---|---|---|
| INSOMNIA WITH AN INABILITY TO RELAX | ❑ Overactive mind ❑ Eventually falls asleep, but tosses and turns in anguish. | • *Sudden emotions as a result of receiving either good or bad news* |
| INSOMNIA WITH IRRITABILITY | ❑ Falls asleep easily but there is a tendency to wake up between 3 a.m. and 4 a.m. and remains awake for a few hours, before falling asleep just as it is time to get up ❑ Sleep pattern may be associated with nightmares ❑ Irritable ❑ Miserable outlook ❑ Extremely critical of others. | • *Overexcitement* • *Exhaustion and stress* |
| INSOMNIA WITH GREAT FEAR | ❑ Nervousness and restlessness ❑ A strong fear of dying, even to the point of predicting the time of death ❑ Nightmares and tossing and turning in sleep. | • *Shock or scare* • *Exposure to dry, cold, windy weather* |
| INSOMNIA WITH A FEAR THAT YOU WILL NEVER SLEEP AGAIN | ❑ Continual yawning, but cannot get to sleep and comes to fear bedtime ❑ Rapid changes of mood, from laughing to crying and hysterical behavior ❑ Possible nightmares. | • *Emotional stress* • *Grief* |

| YOU FEEL BETTER | YOU FEEL WORSE | REMEDY & DOSAGE |
|---|---|---|
| ◆ After urinating<br>◆ From perspiring<br>◆ From alcohol | ◆ From excitement<br>◆ Hearing bad news<br>◆ With heat | **Gelsemium – see p. 99**<br>*Take 30c every 30 minutes for up to 10 doses.*  |
| ◆ From eating<br>◆ From walking<br>◆ With heat | ◆ If cold<br>◆ When warmly dressed<br>◆ From coffee and stimulants<br>◆ Near strong smells | **Ignatia – see pp. 58–9**<br>*Take 6c 3 times a day for up to 14 days.* 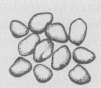 |
| ◆ From crying<br>◆ From gentle exercise<br>◆ From fresh air<br>◆ From cold drinks | ◆ With heat<br>◆ In stuffy rooms<br>◆ From eating rich, fatty foods<br>◆ At twilight | **Pulsatilla – see pp. 68–9**<br>*Take 6c 3 times a day for up to 14 days.*  |
| ◆ With warmth<br>◆ Lying down<br>◆ Sucking ice | ◆ Using sleeping pills<br>◆ Near strong smells<br>◆ Near noise<br>◆ From fresh air and cold | **Coffea – see p. 125**<br>*Take 30c 1 hour before bed for 10 nights. Repeat the dose if you wake up and cannot get back to sleep.*  |
| ◆ With warmth<br>◆ With sleep<br>◆ In the evening<br>◆ From being left alone | ◆ From overeating, especially spicy foods<br>◆ In cold, windy weather<br>◆ Near noise | **Nux vomica – see pp. 74–5**<br>*Take 30c 1 hour before bed for 10 nights. Repeat the dose if you wake up and cannot get back to sleep.* |
| ◆ From fresh air | ◆ In warm rooms<br>◆ Near tobacco smoke<br>◆ Near music<br>◆ In the evening | **Aconite – see p. 82**<br>*Take 30c 1 hour before bed for 10 nights. Repeat the dose if you wake up and cannot get back to sleep.* 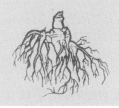 |
| ◆ From eating<br>◆ After urinating<br>◆ From walking around | ◆ From fresh air<br>◆ If cold<br>◆ When warmly dressed<br>◆ From coffee and alcohol | **Ignatia – see pp. 58–9**<br>*Take 30c 1 hour before bed for 10 nights. Repeat the dose if you wake up and cannot get back to sleep.*  |

# FATIGUE

Common tiredness responds to rest and extra sleep. By contrast, chronic fatigue syndrome is a long-lasting condition and is diagnosed only after months of continuous fatigue and illness.

**TIREDNESS** is usually due to lack of sleep, physical or emotional stress, or overwork, and is common premenstrually and during early pregnancy, childbirth, and menopause. It can be related to anemia, which is normally due to iron deficiency, but can also be caused by a deficiency of other vitamins and minerals, particularly vitamin $B_{12}$. Tiredness can be a side effect of drugs, alcohol, caffeine, nicotine, and too much vitamin A. It may also follow illness, physical injury, or an operation.

**CHRONIC FATIGUE SYNDROME**, also known as postviral fatigue syndrome or ME (myalgic encephalomyelitis), is of no known cause, although there are many theories to explain its occurrence. A persistent viral infection, stress, and nervous exhaustion are thought to be possible causes of ME. It is diagnosed if fatigue is the main symptom, is experienced 50 percent of the time, and has been present for more than

## TIREDNESS

| AILMENT | SYMPTOMS | CAUSE & ONSET |
|---|---|---|
| **FATIGUE WITH GREAT ANXIETY** | ❑ Swollen glands in the groin and neck ❑ Joint pain ❑ Burning pain inside the head ❑ Abdominal cramps and a bloated stomach ❑ Candidiasis ❑ Inability to sleep ❑ Weakness after the slightest physical exertion ❑ Panic attacks because of poor memory ❑ A feeling of not being able to function and concern that others will notice ❑ Fear of insanity. | • *Overwork* |
| **FATIGUE WITH RESTLESSNESS** | ❑ Constantly feeling cold with joint and muscle pain ❑ Aching and burning all over from stiffness ❑ Numb fingers and toes ❑ Weakness and dizziness from the slightest exertion ❑ Feeling faint in the morning ❑ Tendency to migraines, loose bowels, tired eyes, and blurred vision ❑ Anxiety and panic attacks with a poor memory, sleeplessness, and breathlessness. | • *Stress from worry* |
| **FATIGUE WITH IRRITABILITY** | ❑ Extreme chilliness ❑ Aching all over with joint pain ❑ Tense muscles ❑ Indigestion, especially 30 minutes after eating, with gas and constipation ❑ Frequent waking in the early hours of the morning and difficulty returning to sleep ❑ Feeling faint on waking ❑ Difficulty concentrating ❑ Critical of others. | • *Lack of sleep*<br>• *Stress*<br>• *Overwork* |

## CHRONIC FATIGUE SYNDROME

| | | |
|---|---|---|
| **FATIGUE WITH TREMBLING** | ❑ Anxiety, irritability, and a feeling of being unable to cope ❑ Fear of losing control and screaming ❑ Nervous anticipation ❑ Severe muscle fatigue on exertion ❑ Pale complexion that flushes due to stress or excitement ❑ Sensitivity to touch. | • *Stress*<br>• *Nervous exhaustion from overwork* |

six months. The fatigue has a definite onset and is severely physically and mentally disabling, and there are other symptoms, especially muscle pain, fluctuation in weight, sleep disturbance, and temperature variation. Recurrent acute attacks that resemble viral infections are characteristic, and there is rarely a return to full health between attacks. Before accepting a diagnosis of chronic fatigue syndrome have a thorough checkup to rule out any other causes.

## PRECAUTION

**Tiredness** If it is associated with any other symptoms in addition to those listed here, see a doctor.

## SELF-HELP TREATMENTS

**Tiredness** *Increase the amount of sleep you get at night, and, if possible, take an afternoon nap. If fatigue is due to overwork and stress, take some time off. Avoid caffeine. Take extra iron, a multivitamin and mineral supplement, and vitamin B$_{12}$ (see p. 225–6).*

**Chronic Fatigue Syndrome** *In the early stages of the illness make sure you get frequent periods of bed rest to improve your energy stores. Gradually increase exercise levels, but keep some energy in reserve. Prevent low blood sugar by eating small meals regularly. Take beta-carotene, copper, EPA marine oils, evening primrose oil, iron, magnesium, selenium, vitamins B$_5$, C, D, and E, and zinc (see pp. 224–6).*

| YOU FEEL BETTER | YOU FEEL WORSE | REMEDY & DOSAGE |
|---|---|---|
| • In the morning<br>• When slightly constipated<br>• Lying on the painful side | • In a draft<br>• In cool surroundings<br>• In cold, damp, windy weather<br>• Between 2 a.m. and 3 a.m. | **Calc. carb. – see pp. 54–5**<br>*Take 30c twice a day for up to 14 days. If beneficial, repeat dose.* 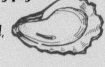 |
| • With warmth<br>• From hot drinks<br>• Lying down with the head propped up | • From the sight or the smell of food<br>• From cold food and drinks<br>• In cold, dry, windy weather<br>• Between midnight and 2 a.m. | **Arsen. alb. – see pp. 52–3**<br>*Take 30c twice a day for up to 14 days. If beneficial, repeat dose.*  |
| • With warmth<br>• With sleep<br>• From firm pressure<br>• From washing<br>• In the evening<br>• When left alone | • In cold, dry, windy weather<br>• Around noise<br>• From spices and stimulants<br>• From eating | **Nux vomica – see pp. 74–5**<br>*Take 30c twice a day for up to 14 days. If beneficial, repeat dose.*  |
| • With warmth<br>• From eating | • From physical and mental exertion<br>• From excitement<br>• In cool surroundings<br>• Between 3 a.m. and 5 a.m. | **Kali phos. – see p. 104**<br>*Take 30c twice a day for up to 14 days. If beneficial, repeat dose.* 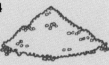 |

# CIRCULATORY COMPLAINTS

Circulatory problems are common later in life, as the arteries clog up with cholesterol and the veins lose their elasticity. Blood flow is also controlled by the nervous system, so stress can affect it. A low-fat diet, exercise, relaxation, and stopping smoking all help to reduce problems. Constitutional treatment (see pp. 24–5) may help circulatory conditions by reducing stress and improving the body's metabolic function.

**COLD HANDS & FEET** may be the result of a poor diet, nervous tension, or a genetic disease. It may also be due to Raynaud's disease, in which

exposure to cold makes the arteries that supply blood to the fingers and toes contract rapidly. Raynaud's disease is aggravated by stress or the repeated use of vibrating machinery and equipment, such as pneumatic drills, and it may be a side effect of certain drugs.

**CHILBLAINS** occur on the fingers and toes and are caused by extreme sensitivity to the cold. The small blood vessels below the skin's surface go into spasm, causing the skin to become pale and numb, then red, swollen, and itchy. Eventually the skin may break.

## COLD HANDS & FEET

| AILMENT | SYMPTOMS | CAUSE & ONSET |
|---|---|---|
| COLD HANDS AND FEET WITH A BURNING SENSATION | ❑ Fingers and toes are cold but with a burning sensation ❑ Rest of the body also feels cold ❑ Fingers and toes are blue or white. | • *Raynaud's disease* |
| COLD HANDS AND FEET WITH MOTTLING OF THE SKIN | ❑ Skin feels ice-cold and appears blue, with prominent veins ❑ Blotchy skin ❑ Skin itches on going to bed. | • *Spasms in the blood vessel walls leading to poor blood flow* |

## CHILBLAINS

| | | |
|---|---|---|
| BURNING, ITCHY CHILBLAINS | ❑ The skin on affected areas is red, prickly, and swollen. | • *Exposure to cold* |
| CHILBLAINS WITH SWOLLEN VEINS | ❑ Burning, throbbing pain is severe enough to cause tears ❑ Bluish inflamed swelling ❑ A desire for sympathy. | • *Exposure to cold* |

## VARICOSE VEINS

| | | |
|---|---|---|
| VARICOSE VEINS THAT FEEL BRUISED | ❑ Extremely tender, sore, and swollen veins, with slight bruising and possibly a burning sensation ❑ Inflammation ❑ Possible bleeding. | • *Pregnancy*<br>• *Injury* |

**VARICOSE VEINS** are swollen and lumpy. They usually occur in the legs and develop as a result of weakness of the valves in the veins. Weak valves may be due to being overweight or pregnant, prolonged sitting or standing, or constipation.

## PRECAUTIONS

**Cold hands & feet** If the fingers and toes frequently become numb and cold, see a doctor.

**Varicose veins** If there is no improvement within 3 weeks of taking a remedy, see a doctor. If there are pains deep in the calves with swelling and dark red discoloration of the skin, see a doctor within 12 hours.

## SELF-HELP TREATMENTS

**Cold hands & feet** *Avoid wearing tight gloves and socks. Stop smoking. Eat a low-fat diet.*

**Chilblains** *Keep the affected areas as warm and dry as possible and do not scratch the chilblains. Apply tamus ointment or, if the skin is broken, calendula cream (see p. 227). Get regular exercise to improve circulation.*

**Varicose veins** *Avoid standing for long periods and wear support stockings. Sit with the feet raised above hip level whenever possible. Raise the foot of the bed by 4 in (10 cm). Get regular exercise, eat a high-fiber diet, and avoid gaining too much weight. Take bioflavonoids and vitamins C and E (see pp. 224–6).*

| YOU FEEL BETTER | YOU FEEL WORSE | REMEDY & DOSAGE |
|---|---|---|
| ◆ From cool, circulating air<br>◆ From uncovering, rubbing, and stretching out the fingers and toes | ◆ With heat and warmth | **Secale – see pp. 144–5**<br>*Take 6c every 30 minutes for up to 10 doses.*  |
| ◆ From cool, circulating air | ◆ In the evening<br>◆ From rich, fatty foods<br>◆ In warm, humid weather | **Carbo veg. – see p. 90**<br>*Take 6c every 30 minutes for up to 10 doses.* 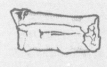 |
| ◆ With slow movement | ◆ In cold weather<br>◆ Before a thunderstorm | **Agaricus – see p. 114**<br>*Take 6c every 30 minutes for up to 6 doses.* 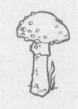 |
| ◆ Raising the hands above the head<br>◆ From gentle exercise | ◆ With heat<br>◆ With extremes of temperature<br>◆ In the evening and at night | **Pulsatilla – see pp. 68–9**<br>*Take 6c every 30 minutes for up to 6 doses.*  |
| ◆ With rest<br>◆ Lying down quietly | ◆ In warm, humid weather<br>◆ With movement<br>◆ With pressure | **Hamamelis – see p. 100**<br>*Take 30c every 12 hours for up to 7 days.* 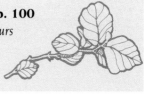 |

# URINARY DISORDERS

In homeopathy, urinary disorders are viewed not just as problems in the kidneys and urinary system but as a mirror of the body's functioning and diet. Stress increases chemicals in the body, which must be excreted, while a poor diet strains the whole metabolism and the kidneys in particular. To prevent urinary disorders, avoid too much stress, eat a good diet, exercise, and drink plenty of fluids to cleanse the kidneys.

**CYSTITIS** can be caused by an infection, which results in painful urination with increased frequency. It can also be due to an irritation of the bladder resulting from antibiotics. Stress, a bad diet, a food allergy, poor hygiene, nylon tights and underwear, oral and barrier methods of contraception, and sexual intercourse all aggravate cystitis. Without treatment, it can develop into a serious kidney infection.

**PROSTATE ENLARGEMENT** is extremely common in men over 45, although the cause is not known. Symptoms include difficulty in starting to urinate, especially in the morning, and needing to urinate frequently at night. The stream of urine also becomes weaker than usual.

## CYSTITIS

| AILMENT | SYMPTOMS | CAUSE & ONSET |
|---|---|---|
| CYSTITIS WITH A NONSTOP DESIRE TO URINATE | ❑ Burning, cutting pains in the lower abdomen ❑ Aching in the small of the back ❑ Continuous urge to urinate ❑ Sensation that the bladder cannot be emptied properly ❑ Only small amounts of urine with some blood in it may be passed. | • *Infection* |
| CYSTITIS WITH PAINFUL URGING | ❑ Despite a frequent need to urinate, little urine is produced ❑ Chills ❑ Irritability ❑ Extremely critical of others ❑ A desire to be left alone. | • *Stress* <br> • *Too much spicy food, alcohol, and caffeine* <br> • *Lack of sleep* |
| CYSTITIS WITH A CONTINUOUS BURNING SENSATION | ❑ Sensation that a drop of urine is constantly trickling through the urethra ❑ Resentfulness and anger. | • *Sexual intercourse or catheterization* |

## PROSTATE ENLARGEMENT

| | | |
|---|---|---|
| ENLARGED PROSTATE WITH A CONSTANT DESIRE TO URINATE | ❑ Urination is difficult ❑ There may be a discharge from the penis ❑ Spasms in the bladder or urethra ❑ Sensation of coldness from the prostate gland to the genitals. | • *Enlarged prostate* |

## STRESS INCONTINENCE

| | | |
|---|---|---|
| INVOLUNTARY LEAKAGE OF URINE | ❑ Urine leaks unnoticed when pressure in the abdomen rises, as a result of coughing, sneezing, or walking. | • *Weakened pelvic floor muscles* |

**STRESS INCONTINENCE** is a condition in which trickles of urine are passed involuntarily when pressure in the abdomen rises as a result of coughing, sneezing, laughing, or lifting. It is caused by weakened pelvic floor muscles (which support the uterus, vagina, and bladder), due to childbirth, being overweight, or the loss of muscle tone that occurs after menopause.

## PRECAUTIONS

**Cystitis** If there is pain in the kidneys or blood in the urine, see a doctor.

**Prostate enlargement** Prostate problems should always be referred to a doctor.

## SELF-HELP TREATMENTS

**Cystitis** *Increase fluid intake to 5 pints (10 liters) a day. Drink an alkaline solution (1 teaspoon sodium bicarbonate in 1½ pints [900 ml] water) every hour for up to 3 hours. Drink cranberry juice, try an alkaline diet, and avoid alcohol, coffee, meat, and dairy products (see pp. 225–9). Avoid using tampons, vaginal douches, and medicated or perfumed bath products, and use a lubricant for sexual intercourse. Never suppress the urge to urinate.*

**Prostate enlargement** *Take calcium, lecithin, and magnesium (see pp. 224–5).*

**Stress incontinence** *To strengthen the pelvic floor muscles, alternately tighten and relax them as you urinate.*

| YOU FEEL BETTER | YOU FEEL WORSE | REMEDY & DOSAGE |
|---|---|---|
| • With warmth<br>• With a gentle massage<br>• At night<br>• In the morning | • With movement<br>• From drinking coffee or cold water<br>• In the afternoon | **Cantharis – see p. 107** *Take 30c every 30 minutes for up to 10 doses, until you see a doctor.* 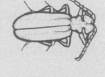 |
| • With warmth and sleep<br>• From pressing the bladder<br>• From washing<br>• In the evening | • In cold, windy weather<br>• From noise, spicy foods, stimulants, and eating<br>• Between 3 a.m. and 4 a.m. | **Nux vomica – see pp. 74–5** *Take 6c every 30 minutes for up to 10 doses.*  |
| • With warmth<br>• From a good night's sleep | • From pressing the bladder<br>• From not drinking enough fluids | **Staphysagria – see p. 127** *Take 6c every 30 minutes for up to 10 doses.*  |
| • With warmth | • From sympathy<br>• From cold<br>• In damp, cloudy weather | **Sabal – see p. 143** *Take 6c 4 times a day for up to 21 days.* 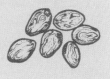 |
| • From cold drinks<br>• From washing<br>• Sitting down | • From sneezing, coughing, walking, or blowing the nose<br>• From cold<br>• After the first hours of sleep | **Causticum – see p. 123** *Take 6c 4 times a day for up to 21 days.*  |

# WOMEN'S HEALTH

A woman's reproductive cycle begins with the onset of menstruation and ends with menopause, when menstruation ceases. Physical and emotional problems associated with this cycle are generally due to a hormonal imbalance. The homeopathic approach to women's problems not only takes into account specific symptoms, but assesses lifestyle factors such as diet and exercise in order to restore hormonal balance and improve overall well-being.

**CANDIDIASIS** is a fungal infection, and the main symptom is an itchy, white vaginal discharge. Causes include stress, overwork, a hormonal imbalance, pregnancy, and drugs such as antibiotics and oral contraceptives. Wearing tight trousers or nylon underwear and lack of lubrication before sex aggravate the condition.

**PREMENSTRUAL SYNDROME (PMS)** is the name given to a range of physical and mental symptoms, such as bloating, swollen breasts, anxiety, tearfulness, and irritability that affect women 2–14 days before menstruation. PMS can be caused by many factors, including stress, overwork, a hormonal imbalance, and weight gain.

**HEAVY MENSTRUATION** is the loss of more than 3 fl oz (90 ml) of blood during one menstrual cycle (the average is 2 fl oz or 60 ml). It may be due to a hormonal imbalance, stress, overwork, or the approach of menopause.

**PAINFUL MENSTRUATION** is common in teenage girls and young women. It tends to disappear after childbirth, though many older women have some discomfort during menstruation. In a few women, the pain may be severe enough to cause nausea and vomiting. Pain may be due to a hormonal imbalance and stress makes it worse.

**ABSENT MENSTRUATION** sometimes occurs if menstrual periods begin but then stop because of anorexia nervosa, excessive weight loss or

## CANDIDIASIS (YEAST INFECTION)

| AILMENT | SYMPTOMS | CAUSE & ONSET |
|---------|----------|---------------|
| CANDIDIASIS WITH AN ITCHY, MILKY DISCHARGE | ❑ Itching is worse before menstruation and after urination ❑ May be associated with vaginal warts or cervical erosion (wearing away of the cells lining the cervix) ❑ Candidiasis may be accompanied by a chronic headache, an increased appetite, anxiety, and depression. | • *Stress*<br>• *Overwork*<br>• *Pregnancy* |
| CANDIDIASIS WITH A VERY OFFENSIVE DISCHARGE | ❑ Marked vaginal and vulval itching ❑ Soreness and burning in the vagina ❑ Possible ulcers on the labia ❑ White discharge that is worse after sexual intercourse ❑ Associated tearfulness, irritability, and indifference toward loved ones. | • *Menopause*<br>• *Hormonal imbalance* |
| CANDIDIASIS WITH BURNING PAINS | ❑ Offensive yellowish or white discharge causes itching and vaginal soreness ❑ Pain in the vagina during sex ❑ Alternating constipation and diarrhea ❑ Offensive gas ❑ Anal itching with irritation of the skin around the anus ❑ Candidiasis may be associated with increased appetite. | • *Stress*<br>• *After another illness* |

exercise, stress, stopping oral contraceptives, shock, or problems in the uterus. Menstruation should start by the age of 16 but may be delayed. If menstruation stops or does not start, seek advice from a medical practitioner.

**MENOPAUSE** is the cessation of menstruation and usually occurs in women aged 45–55. Symptoms, which include hot flashes, sweats, vaginal dryness, and anxiety, can be especially severe if menstruation stops abruptly, either naturally or following the removal of the ovaries.

## PRECAUTIONS

**Candidiasis** If the discharge does not clear up within 5 days, see a doctor.

**Menstruation** See a doctor if there is a sudden, unusual change in menstrual flow or if menstruation stops and does not restart after 2 months. If you might be pregnant, bleed more than usual, or have severe pain, see a doctor.

**Menopause** If there is prolonged or irregular bleeding, see a doctor.

## SELF-HELP TREATMENTS

**Candidiasis** *Eat live yogurt or take acidophilus (see p. 224). The infection can be passed during sex, so use condoms. Avoid sweet foods and foods that contain yeast.*

**Premenstrual syndrome** *Avoid salty and fatty foods, tea, and coffee. Eat small, protein-rich snacks and raw vegetables and salads, rather than large meals. Cut refined carbohydrates and dairy products out of the diet. Take evening primrose oil, vitamins B6 and E, and a multivitamin and mineral supplement (see pp. 225–6).*

**Heavy menstruation** *Avoid tea, coffee, and alcohol. Try the liver diet (see p. 229). Take bioflavonoids, calcium, iron, vitamins A and B6, and zinc (see pp. 224–6).*

**Painful menstruation** *Try the liver diet (see p. 229). Take calcium, evening primrose oil, magnesium, vitamins B complex, C, and E, and zinc (see pp. 224–6).*

**Absent menstruation** *Take multivitamins (see p. 225).*

**Menopause** *Avoid sweet foods and caffeine. Take calcium, selenium, vitamins B complex, C, and E (see pp. 224–6).*

| YOU FEEL BETTER | YOU FEEL WORSE | REMEDY & DOSAGE |
|---|---|---|
| ◆ In the morning<br>◆ When slightly constipated | ◆ Before and after menstruation<br>◆ From applying heat to the vulval area<br>◆ During pregnancy<br>◆ In cold, damp, windy weather<br>◆ From exertion<br>◆ Between 2 a.m. and 3 a.m. | **Calc. carb. – see pp. 54–5**<br>*Take 6c 6 times a day for up to 5 days.* 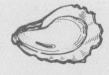 |
| ◆ From eating<br>◆ With sleep<br>◆ From exercise<br>◆ From applying heat to the vulval area | ◆ From cold<br>◆ Near tobacco smoke<br>◆ From being overtired<br>◆ In the early morning and evening | **Sepia – see pp. 70–1**<br>*Take 6c 6 times a day for up to 5 days.* 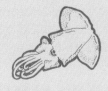 |
| ◆ From fresh air<br>◆ From dry warmth | ◆ From prolonged standing<br>◆ From wearing too many clothes<br>◆ From cold and dampness<br>◆ From washing<br>◆ From being too warm in bed<br>◆ From drinking alcohol<br>◆ In the morning and at night | **Sulfur – see pp. 76–7**<br>*Take 6c 6 times a day for up to 5 days.* 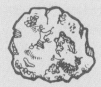 |

# PREMENSTRUAL SYNDROME (PMS)

| AILMENT | SYMPTOMS | CAUSE & ONSET |
|---|---|---|
| PMS WITH MARKED INDIFFERENCE TO LOVED ONES | ❑ Irritability ❑ Tearfulness ❑ Difficulty in concentrating ❑ A desire to get away from everything ❑ Fits of screaming ❑ Extreme anger ❑ Aversion to sex ❑ A feeling that the uterus may fall out ❑ PMS may be accompanied by oily skin, acne, and a craving for sweet and salty food ❑ Associated sinus problems, hot flashes, and sore throat ❑ Weariness, especially in the morning. | • *Hormonal imbalance*<br>• *Approach of menopause*<br>• *Stress* |
| PMS WITH FLUID RETENTION, PARTICULARLY SWOLLEN, TENDER BREASTS | ❑ Painful joints ❑ Weakness and lack of energy ❑ Possible vaginal discharge or candidiasis ❑ Depression ❑ Indifference ❑ Tearfulness ❑ Irritability ❑ Loss of concentration ❑ Anxiety that symptoms have been observed, or fear of insanity. | • *Hormonal imbalance*<br>• *Being overweight*<br>• *Overwork* |
| PMS WITH EXTREME TEARFULNESS | ❑ Depression, self-pity, and bursting into tears for no reason ❑ Anxiety about the future ❑ Fearfulness in crowds ❑ Possible swelling of the upper eyelids and face ❑ A desire for candy, a bloated stomach, and vaginal discharge ❑ A tendency to gain weight before menstruation ❑ Associated headaches, nausea, and dizziness. | • *Hormonal imbalance* |

# HEAVY MENSTRUATION

| AILMENT | SYMPTOMS | CAUSE & ONSET |
|---|---|---|
| HEAVY MENSTRUATION WITH MARKED WEIGHT GAIN BEFOREHAND | ❑ Chilliness before menstruation ❑ Cramps in the uterus ❑ Bright red blood ❑ Irregular menstruation ❑ Confusion and difficulty concentrating ❑ Anxiety that symptoms have been observed, or fear of insanity ❑ May be associated with backache, clumsiness, and clammy sweats, especially if overweight. | • *Stress*<br>• *Overwork* |
| HEAVY MENSTRUATION WITH FAINTNESS AND IRRITABILITY | ❑ Cramps are severe enough to cause fainting ❑ Irregular menstruation ❑ Visual disturbances ❑ Itchy vaginal discharge ❑ Sweating during menstruation ❑ Tearfulness ❑ Indifference, even to loved ones. | • *Approach of menopause*<br>• *Hormonal imbalance*<br>• *Stress* |

# PAINFUL MENSTRUATION

| AILMENT | SYMPTOMS | CAUSE & ONSET |
|---|---|---|
| PAINFUL CRAMPS WITH MARKED TEARFULNESS | ❑ Pains in the uterus severe enough to cause nausea or vomiting ❑ Tenderness in the stomach ❑ Tearing pain in the lower abdomen ❑ Possible associated migraine or diarrhea ❑ Menstruation is heavy with clots, or it may be scanty ❑ Tearfulness at the slightest excuse ❑ Depression and self-pity. | • *Hormonal imbalance* |

| YOU FEEL BETTER | YOU FEEL WORSE | REMEDY & DOSAGE |
|---|---|---|
| ◆ From eating<br>◆ With sleep<br>◆ From vigorous exercise<br>◆ With heat | ◆ From cold<br>◆ Near tobacco smoke<br>◆ From mental stimulation<br>◆ In the early morning and evening<br>◆ Before a thunderstorm | **Sepia – see pp. 70–1**<br>*Take 30c every 12 hours for up to 3 days, starting a day before PMS usually occurs.*  |
| ◆ In the morning<br>◆ When slightly constipated | ◆ In a draft<br>◆ In cold, damp, windy weather<br>◆ From cold<br>◆ From overexertion<br>◆ Between 2 a.m. and 3 a.m. | **Calc. carb. – see pp. 54–5**<br>*Take 30c every 12 hours for up to 3 days, starting a day before PMS usually occurs.*  |
| ◆ From crying<br>◆ From sympathy<br>◆ From exercise<br>◆ From fresh air<br>◆ From cold drinks | ◆ In sun and with warmth<br>◆ From eating rich, fatty foods<br>◆ In the evening and at night | **Pulsatilla – see pp. 68–9**<br>*Take 30c every 12 hours for up to 3 days, starting a day before PMS usually occurs.*  |
| ◆ In the morning<br>◆ When slightly constipated | ◆ In a draft<br>◆ In cold, damp, windy weather<br>◆ From exercise<br>◆ Between 2 a.m. and 3 a.m. | **Calc. carb. – see pp. 54–5**<br>*Take 30c every 8 hours for up to 10 doses.*  |
| ◆ From eating and sleeping<br>◆ From exercise<br>◆ From applying hot compresses to the lower abdomen | ◆ From cold<br>◆ Near tobacco smoke<br>◆ From mental exertion<br>◆ In the early morning and evening | **Sepia – see pp. 70–1**<br>*Take 30c every 8 hours for up to 10 doses.* 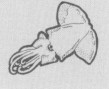 |
| ◆ From crying and sympathy<br>◆ Raising your hands above your head<br>◆ From gentle exercise<br>◆ From fresh air<br>◆ From cold drinks<br>◆ From cold compresses | ◆ With heat<br>◆ With extremes of temperature<br>◆ From rich, fatty foods<br>◆ Lying on the more painful side<br>◆ In the evening and at night | **Pulsatilla – see pp. 68–9**<br>*Take 30c every hour for up to 10 doses.*  |

**PAINFUL MENSTRUATION** *continued*

## PAINFUL MENSTRUATION *continued*

| AILMENT | SYMPTOMS | CAUSE & ONSET |
|---|---|---|
| CRAMPS WITH INDIFFERENCE TO LOVED ONES | ❑ Sharp, piercing pain in the lower abdomen ❑ Irritability ❑ Tearfulness with a desire to be left alone ❑ Cramps may be accompanied by migraine, acne, weakness, fainting, and sweating. | • *Hormonal imbalance* |

## ABSENT MENSTRUATION

| AILMENT | SYMPTOMS | CAUSE & ONSET |
|---|---|---|
| MENSTRUATION STOPS SUDDENLY | ❑ Heaviness and aching pains in the ovaries ❑ Sharp, shooting pain in the uterus ❑ Fear and anxiety ❑ Nervousness to the point of being afraid of death and even predicting the time of death. | • *Great emotional shock* • *Stress from exposure to cold, dry, windy weather* |
| ABSENT MENSTRUATION WITH MARKED CHANGE IN BEHAVIOR | ❑ Suppressed emotion with a fear that feelings will be displayed at inappropriate times ❑ Very changeable moods, crying and laughing at unexpected times ❑ Possible hysteria. | • *Acute onset after the death of a loved one* |

## MENOPAUSE

| AILMENT | SYMPTOMS | CAUSE & ONSET |
|---|---|---|
| MENOPAUSE WITH AVERSION TO SEXUAL INTERCOURSE | ❑ Vaginal pain during sexual intercourse due to vaginal dryness ❑ Anxiety during hot flashes ❑ Left-sided headache ❑ Anxiety about sex ❑ Sinking feeling in the pit of the stomach ❑ Heavy menstruation with flooding ❑ Irregular menstruation ❑ A tendency to candidiasis ❑ Sudden fainting spells ❑ Chills ❑ Tearfulness ❑ Irritability ❑ Indifference to loved ones ❑ Hair loss. | • *Hormonal imbalance* |
| MENOPAUSE WITH WEIGHT GAIN AND PANIC ATTACKS | ❑ Anxiety and fear that memory loss and lack of cencentration will be observed ❑ Possible fear of insanity ❑ Phobias ❑ Noises in the ears ❑ Perspiration on the face ❑ A craving for sweet foods ❑ A tendency to candidiasis ❑ Backache ❑ Swelling of the finger joints ❑ Varicose veins. | • *Overwork* |
| MENOPAUSE WITH SUSPICIOUSNESS AND A TENDENCY TO TALK TOO MUCH | ❑ Overexcitement ❑ A feeling of congestion all over the body, as if something needs to come out ❑ Dizziness and a tendency to faint ❑ Headache, worse on waking and on the left side ❑ Left-sided migraines ❑ A constricted feeling in the abdomen ❑ Difficulty breathing ❑ Sleeplessness. | • *Suppressed menstruation, especially before early menopause due to emotional or physical shock* |

| YOU FEEL BETTER | YOU FEEL WORSE | REMEDY & DOSAGE |
|---|---|---|
| ◆ Lying on the right side with the knees tucked up under the chin<br>◆ From eating and sleeping<br>◆ From exercise<br>◆ From hot compresses | ◆ From cold<br>◆ Near tobacco smoke<br>◆ From mental exertion<br>◆ In the early morning and evening | **Sepia – see pp. 70–1**<br>*Take 30c every hour for up to 10 doses.* |
| ◆ From fresh air | ◆ In warm rooms<br>◆ Near tobacco smoke<br>◆ In the evening and at night | **Aconite – see p. 82**<br>*Take 30c every 12 hours for up to 14 days.* |
| ◆ From eating<br>◆ After urinating<br>◆ With heat | ◆ From fresh air<br>◆ From cold<br>◆ From being overdressed<br>◆ From coffee, alcohol, and tobacco smoke<br>◆ Near strong smells<br>◆ In the morning<br>◆ After meals | **Ignatia – see pp. 58–9**<br>*Take 30c every 12 hours for up to 14 days.* |
| ◆ From eating<br>◆ With sleep<br>◆ From exercise<br>◆ From hot compresses applied to the affected area<br>◆ In stormy weather | ◆ Before menstruation<br>◆ From cold<br>◆ Near tobacco smoke<br>◆ From mental fatigue<br>◆ In hot, damp conditions<br>◆ In the early morning and evening<br>◆ Before a thunderstorm | **Sepia – see pp. 70–1**<br>*Take 30c every 12 hours for up to 7 days.* |
| ◆ In the morning<br>◆ When slightly constipated | ◆ In a draft<br>◆ In cold, damp, windy weather<br>◆ From exertion<br>◆ Between 2 a.m. and 3 a.m. | **Calc. carb. – see pp. 54–5**<br>*Take 30c every 12 hours for up to 7 days.* |
| ◆ At the onset of menstruation | ◆ From touch<br>◆ After a hot or warm bath<br>◆ From hot drinks<br>◆ With sleep<br>◆ On waking | **Lachesis – see pp. 78–9**<br>*Take 30c every 12 hours for up to 7 days.* |

# PREGNANCY & BIRTH

It is good to treat the baby inside you as a person right from the start. Eat well, get regular exercise, avoid becoming stressed and tired, and do not smoke or drink alcohol. Avoid all drugs and nutritional supplements during the first 14 weeks of pregnancy. There is no evidence that homeopathic remedies can cause the slightest problem in pregnancy, but it is safer to take them only if necessary.

**MORNING SICKNESS** is very common and is due to changes in hormone levels in pregnancy. It ends by weeks 14–16, although a few women go on to develop severe vomiting that can be harmful to both mother and baby.

**HEARTBURN** is a burning pain in the center of the chest and is due to hormones that cause the muscles around the entrance of the stomach to relax, allowing acid to back up into the esophagus. Heartburn is worse in late pregnancy when the uterus presses on the stomach.

**CRAMPS** that mainly affect the legs are common during pregnancy and may occur during the day as well as at night. They may interfere with sleep, which can lead to exhaustion.

**BREAST PAIN** and swelling of the breasts is very common in the first few months of pregnancy as hormone levels increase, and in the last two or three months as the milk comes in. Inflammation of the breast tissue (mastitis) may occur because of an infection.

**FREQUENT URINATION** is caused by pressure from the uterus on the bladder, urethra, and pelvic floor muscles, and is aggravated if the pelvic floor muscles are weak and by wearing tight clothes.

**LABOR PAIN** varies enormously and women react to it in different ways. Homeopathy helps to allay the pain and exhaustion of labor and to calm emotions such as fear, anger, and anxiety that occur during the various stages of labor.

## MORNING SICKNESS

| AILMENT | SYMPTOMS | CAUSE & ONSET |
|---|---|---|
| **NAUSEA WITH IRRITABILITY** | ❑ Nausea worse in the morning ❑ Small amounts of food with mucus in it are vomited ❑ Dry mouth and thickly coated tongue ❑ Spasms of retching ❑ A craving for very fresh food or fatty, spicy, sour foods, or alcohol, and a particular dislike of bread, meat, coffee, and tobacco. | • *Comes on in the morning* |
| **NAUSEA WITH TEARFULNESS** | ❑ Nausea worse during early evening, but wears off later in the night ❑ Dry mouth with lack of thirst ❑ Rich or fatty foods, especially pork, cause digestive upset ❑ A sensation of pressure under the breastbone after meals ❑ A craving for sweet foods ❑ Rumbling and gurgling in the stomach. | • *Comes on in the evening* |
| **CONSTANT NAUSEA WITH VOMITING** | ❑ Liquids and solids alike are vomited ❑ Nausea is not eased by vomiting ❑ Tongue feels clean rather than thickly coated ❑ Excessive saliva production ❑ Lack of thirst ❑ Possible fainting spells. | • *Bending forward* |

**BREASTFEEDING PROBLEMS** can result from painful, distended breasts that develop if the baby suddenly stops feeding. The pain may also be due to inflammation of breast tissue (mastitis) caused by a blocked milk duct or an infection, an abscess, or breast engorgement.

## PRECAUTIONS

During pregnancy, take homeopathic remedies or tissue salts only if absolutely necessary and do not take remedies in potencies less than 6c, for example 3c. Avoid the *Apis* remedy below 30c during pregnancy.

**Morning sickness** If vomiting occurs after nearly every meal, see a doctor.

**Breast pain** If there is a fever and/or swollen, tender glands under the arms, see a doctor.

**Frequent urination** If this is associated with pain for more than 48 hours or frequency continues for more than 3 days, see a doctor.

**Breastfeeding problems** If there is engorgement and/or hard breasts, pain, fever, and tender glands under the arms, see a doctor.

## SELF-HELP TREATMENTS

**Morning sickness** *Eat small meals frequently and avoid fatty foods. Try a dry cracker first thing in the morning and use fresh ginger in cooking. Get plenty of rest.*

**Heartburn** *Eat small meals often and avoid spicy and fried foods, tea, and coffee. If heartburn is worse at night raise the head of the bed by 4 in (10 cm) unless you have swollen ankles.*

**Cramps** *Take calcium, magnesium, potassium, and Mag. phos. tissue salts (see pp. 224–7).*

**Frequent urination** *Never suppress the urge to urinate. Urinate twice each time to ensure the bladder is empty. In late pregnancy, rocking backward and forward while urinating can help empty the bladder more fully.*

**Breastfeeding problems** *If the nipples are sore and cracked, bathe them after each feeding with arnica solution (10 drops arnica tincture to half a pint [300 ml] of boiled, cooled water). Dry the nipples thoroughly and apply calendula cream (see p. 227). Expose the nipples to air regularly and never wash them with soap.*

| YOU FEEL BETTER | YOU FEEL WORSE | REMEDY & DOSAGE |
|---|---|---|
| ◆ From warmth, sleep, and firm pressure on the stomach<br>◆ From washing or wet compresses on the stomach<br>◆ In the evening<br>◆ When left alone | ◆ In cold, windy weather<br>◆ From eating spicy foods<br>◆ From stimulants<br>◆ From stress<br>◆ Between 3 a.m. and 4 a.m. | **Nux vomica – see pp. 74–5**<br>*Take 6c every 2 hours for up to 3 days.*  |
| ◆ From cold drinks or a cold compress placed over the stomach<br>◆ From crying and sympathy<br>◆ Raising the hands above the head<br>◆ From gentle exercise<br>◆ From fresh air | ◆ In hot, stuffy rooms<br>◆ In the evening<br>◆ From rich, fatty foods<br>◆ Lying on the left side | **Pulsatilla – see pp. 68–9**<br>*Take 6c every 2 hours for up to 3 days.* |
| ◆ From fresh air | ◆ With movement<br>◆ With warmth<br>◆ Lying down<br>◆ From embarrassment or stress | **Ipecac. – see p. 91**<br>*Take 6c every 2 hours for up to 3 days.*  |

# HEARTBURN

| AILMENT | SYMPTOMS | CAUSE & ONSET |
|---|---|---|
| **HEARTBURN WITH A BURNING SENSATION BEHIND THE BREASTBONE** | ❏ Extreme thirst, but very trembly after drinking ❏ Marked passing of gas ❏ Burning on the tip of the tongue ❏ A craving for stimulants ❏ A sinking feeling in the pit of the stomach. | • *Drinking and eating* |
| **HEARTBURN WITH NAUSEA AND VOMITING** | ❏ A cold feeling in the pit of the stomach with a craving for carbonated drinks ❏ Mucus, bile, and food are vomited. | • *Sight or smell of food* |

# CRAMPS

| | | |
|---|---|---|
| **CRAMPS RELIEVED BY WALKING** | ❏ Cramps in the calves ❏ Associated vomiting and diarrhea ❏ Exhaustion. | • *Comes on during the daytime* |
| **CRAMPS RELIEVED BY REST** | ❏ Cramps in the calves and soles of the feet ❏ Numbness in the arms and hands ❏ Irritability ❏ Extremely critical of others. | • *Comes on in the morning* |

# BREAST PAIN

| | | |
|---|---|---|
| **BREAST PAIN DUE TO SWELLING** | ❏ Breasts are tender when touched ❏ Stitchlike pain in the nipples ❏ A desire to press the breasts hard with the hand ❏ Legs feel heavy. | • *Hormonal changes associated with early pregnancy* |
| **BREAST DISCOMFORT, WORSE WITH THE SLIGHTEST MOTION** | ❏ Breasts may be hard and inflamed, as if there is an abscess forming ❏ Associated splitting headache. | • *Hormonal changes associated with late pregnancy* • *Threatening breast abscess* |

# FREQUENT URINATION

| | | |
|---|---|---|
| **SMALL DRIBBLES OF URINE PASSED FREQUENTLY WITH GREAT DIFFICULTY** | ❏ Blood in urine due to straining ❏ Urethra and vulva feel itchy ❏ Irritability ❏ The greater the strain to pass urine, the less comes. | • *Spasm of the muscle at the neck of the bladder* |

| YOU FEEL BETTER | YOU FEEL WORSE | REMEDY & DOSAGE |
|---|---|---|
| ◆ With heat<br>◆ From eating, but it gives you heartburn | ◆ From fresh air<br>◆ After undressing<br>◆ In a draft<br>◆ After eating | **Capsicum – see pp. 122–3**<br>*Take 6c four times a day for up to 7 days.*  |
| ◆ Bending forward | ◆ At night<br>◆ With movement<br>◆ From lack of sleep<br>◆ From mental exertion | **Causticum – see p. 123**<br>*Take 6c four times a day for up to 7 days.*  |
| ◆ With warmth<br>◆ From walking | ◆ At night<br>◆ In wet, damp weather | **Verat. alb. – see p. 148**<br>*Take 6c every four hours for up to 7 days.* 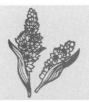 |
| ◆ With warmth, sleep, and firm pressure<br>◆ From washing or wet compresses over the calves and feet<br>◆ With rest<br>◆ In the evening | ◆ From cold<br>◆ From stimulants<br>◆ From eating<br>◆ If touched<br>◆ Between 3 a.m. and 4 a.m. | **Nux vomica – see pp. 74–5**<br>*Take 6c every four hours for up to 7 days.*  |
| ◆ From fasting<br>◆ From expressing emotion<br>◆ Letting the arms hang down | ◆ Lying down<br>◆ From turning over in bed<br>◆ From cold | **Conium – see p. 125**<br>*Take 6c every four hours for up to 5 days.*  |
| ◆ From cool air<br>◆ From firm, cool pressure applied to the breasts | ◆ With the slightest movement<br>◆ In the morning<br>◆ At 9 p.m. and 3 a.m.<br>◆ In cold, dry, windy weather | **Bryonia – see p. 88**<br>*Take 6c every four hours for up to 5 days.* 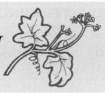 |
| ◆ From warmth, sleep, and firm pressure<br>◆ From washing or wet compresses over the bladder<br>◆ In the evening | ◆ In cold, windy weather<br>◆ From spicy food<br>◆ From stimulants<br>◆ Between 3 a.m. and 4 a.m. | **Nux vomica – see pp. 74–5**<br>*Take 6c every two hours for up to 3 days.*  |

**FREQUENT URINATION** *continued*

REMEDIES FOR COMMON AILMENTS

## FREQUENT URINATION *continued*

| AILMENT | SYMPTOMS | CAUSE & ONSET |
|---|---|---|
| **FREQUENT URINATION DUE TO WEAKENED PELVIC FLOOR MUSCLES** | ❏ Scalding sensation during and after urination ❏ Possible lack of thirst ❏ Tearfulness and self-pitying attitude. | • *Coughing or passing gas* |

## LABOR PAIN

| AILMENT | SYMPTOMS | CAUSE & ONSET |
|---|---|---|
| **UNBEARABLE PAIN THAT CAUSES UNCONTROLLABLE CRYING** | ❏ Contractions so painful that they cause involuntary screaming ❏ Nervousness and restlessness between contractions. | • *Particular sensitivity to pain* |
| **PAIN ASSOCIATED WITH A FREQUENT URGE TO PASS URINE OR A STOOL** | ❏ Contractions are ineffectual ❏ Pain extends into the rectum ❏ Irritability ❏ Impatience ❏ Extremely critical of others. | • *Spasm in the cervix because it will not dilate properly* |
| **LABOR PAIN WITH GREAT TEARFULNESS** | ❏ Labor that progresses slowly ❏ Restlessness ❏ Chills ❏ Apologetic attitude ❏ A tendency to whine. | • *Poor position of baby* <br> • *Maternal exhaustion* |

## BREASTFEEDING PROBLEMS

| AILMENT | SYMPTOMS | CAUSE & ONSET |
|---|---|---|
| **ENGORGEMENT OR HARDNESS OF THE BREASTS, WITH RED STREAKS ON THE SKIN** | ❏ Breasts are throbbing, swollen, and red ❏ Breasts feel heavy ❏ Skin is hot and dry. | • *Mastitis with possible developing breast abscess* |
| **SORE, CRACKED NIPPLES** | ❏ Nipples inflamed and very tender to the touch ❏ Baby's suckling unbearable, and mother becomes angry, spiteful, rude, and complaining. | • *Not cleaning nipples properly* <br> • *Baby does not latch on correctly* |

| YOU FEEL BETTER | YOU FEEL WORSE | REMEDY & DOSAGE |
|---|---|---|
| • Raising the hands above the head<br>• From gentle exercise<br>• From fresh air<br>• From cold drinks or cold compresses<br>• From crying and sympathy | • With heat<br>• Lying down<br>• In the evening<br>• At night | **Pulsatilla – see pp. 68–9**<br>*Take 6c every 2 hours for up to 3 days.*  |
| • With warmth<br>• Lying down<br>• From sucking ice | • From excessive emotions, even joy<br>• Near strong smells<br>• Near noise<br>• From fresh air<br>• From cold<br>• At night | **Coffea – see p. 125**<br>*Take 30c every 5 minutes for up to 10 doses.*  |
| • With warmth, sleep, and firm pressure<br>• From washing, a warm bath, or wet compresses<br>• In the evening<br>• When left alone | • From cold<br>• Near noise<br>• From stimulants<br>• From eating<br>• From stress | **Nux vomica – see pp. 74–5**<br>*Take 30c every 5 minutes for up to 10 doses.*  |
| • From crying and sympathy<br>• Raising the hands above the head<br>• With gentle movement<br>• From fresh air<br>• From cold drinks<br>• From cold compresses | • With heat<br>• With extremes of temperature<br>• Lying on the painful side<br>• In the evening and at night | **Pulsatilla – see pp. 68–9**<br>*Take 30c every 5 minutes for up to 10 doses.*  |
| • Standing or sitting upright<br>• In warm rooms<br>• From warm compresses applied to the breasts | • With jarring or movement<br>• Near noise<br>• From pressure<br>• Lying down, especially on the right side<br>• At night | **Belladonna – see p. 86**<br>*Take 30c every hour for up to 10 doses.* 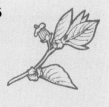 |
| • No specific factors | • With heat<br>• At night | **Chamomilla – see pp. 134–5**<br>*Take 30c every 4 hours for up to 6 doses.*  |

# CHILDHOOD COMPLAINTS

Homeopathy is extremely popular with parents, since it offers them a way to treat their children for common illnesses without the side effects of some orthodox medicines. Homeopathy works very well in children because their immune system is so responsive and generally, they are not worn down by stress, chronically bad diet, or too many antibiotics or other drugs. Childhood illnesses test the vital force (see pp. 18–19), thereby preparing the immune system to cope with more serious illnesses later.

COLIC (spasm in the intestines) is most common in the first three months. Colicky babies pull up their legs, scream, and turn red. The problem is thought to be caused by swallowing air, dehydration, a mother's anxiety, or something passed through the breast milk (wheat, cabbage, dairy products, and citrus fruits are common culprits).

SLEEPLESSNESS in babies may be due to hunger, gas, colic, a dirty diaper, teething, anger, overstimulation, or being cold. In older children it may be due to irregular bedtimes, being too hot or cold, a stuffy bedroom, overtiredness, too much caffeine from cola drinks, food allergy, noise, stress, or anxiety.

TEETHING PROBLEMS result in sore gums, fever, irritability, and diarrhea caused by the stress of pain. Never assume that fever is due to teething pain rather than an infection.

DIAPER RASH is often due to irritation from ammonia released as a result of the reaction between urine and feces, or detergent residue in cloth diapers. The skin on the buttocks, thighs, and genitals becomes sore, red, blotchy, and oozing.

BEDWETTING can occur because the nervous system function that regulates bladder control is not yet fully developed. A child who has been dry during the night may start to wet the bed again because of anxiety, a scare or shock, food allergy, coughing, or a urinary tract infection.

## COLIC IN BABIES

| AILMENT | SYMPTOMS | CAUSE & ONSET |
|---|---|---|
| BABY'S KNEES ARE PULLED UP TO THE CHIN | ❏ Irritability ❏ Angry crying. | • *Swallowing air during feeding* |
| SUDDEN SHOOTING PAINS MANIFESTED BY SHARP MOVEMENTS AND CRYING | ❏ Bloated stomach ❏ Pain not relieved by burping. | • *Gas*<br>• *Sudden onset* |
| COLIC WITH SCREAMING AT THE SLIGHTEST MOVEMENT | ❏ Sudden sharp pains brought on by the slightest movement ❏ Stools are dry ❏ Mouth is dry. | • *Dehydration* |
| VIOLENT COLIC WITH ANGRY CRYING | ❏ Irritability ❏ The baby is impossible to calm unless picked up and carried. | • *Anger* |

**FEVER** is usually a sign that the body is fighting an infection. Symptoms include restlessness, hot skin, and a raised temperature. Anything that weakens the immune system, such as exposure to cold, makes infection more likely.

**GLUE EAR** is a buildup of sticky fluid in the middle ear, which can impair hearing. It is usually caused by a chronic infection, but may be due to allergies or exposure to drafts.

## PRECAUTIONS

**Colic** If the baby cries abnormally, becomes pale, limp, or develops vomiting or diarrhea, see a doctor.

**Bedwetting** If you suspect a urinary infection, see a doctor within 48 hours.

**Fever** If associated with breathing difficulties, coughing, convulsions, irritability, unusual drowsiness, high-pitched crying, headache, or intolerance of light, or if the temperature does not drop below 102° F (39° C), see a doctor.

If there is diarrhea, vomiting, a stiff neck, or a purple rash, or the child is pulling on the ear, see a doctor immediately.

## SELF-HELP TREATMENTS

**Colic** *If bottlefeeding, enlarge the hole in the nipple. If the mother is exhausted from breastfeeding, she should increase her fluid intake and get some rest.*

**Sleeplessness** *Try to put the baby to bed at roughly the same time each day. The room temperature should be around 64–68° F (16–20° C). Avoid overexcitement before bedtime and give the baby a feeding.*
*If an older child seems tired and then becomes very energetic and wakes frequently during the night, make the bedtime earlier by 15 minutes every 3 nights. Avoid late meals and give the child a relaxing, warm bath before bed.*

**Teething problems** *Give Calc. fluor. and Calc. phos. or Combination R tissue salts throughout the teething period (see p. 227).*

**Diaper rash** *Wash the affected area with calendula and hypericum solution, dry well, and then apply calendula cream (see p. 227). Change the diaper more frequently.*

**Fever** *Sponge the child's face, arms, legs, and body with tepid water, then pat dry with a towel. Repeat 6 times and again after 2 hours. Give the child plenty to drink.*

| CHILD FEELS BETTER | CHILD FEELS WORSE | REMEDY & DOSAGE |
|---|---|---|
| • From gentle pressure on the stomach<br>• With warmth and sleep<br>• From passing gas | • From being fed<br>• Around 4 p.m. | **Colocynthis – see p. 94** *Give 6c every 5 minutes for up to 10 doses.* 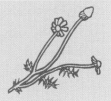 |
| • With warmth<br>• From gentle pressure on the stomach | • Lying on the right side<br>• At night and if touched<br>• After being undressed<br>• If the stomach gets cold | **Mag. phos. – see p. 134** *Give 6c every 5 minutes for up to 10 doses.* 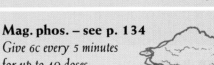 |
| • With rest<br>• From cool air<br>• With cold compresses | • From noise and bright light<br>• In the morning<br>• At 9 p.m. and 3 a.m. | **Bryonia – see p. 88** *Give 30c every 5 minutes for up to 30 doses.* 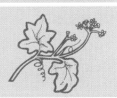 |
| • With movement | • From heat<br>• After burping<br>• At night | **Chamomilla – see pp. 134–5** *Give 6c every 5 minutes for up to 10 doses.* 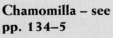 |

## SLEEPLESSNESS

| AILMENT | SYMPTOMS | CAUSE & ONSET |
|---|---|---|
| SLEEPLESSNESS WITH IRRITABILITY AND ANGER IN BABIES | ❑ Eyes are half open when asleep ❑ Moaning during sleep ❑ The baby is impossible to calm when awake. | • *Anger*<br>• *Teething* |
| SLEEPLESSNESS DUE TO OVER-EXCITEMENT IN OLDER CHILDREN | ❑ Overstimulated state that prevents sleep ❑ Waking up in excited state and starting to play with toys. | • *Too much stimulation and excitement* |

## TEETHING PROBLEMS

| AILMENT | SYMPTOMS | CAUSE & ONSET |
|---|---|---|
| TEETHING WITH ONE CHEEK HOT AND RED AND THE OTHER PALE | ❑ Irritability and anger ❑ The baby is soothed only by being carried ❑ The baby is fussy when put back in the crib ❑ Acutely inflamed gums that are sore when touched ❑ Offensive diarrhea may be caused by the pain. | • *Teething pain* |
| TEETHING WITH HOT FLUSHED FACE AND WIDE STARING PUPILS | ❑ Restlessness ❑ High fever indicated by wide, staring eyes and hot, flushed face ❑ Swollen gums ❑ Hot, dry mouth. | • *Inflamed gums*<br>• *Sudden onset* |
| TEETHING WITH ACUTE PAIN | ❑ The baby seems frightened by the severity of the pain ❑ Sore, inflamed gums ❑ Restlessness ❑ Tossing and turning even when asleep. | • *Sudden onset* |

## DIAPER RASH

| AILMENT | SYMPTOMS | CAUSE & ONSET |
|---|---|---|
| DRY, RED, SCALY DIAPER RASH | ❑ The baby may generally suffer from dry skin ❑ Skin around the diaper area is dry, red and irritated. | • *Sensitive skin with a reaction to the germs on the skin in the diaper area* |
| DIAPER RASH WITH LITTLE BLISTERS | ❑ Skin is very itchy ❑ Blisters around the diaper area ❑ Restlessness. | • *A reaction to the detergent used to clean diapers* |

| CHILD FEELS BETTER | CHILD FEELS WORSE | REMEDY & DOSAGE |
|---|---|---|
| ◆ Being carried<br>◆ In warm, wet weather | ◆ From being overheated<br>◆ In cold, windy weather<br>◆ After burping<br>◆ At night, from 9 p.m. onward | **Chamomilla – see pp. 134–5**<br>*Give 30c every 30 minutes starting one hour before bedtime, and every 30 minutes if the child wakes up, for up to 10 doses.* 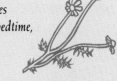 |
| ◆ With warmth<br>◆ Lying down | ◆ From too much excitement<br>◆ From sleeping in a draft<br>◆ Near noise<br>◆ From cold<br>◆ Near strong smells | **Coffea – p. 125**<br>*Give 6c every 30 minutes starting one hour before bedtime, and every 30 minutes if the child wakes up, for up to 10 doses.*  |
| ◆ Being carried | ◆ From anger<br>◆ From heat<br>◆ From fresh air<br>◆ At night, from 9 p.m. onward | **Chamomilla – see pp. 134–5**<br>*Give 30c every 30 minutes, or more frequently if pain is severe, for up to 10 doses.* 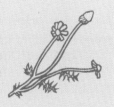 |
| ◆ With warmth | ◆ From jarring, motion, light, and noise<br>◆ From pressure on the gums<br>◆ Lying down<br>◆ At night | **Belladonna – see p. 86**<br>*Give 30c every 30 minutes or more frequently if pain is severe, for up to 10 doses.*  |
| ◆ From fresh air | ◆ In warm rooms<br>◆ Lying on the painful side<br>◆ In the evening and at night | **Aconite – see p. 82**<br>*Give 30c every 30 minutes or more frequently if pain is severe, for up to 10 doses.* 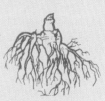 |
| ◆ From fresh air<br>◆ When warm and dry | ◆ From wearing too many clothes<br>◆ From being washed<br>◆ From being too warm and from heat | **Sulfur – see pp. 76–7**<br>*Give 6c 4 times a day for up to 5 days.* 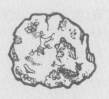 |
| ◆ Changing position<br>◆ When warm and dry | ◆ From being undressed | **Rhus tox. – see p. 108**<br>*Give 6c 4 times a day for up to 5 days.* 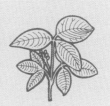 |

## BEDWETTING

| AILMENT | SYMPTOMS | CAUSE & ONSET |
|---|---|---|
| **BEDWETTING DURING DREAMS** | ❑ Urination during dreams or nightmares. | • *Nervous system function not yet fully developed (see p. 214)* |
| **BEDWETTING SOON AFTER FALLING ASLEEP** | ❑ Bedwetting often occurs in excitable, outgoing children who get very involved with everything and are oversensitive and deeply concerned about injustice. | • *Coughing*<br>• *Emotional stress*<br>• *After the death of a loved one*<br>• *A severe scare* |

## FEVER

| AILMENT | SYMPTOMS | CAUSE & ONSET |
|---|---|---|
| **FEVER WITH ASSOCIATED FEAR** | ❑ Pale face ❑ Restlessness ❑ Thirst. | • *Exposure to cold, dry, windy weather*<br>• *Sudden onset* |
| **FEVER WITH HOT, FLUSHED FACE AND STARING EYES** | ❑ Violent fever with pounding pulse<br>❑ Dry, hot skin. | • *Sudden onset* |
| **FEVER IN THE EARLY STAGES OF INFECTION** | ❑ Red cheeks ❑ Weak, rapid pulse ❑ Profuse sweating ❑ Shivering ❑ Throbbing headache. | • *Gradual onset* |
| **FEVER WITH ASSOCIATED ANXIETY** | ❑ Restlessness ❑ Chills and exhaustion ❑ Burning pain in the limbs ❑ Thirst for small, frequent sips of warm drinks. | • *Especially found in infections involving the gastrointestinal system* |

## GLUE EAR

| AILMENT | SYMPTOMS | CAUSE & ONSET |
|---|---|---|
| **GLUE EAR WITH SWOLLEN NECK GLANDS** | ❑ Possible discharge from the ear ❑ Pain or sensation of fullness in the ear ❑ Swollen neck glands ❑ A tendency to occur in overweight children. | • *Exposure to a draft and cold, windy weather* |
| **GLUE EAR WITH THICK, STRINGY MUCUS** | ❑ Mucus drips down the throat from the sinuses ❑ Pain or sensation of fullness in the ear ❑ Dull ache at the top of the nose. | • *Tendency to catch cold* |

| CHILD FEELS BETTER | CHILD FEELS WORSE | REMEDY & DOSAGE |
|---|---|---|
| ◆ From a nap | ◆ Lying on the right side<br>◆ With movement<br>◆ With pressure<br>◆ From being touched | **Equisetum – see p. 128**<br>*Give 6c once at bedtime for up to 14 nights.* |
| ◆ In warm, damp weather | ◆ In cold, dry weather<br>◆ From eating candy | **Causticum – see p. 123**<br>*Give 6c once at bedtime for up to 14 nights.* |
| ◆ From fresh air | ◆ In warm rooms<br>◆ Near tobacco smoke<br>◆ At midnight | **Aconite – see p. 82**<br>*Give 30c every hour for up to 10 doses.* |
| ◆ Standing or sitting upright<br>◆ With warmth | ◆ With jarring and movement<br>◆ From light, noise, and pressure<br>◆ Lying on the right side<br>◆ At night | **Belladonna – see p. 86**<br>*Give 30c every hour for up to 10 doses.* |
| ◆ From applying cold compresses to the head<br>◆ From gentle exercise | ◆ With jarring, movement, and touch<br>◆ Lying on the right side<br>◆ From being overheated<br>◆ Between 4 a.m. and 6 a.m. | **Ferrum phos. – see p. 98**<br>*Give 30c every hour for up to 10 doses.* |
| ◆ From being hot<br>◆ From applying cold compresses to the head<br>◆ From warm drinks<br>◆ Lying down with the head propped up | ◆ Near the smell or sight of food<br>◆ From cold food and drinks<br>◆ In cold, windy weather<br>◆ Between midnight and 2 a.m. | **Arsen. alb. – see pp. 52–3**<br>*Give 6c every hour for up to 10 doses.* |
| ◆ When slightly constipated<br>◆ Lying on the affected side | ◆ From exertion<br>◆ Between 2 a.m. and 3 a.m. | **Calc. carb. – see pp. 54–5**<br>*Give 6c 3 times a day for up to 14 days.* |
| ◆ With warmth | ◆ In the morning<br>◆ In hot weather | **Kali bich. – see p. 103**<br>*Give 6c 3 times a day for up to 14 days.* |

# FIRST AID

Homeopathic remedies can play an important part in accidents and emergencies, especially in the treatment of minor flesh wounds. Their purpose is to relieve pain, calm the mind, and help the body heal itself.

For minor injuries, follow the guidelines for essential treatment and choose the appropriate remedy from the alternatives given, but in a serious accident, the overriding priority is to get expert help as soon as possible.

## HOMEOPATHIC FIRST-AID KIT

If stored in a dark, dry, cool place, homeopathic remedies will keep their strength for years. Always keep them out of the reach of children.

**FIRST-AID REMEDIES**
**Dosage** For acute first-aid complaints use 30c potency remedies. For less acute first-aid ailments use 6c potency. Dosages are suitable for babies, children, and adults. Before taking a remedy, rinse the mouth with water.

Keep the following homeopathic remedies for minor first-aid emergencies.

• Arnica 6c, 30c
*Arnica* is the most valuable remedy to have in the first-aid kit. It is available as

## FIRST-AID PROCEDURE

| CUTS & ABRASIONS | KEY FEATURES | REMEDY & DOSAGE |
|---|---|---|
| If there is bleeding from a minor cut or abrasion, infection may occur because of the break in the skin. There may also be bruising. | ❑ Wound has moderate to severe bruising. | **Arnica – see p. 85** *Take 30c every 2 hours for up to 6 doses, then 3 times a day for up to 3 days.*  |
| **ESSENTIAL TREATMENT** • Clean the wound well with sterile gauze soaked in calendula and hypericum solution • Apply calendula cream • Cover minor cuts and abrasions with a sterile dressing; leave in place for 2–3 days. | ❑ Wound feels numb and cold ❑ Applying a cold compress soothes the wound. | **Ledum – see p. 105** *Take 6c every 2 hours for up to 6 doses, then 3 times a day for up to 3 days.* 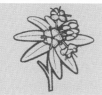 |
| | ❑ Wound with shooting nerve pain. | **Hypericum – see p. 102** *Take 30c every 2 hours for up to 3 days.* 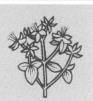 |

| MINOR BURNS & SCALDS | KEY FEATURES | REMEDY & DOSAGE |
|---|---|---|
| Minor burns and scalds are painful; avoid touching them more than necessary. | ❑ Burn may form a blister ❑ Searing, smarting pain ❑ Applying a cold compress soothes the burn or scald. | **Arnica – see p. 85** *Take 30c every 15 minutes for up to 3 doses.*  FOLLOWED BY |
| **ESSENTIAL TREATMENT** • Immerse the wound in cold running water to cool the skin and reduce pain • Apply urtica ointment to soothe superficial burns. | | **Cantharis – see p. 107** *Take 30c every 15 minutes for up to 6 doses.* 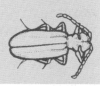 |
| **CAUTION** If a burn is bigger than the palm of a hand, see a doctor immediately. | ❑ Continuous stinging pain from the burn or scald. | **Urtica – see p. 111** *Take 6c every 15 minutes for up to 10 doses.*  |

tablets, a cream, or tincture. Emotionally, it helps steady the nerves after injury and physically, it reduces swelling and heals bruised tissues.
• **Apis** 30c (*Do not take the Apis remedy below 30c during pregnancy.*)
• **Bryonia** 30c
• **Cantharis** 6c, 30c
• **Euphrasia** 6c
• **Gloinon.** 30c
• **Hypericum** 30c
• **Ledum** 6c

• **Nux vomica** 6c
• **Phos.** 6c
• **Rhus tox.** 6c
• **Ruta grav.** 6c
• **Silica** 6c
• **Tabacum** 6c
• **Urtica** 6c

### CREAMS & OINTMENTS
Homeopathic and herbal creams and ointments are identical and can be bought ready-made.
• **Arnica** cream (*Do not apply to broken skin.*)

• **Calendula** cream
• **Urtica** ointment.

### TINCTURES
Homeopathic tinctures are the same as herbal tinctures and can be bought ready-made.
• **Arnica** tincture (*Do not apply to broken skin.*)
• **Calendula** tincture and **hypericum** tincture
*To make calendula and hypericum solution, add 10 drops each of calendula and hypericum*

*tinctures to 2 pints (1.25 liters) of boiled, cooled water.*
• **Euphrasia** tincture
*To make euphrasia solution, add 10 drops euphrasia tincture to 2 pints (1.25 liters) of boiled, cooled water.*
• **Pyrethrum** tincture

### BACH RESCUE REMEDY
Rescue Remedy is a tincture that is good for nervousness and trembling, worry or panic. Take the dose recommended on the pack.

## FIRST-AID PROCEDURE

| INSECT STINGS | KEY FEATURES | REMEDY & DOSAGE |
|---|---|---|
| Insect stings cause pain, swelling, and sometimes infection. | ❏ Sting is swollen, bruised, and painful. | **Arnica – see p. 85** *Take 30c every 5 minutes for up to 10 doses* 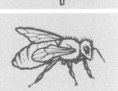 |
| **ESSENTIAL TREATMENT** • Remove wasp or bee stingers with sterilized tweezers • Apply pyrethrum tincture to the sting. | | FOLLOWED BY <br> **Ledum – see p. 105** *Take 6c every 8 hours for up to 3 days.* 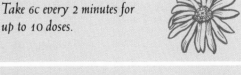 |
| **CAUTION** If a sting is inside the mouth, rinse the mouth with ice water to prevent swelling and see a doctor. | ❏ Sting is hot, red, and swollen. | **Apis – see p. 84** *Take 30c every 15 minutes for up to 6 doses.*  |

| NOSEBLEEDS | KEY FEATURES | REMEDY & DOSAGE |
|---|---|---|
| Nosebleeds occur after an injury to the nose or may be brought on by blowing the nose violently. | ❏ Nosebleed after an injury. | **Arnica – see p. 85** *Take 6c every 2 minutes for up to 10 doses.* |
| **ESSENTIAL TREATMENT** • To stop bleeding, sit down with the head well forward and pinch the lower part of the nostrils firmly for 10 minutes, then release slowly. | ❏ Nosebleed brought on by blowing the nose violently. | **Phos. – see pp. 66–7** *Take 6c every 2 minutes for up to 10 doses.* |
| **CAUTION** If bleeding persists, see a doctor. | | |

# FIRST-AID PROCEDURE

## HEAT EXHAUSTION

Heat exhaustion is caused by excessive fluid loss in hot, humid weather.

**ESSENTIAL TREATMENT**
• Lay the person in a cool place
• Give frequent sips of salty water (1 teaspoon/5ml of salt per 1 ³/₄ pints/liter water).

### KEY FEATURES

❑ Severe headache that is aggravated by the slightest movement ❑ Nausea.

❑ Throbbing, splitting headache ❑ Hot face ❑ Sweaty skin.

### REMEDY & DOSAGE

**Bryonia – see p. 88**
*Take 30c every 5 minutes for up to 10 doses.*

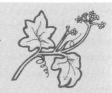

**Glonoin. – see pp. 129–30**
*Take 30c every 5 minutes for up to 10 doses.*

## MOTION SICKNESS

The balance mechanism of the inner ear can be upset by the motion of a car, boat, train, or airplane, causing motion sickness. Children are especially vulnerable.

**Note** Homeopathic remedies can also be taken one hour before starting a journey to help prevent motion sickness.

### KEY FEATURES

❑ Nausea ❑ Dizziness and faintness ❑ Chills ❑ Sweating ❑ Sensation of a tight band around the head ❑ Worse near tobacco smoke.

❑ Queasiness ❑ Chills ❑ Headache at the back of the head or over one eye ❑ Worse from food, tobacco smoke, and coffee.

### REMEDY & DOSAGE

**Tabacum – see p. 138**
*Take 6c every 15 minutes for up to 10 doses.*

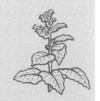

**Nux vomica – see pp. 74–5**
*Take 6c every 15 minutes for up to 10 doses.*

## SPLINTERS

Since splinters break the skin, infection can result.

**ESSENTIAL TREATMENT**
• Remove the splinter with sterilized tweezers.

**CAUTION** If not inoculated against tetanus, see a doctor.

### KEY FEATURES

❑ Stinging, burning pain ❑ Applying a warm compress may help draw the splinter to the skin's surface.

### REMEDY & DOSAGE

**Silica – see pp. 72–3**
*Take 6c 4 times a day for up to 14 days.*

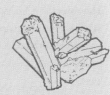

## BLISTERS

Blisters are bubbles of fluid that form under the skin as a result of friction or burns.

**ESSENTIAL TREATMENT**
• If the blister bursts, bathe it with calendula and hypericum solution.

### KEY FEATURES

❑ Blister is burning and itchy ❑ Applying a cold compress soothes affected part.

❑ Blister is extremely itchy, red, and swollen.

### REMEDY & DOSAGE

**Cantharis – see p. 107**
*Take 6c 4 times a day until the pain subsides.*

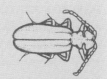

**Rhus tox. – see p. 108**
*Take 6c 4 times a day until the pain subsides.*

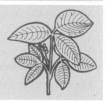

# FIRST-AID PROCEDURE

| EYE INJURIES | KEY FEATURES | REMEDY & DOSAGE |
|---|---|---|

The surface of the eye is very delicate and easily damaged by pressure, injury, and foreign objects.

**ESSENTIAL TREATMENT**
• Gently wash dust and grit from the eye with cold water
• To prevent infection, bathe the eye with calendula and hypericum solution
• If there is still pain after removing an object, bathe the eye with euphrasia solution every four hours.

**CAUTION** All eye injuries should be examined by a doctor. If there is a chemical in the eye or it has been penetrated by a sharp object, call an ambulance.

❑ Bruising around the eye immediately after injury
❑ Black eye.

**Arnica – see p. 85**
*Take 6c every 2 hours for up to 4 doses.*

❑ Black eye ❑ Persistent pain that is eased by applying a cold compress.

**Ledum – see p. 105**
*Take 6c every 2 hours for up to 10 doses.*

❑ Persistent pain after removing a foreign object.

**Euphrasia – see p. 97**
*Take 6c every 2 hours for up to 3 doses.*

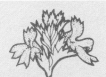

| SPRAINS & STRAINS | KEY FEATURES | REMEDY & DOSAGE |
|---|---|---|

Sprains, caused by over-stretching the ligaments, which bind the joints together, can be mild or severe. Strains (also due to overstretching) affect the muscles. In both, symptoms include swelling, stiffness, and pain whenever the joint or muscle is used.

**ESSENTIAL TREATMENT**
• Support the injury in the most comfortable position
• To reduce swelling, apply a cold compress soaked in cold water and 10 drops arnica tincture
• If the ankle is sprained, bandage it firmly and apply arnica cream.

**CAUTION** If pain and swelling are not relieved, see a doctor.

❑ Pulled tendons and ligaments ❑ Pain and stiffness.

**Arnica – see. p. 85**
*Take 30c every 30 minutes for up to 10 doses.*

**FOLLOWED BY**

**Ruta grav. – see p. 109**
*Take 6c 4 times a day until pain and stiffness subside.*

❑ Torn muscles ❑ Hot, swollen joints ❑ Pain is worse on starting to move, but wears off with continued movement.

**Arnica – see. p. 85**
*Take 30c every 30 minutes for up to 10 doses.*

**FOLLOWED BY**

**Rhus tox. – see p. 108**
*Take 6c 4 times a day until pain and stiffness subside.*

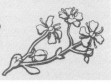

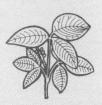

# NUTRITION, SUPPLEMENTS & OTHER USEFUL REMEDIES

*Many ailments can be prevented or improved by alterations to the diet, extra nutrients, and other remedies. In the Remedies for Common Ailments section (see pp. 152–219) nutritional supplements, tissue salts, and herbal and homeopathic ointments and tinctures are recommended in the*

*Self-help Treatment boxes. Profiles of the supplements and other remedies recommended in this section are given on the following pages. Supplements are recommended for specific ailments, and each entry lists information about the source, function, and dosage, where applicable.*

## NUTRITION & SUPPLEMENTS

A well-balanced diet should provide enough of the various nutrients that are normally needed for good health. But when illness occurs, the body may require certain extra nutrients. These are best obtained by increasing the intake of specific foods, but they can also be gained from nutritional supplements. The supplement dosage listed here is for specific ailments; it is not a daily recommended dosage.

## IMPORTANT NOTES
• Never exceed the stated recommended dose of any supplement. Dosage information on supplement packs varies enormously, so be sure to read the packaging carefully and, if in doubt, ask a doctor or a trained nutritionist.
• If taken in excess, water-soluble vitamins, such as vitamins B and C, are naturally excreted, whereas fat-soluble vitamins, namely, A, D, E, and K, accumulate and may cause tissue damage.
• Unless otherwise indicated, the recommended dosages are unsuitable for children.
• Avoid taking nutritional supplements during the first 14 weeks of pregnancy unless recommended to do so by a doctor.
• In general, unless otherwise stated, take a supplement for one month and, if it proves beneficial, continue taking it 5 days a week for another month. After this stop, and consult a doctor or a trained nutritionist.

❑ **ACIDOPHILUS**
**Found in** Live yogurt.
**Function** Provides a colony of healthful bacteria to repopulate the intestinal flora; especially needed when these bacteria have been killed off by antibiotics, resulting in diarrhea or candidiasis.
**Usage and dosage** For diarrhea and thrush, follow the dose recommended on the pack. Children may take half the adult dose for 2 weeks.

**Caution** Long-term use of supplements may be harmful. After 1 month stop taking supplements on weekends and discontinue dosage after 3–4 months.

❑ **BETA-CAROTENE**
**Function** Has the same function and sources as vitamin A; beneficial in the treatment of chronic fatigue syndrome (see *Vitamin A*).
**Usage and dosage** For chronic fatigue syndrome, take 4,500 mcg.

**Caution** If pregnant or planning a pregnancy, do not take beta-carotene except under the supervision of a doctor.

❑ **BIOFLAVONOIDS**
**Found in** Foods containing vitamin C, including raw fruit and vegetables, especially citrus fruit, and new potatoes, kidney, and liver.
**Function** Enhances vitamin C activity and acts as an antiviral agent.
**Usage and dosage** For cold sores, depression, heavy menstruation, anger and irritability, and varicose veins, follow the dose recommended on the pack.

❑ **BIOTIN**
**Found in** Dairy products, whole-grain cereals, and meat.
**Function** Helps prevent growth of fungi.
**Usage and dosage** For depression and insomnia, take 200 mcg a day.

❑ **CALCIUM**
**Found in** Spinach, parsley, milk, cheese, sesame seeds, whole-grain bread, navy beans, almonds, broccoli, turnips, hard water, and fish, including herring roe.
**Function** A component of bones, teeth, muscles, nerves, and blood; particularly needed by growing children, and by older women to prevent osteoporosis.

**Usage and dosage** For anxiety, anger, cramps in pregnancy, depression, heavy or painful menstruation, prostate enlargement, and rheumatism, take 500 mg a day; for menopause, take up to 1,000 mg a day.
**Caution** If pregnant, take calcium supplements only under the supervision of a doctor.

❑ **COD LIVER OIL**
**Found in** Cod liver.
**Function** Supplies vitamin A (q.v.) and vitamin D (q.v.).
**Usage and dosage** For osteoarthritis follow the dose recommended on the pack.

❑ **COPPER**
**Found in** Kidney, liver, nuts, shellfish, cocoa, fruit with pits, for example, cherries, and water.
**Function** Essential for bone growth and healthy blood cells.
**Usage and dosage** Consult a doctor if suffering from osteoarthritis or chronic fatigue syndrome, for which supplements are occasionally recommended. Most people get adequate copper from the many foods that contain it and in the water from copper pipes.
**Caution** Avoid excessive amounts if depressed.

❑ **CRANBERRY JUICE**
**Function** Reduces the ability of bacteria to adhere to the lining of the bladder and urinary tract.
**Usage and dosage** For cystitis, drink a glass daily as long as the condition lasts.

❑ **EPA MARINE OILS**
**Found in** Fish, especially oily fish, such as mackerel.
**Function** Strengthens the cell walls; necessary for the production of prostaglandins (fatty acids), which act against inflammation.
**Usage and dosage** For chronic fatigue syndrome, follow the dose recommended on the pack.
**Caution** Do not take EPA marine oils without a doctor's knowledge if you have a bleeding disorder.

❑ **EVENING PRIMROSE OIL**
**Found in** Vegetables, beans, and whole-grain cereals.
**Function** Strengthens cell walls; necessary for the production of prostaglandins (fatty acids), which act against inflammation.
**Usage and dosage** For chronic fatigue syndrome, eczema, migraine, painful menstruation, and PMS, take up to 2 g a day; for eczema, also break a capsule and rub the oil directly onto skin that is not affected.
**Caution** Always take with multivitamins and minerals; avoid supplements if epileptic.

❑ **FOLIC ACID (Folate)**
**Found in** Liver, spinach, broccoli florets, asparagus, beets, kidney, cabbage, lettuce, avocados, nuts, and wheat germ.
**Function** Essential for the formation and functioning of the nervous system and blood cells; closely linked to vitamin $B_{12}$.
**Usage and dosage** For depression, diarrhea, insomnia, and restless legs, take up to 400 mcg a day.

**Caution** Do not take in conjunction with certain epilepsy drugs, or if you have an estrogen-dependent breast tumor; do not take on its own for more than one month without vitamin $B_{12}$.

❑ **GARLIC**
**Found in** Garlic; also available as an expressed oil in capsules.
**Function** Antibacterial and antifungal; reduces blood pressure and cholesterol.
**Usage and dosage** For infections, such as sore throats, follow the maximum recommended dose on the pack.

❑ **GREEN MUSSEL EXTRACT**
**Found in** New Zealand green-lipped mussels.
**Function** Reduces inflammation associated with joint pain.
**Usage and dosage** For osteoarthritis, follow the recommended dose on the pack.

❑ **IRON**
**Found in** Fish, eggs, liver, red meat, legumes, oatmeal, barley, wheat and whole-grain bread, molasses, green vegetables, nuts, and seeds.
**Function** Protects against anemia; necessary for the formation of hemoglobin, which carries oxygen in the red blood cells.
**Usage and dosage** For phlegm, tiredness, chronic fatigue syndrome, hair loss, heavy menstruation, laryngitis, osteoarthritis, restless legs, sinus congestion, and tonsillitis, take up to 14 mg a day.
**Caution** If supplements cause constipation, take a liquid herbal tonic containing iron instead.

❑ **KELP**
**Found in** Seaweed.
**Function** A source of iodine; essential for thyroid function, which helps maintain a normal metabolic rate.

**Usage and dosage** For osteoarthritis, follow the recommended dose on the pack.

❑ **LECITHIN**
**Found in** Soybeans, vegetable and seed oils, nuts, wheat germ, egg yolk, and liver.
**Function** Emulsifies fats.
**Usage and dosage** For prostate enlargement, take 1.2 g a day.

❑ **LYSINE**
**Found in** Protein, mainly animal.
**Function** One of the eight essential amino acids, it transports fatty acids in cells.
**Usage and dosage** For cold sores, take a maximum of 1.2 g a day.
**Caution** Can increase cholesterol and triglyceride (common fat) levels.

❑ **MAGNESIUM**
**Found in** Soybeans, shrimp, green vegetables, hard water, whole-grain cereals, and nuts.
**Function** Necessary for the metabolism of proteins and carbohydrates.
**Usage and dosage** For anxiety, depression, chronic fatigue syndrome, constipation, cramps in pregnancy, hay fever (or allergic rhinitis), anger and irritability, painful menstruation, prostate enlargement, and rheumatism, take up to 300 mg a day.
**Caution** If pregnant, take magnesium supplements only under the supervision of a doctor.

❑ **MANGANESE**
**Found in** Nuts, tea, whole-grain cereals, and vegetables.
**Function** Helps protect against low fertility and birth defects; involved in growth and nervous system functions; and fat, mineral, and hormonal metabolism.
**Usage and dosage** For chronic fatigue syndrome, cramps in pregnancy, and

osteoarthritis, take up to 500 mg a day.
**Caution** If pregnant, take manganese supplements only under the supervision of a doctor.

❑ **MULTIVITAMINS & MINERALS**
**Found in** all foods.
**Function** Replenish stores of the main vitamins and minerals.
**Usage and dosage** For absent menstruation, tiredness, and PMS, take a daily supplement that does not exceed 25 mg each of vitamins $B_1$, $B_5$, and $B_6$.

❑ **POTASSIUM**
**Found in** Soy flour, fruit, milk, beef, vegetables, and whole-grain cereals.
**Function** Important for nerve and muscle function and body fluid.
**Usage and dosage** For cramps in pregnancy, depression, and headaches, take up to 900 mg a day; it can also be obtained as a salt substitute containing potassium and/or sodium chloride. Use this in the same way and amount as ordinary salt.
**Caution** If pregnant, take potassium supplements only under the supervision of a doctor.

❑ **SELENIUM**
**Found in** Garlic, brewers' yeast, eggs, fish, shellfish, organ meats, and vegetables.
**Function** Necessary for a healthy heart and liver and for the manufacture of white blood cells.
**Usage and dosage** For chronic fatigue syndrome, menopause, and osteoarthritis, take up to 200 mcg a day. Hair loss can be a symptom of either an excess or deficiency of selenium. The ideal recommended dosages are 45–75 mcg for men and 45–60 mcg for women.

## ❑ VITAMIN A
**Found in** Cheese, eggs, butter, margarine, organ meats, oils, and vegetables.
**Function** May increase resistance to certain diseases; important for the function of the eye and cell membranes.
**Usage and dosage** For colds and flu, acne, heavy menstruation, osteoarthritis, poor growth, and scaly skin, take up to 4.5 mg a day. Hair loss can be a symptom of either an excess or a deficiency of vitamin A. The ideal recommended dosages are 700 mcg for men and 600 mcg for women.
**Caution** If pregnant, or planning a pregnancy, do not take vitamin A except under the supervision of a doctor; avoid if you suffer from headaches.

## ❑ VITAMIN B COMPLEX
**Found in** A variety of foods such as whole-grain cereals, nuts, legumes, yeast, fish, organ meats, whole-grain bread, dairy products, and green vegetables.
**Function** Necessary for the metabolism of fats, protein, and carbohydrates, as well as neurotransmitters and blood cell formation.
**Usage and dosage** Take a daily supplement that contains no more than 25 mg each of vitamins $B_1$, $B_5$, and $B_6$ for the following: acne; eczema; anxiety; irritability and anger; depression; sinus congestion, phlegm, hair loss, mouth ulcers, laryngitis, tonsillitis, diarrhea, osteo-arthritis, restless legs, meno-pause, and painful menstruation.

## ❑ VITAMIN $B_1$ (Thiamine)
**Found in** Nuts, beans, peas, legumes, yeast, pork, beef, liver, and whole-grain bread.
**Function** Needed for the metabolism of carbohydrates.
**Usage and dosage** For depression, fatigue, and insomnia, take up to 25 mg a day.

## ❑ VITAMIN $B_2$ (Riboflavin)
**Found in** Milk, cheese, eggs, fish, green vegetables, and yeast extract.
**Function** Helps in the metabolism of fats, proteins, and carbohydrates.
**Usage and dosage** For sore lips or a sore tongue, take up to 25 mg a day.
**Note** Urine usually turns yellow, but this is harmless.

## ❑ VITAMIN $B_3$ (Niacin or Nicotinic acid)
**Found in** Whole-grain cereals, meat, fish, legumes, organ meats, and nuts.
**Function** Needed for general metabolism.
**Usage and dosage** For headaches, take up to 25 mg a day.

## ❑ VITAMIN $B_5$ (Pantothenic acid)
**Found in** Many different foods, especially in meat, eggs, and whole-grain cereals.
**Function** Involved in the metabolism of amino acids, carbohydrates, and fats.
**Usage and dosage** For chronic fatigue syndrome, take up to 25 mg a day.

## ❑ VITAMIN $B_6$ (Pyroxidine)
**Found in** Nuts, seeds, green vegetables, bananas and most other fruit, whole-grain cereals, liver, and avocados.
**Function** Involved in the metabolism of minerals, certain body chemicals, and nutrients.
**Usage and dosage** For heavy menstruation, migraines, PMS, and rheumatism, take up to 25 mg a day.

## ❑ VITAMIN $B_{12}$ (Cobalamine)
**Found in** Organ meats, fish, pork, eggs, cheese, yogurt, milk, and brewers' yeast.
**Function** Necessary for hemoglobin production and the functioning of the nervous system. Deficiency results in anemia, fatigue, and lack of coordination. Deficiency may be due not to diet but an inadequate absorption of the vitamin from the intestine.
**Usage and dosage** For fatigue, follow the dosage recommended on the pack. (In pernicious anemia, a doctor will administer an injection.)

## ❑ VITAMIN C (Ascorbic acid)
**Found in** Raw fruit and vegetables, especially citrus fruit and green, leafy vegetables, sweet peppers, new potatoes, black currants, rosehips, broccoli, milk, liver, and kidney.
**Function** Helps repair injury and prevent infection; vital to cell metabolism; aids iron absorption; the elderly, smokers, women taking oral contraceptives, heavy drinkers, and those on certain types of medication, including aspirin, steroids, and antibiotics, may need extra vitamin C.
**Usage and dosage** Take 500 mg a day for acne, anxiety, phlegm, hay fever (or allergic rhinitis), cold sores, constipation, depression, eczema, hair loss, insomnia, irritability and anger, menopause, migraine, osteoarthritis, painful menstruation, sore throats, and varicose veins; take up to 2,000 mg a day for chronic fatigue syndrome, acute sinus congestion, colds, flu, laryngitis, and tonsillitis. If diarrhea occurs, reduce the dose by 500 mg.

## ❑ VITAMIN D (Calciferol)
**Found in** Dairy products, vegetable oils, animal fats, and fish liver oils. It is also produced by the body when skin is exposed to sunlight.
**Function** Vital for the absorption and metabolism of calcium; a deficiency may lead to rickets in children.
**Usage and dosage** For chronic fatigue syndrome, take up to 400 mcg a day.
**Caution** Avoid if suffering from diarrhea or if depressed.

## ❑ VITAMIN E (Tocopheral)
**Found in** Butter, whole-grain cereals, vegetable oil, wheat germ, sunflower seeds, and eggs.
**Function** Involved in the breakdown of fats; essential for women taking oral contraceptives.
**Usage and dosage** For migraine, osteoarthritis, painful menstruation, and restless legs, take up to 100 IU a day; for chronic fatigue syndrome, PMS, menopause, and varicose veins, take up to 400 IU a day, but for no longer than 1 month.
**Caution** If you have high blood pressure do not take more than 100 IU a day without consulting a doctor; diabetics should avoid doses over 50 IU a day.

## ❑ ZINC
**Found in** Yeast, legumes, green vegetables, oysters, meat, ginger, milk, eggs, nuts, and seeds.
**Function** Involved in the absorption and metabolism of vitamins, carbohydrates, and phosphorus; a deficiency can cause slow growth, infertility, skin disorders, white spots on the nails, and loss of hearing, taste, or smell.
**Usage and dosage** For acne, phlegm, cold sores, eczema, hair loss, heavy and painful menstruation, colds, flu, insomnia, and osteoarthritis, take up to 15 mg a day; for chronic fatigue syndrome, laryngitis, sinus congestion, sore throat, and tonsillitis, take up to 30 mg a day.
**Caution** Take supplements last thing at night, several hours after eating or taking other supplements. If stomach irritation occurs, take zinc supplement with food.

# HOMEOPATHIC/HERBAL REMEDIES & TISSUE SALTS

The following tinctures, creams, ointments, tissue salts, and herbal remedies are widely available from health food stores and homeopathic pharmacies.

The biochemic tissue salt system was introduced by a German doctor, Wilhelm Schussler, between 1872 and 1898. He believed that many diseases were associated with a deficiency of inorganic substances, or vital minerals. According to Schussler, each deficiency was characterized by certain symptoms and, in turn, each disease could be cured by replacing the missing vital mineral, or tissue salt, in a minute dose. Schussler identified 12 vital tissue salts. Those recommended for use in *Remedies for Common Ailments* (pp. 152–219) are listed here.

Taken singly or in combinations of three or more minerals (for example, Combination H), tissue salts are an effective and safe means of self-treating common ailments.

## IMPORTANT NOTES

• It is not advisable to take tissue salts during the first 14 weeks of pregnancy; thereafter take them if absolutely necessary during pregnancy (see pp. 208–9).

• Tissue salt dosage is suitable for adults and children unless otherwise specified

## ❑ ARNICA SOLUTION
**Source** *Arnica montana.*
**Uses** Aids recovery from injury or trauma where there is bruising and swelling.
**How to use** Add 10 drops tincture to half a pint (300 ml) of boiled, cooled water. Bathe the affected part.
**Caution** Do not use on broken skin.

## ❑ CALENDULA CREAM
**Source** *Calendula officinalis.*
**Uses** Its antiseptic properties are good for injuries where the skin is broken or infected.
**How to use** Apply to the affected area every 4 hours or more often if required.

## ❑ CALENDULA & HYPERICUM SOLUTION
**Sources** *Calendula officinalis* and *Hypericum perforatum.*
**Uses** Acts as an antiseptic and pain reliever.
**How to use** Add 5 drops each of calendula and hypericum tinctures to half a pint (300 ml) of boiled, cooled water. Gargle or apply to affected areas 4 times a day.

## ❑ DEVIL'S CLAW CAPSULES
**Source** *Harpageophytym procumbens.*
**Uses** Reduces inflammation and relieves pain.
**How to use** For osteoarthritis, follow the recommended dose on the pack.

## ❑ EUPHRASIA TINCTURE
**Source** *Euphrasia officinalis.*
**Uses** Relieves eye inflammation; used to flush foreign objects from the eye.
**How to use** Mix 1 level teaspoon of table salt to half a pint (300 ml) of boiled, cooled water. Add 2 drops of euphrasia tincture.

Irrigate the eye every 4 hours up to 4 times a day.

## ❑ HAMAMELIS SUPPOSITORIES
**Source** *Hamamelis virginiana.*
**Uses** Reduces inflammation.
**How to use** For hemorrhoids, insert a suppository at bedtime.

## ❑ PEONY OINTMENT
**Source** *Peonia officinalis.*
**Uses** Reduces inflammation.
**How to use** Apply to the affected area twice a day.

## ❑ TAMUS OINTMENT
**Source** *Tamus communis.*
**Uses** Specific soothing action on chilblains.
**How to use** Apply up to 4 times a day.
**Caution** Do not use on broken skin.

## ❑ THUJA TINCTURE
**Source** *Thuja occidentalis.* (see p. 110).
**Uses** Removes warts.
**How to use** Apply 2 drops to a cloth bandage, cover the wart, and apply an extra drop every night and morning until the bandage needs changing, then repeat the process.

## ❑ URTICA OINTMENT
**Source** *Urtica urens.* (see p. 111).
**Uses** Reduces skin irritation and relieves pain.
**How to use** Apply directly to affected area up to 4 times a day.

## ❑ CALC. FLUOR.
**Source** *Calcarea fluorica.*
**Uses** Helps alleviate teething problems and problems associated with sluggish circulation, such as varicose veins.
**Dosage** In acute conditions, take 2 tablets every 30 minutes until relief is obtained; then reduce dosage to 3 times a day.

## ❑ CALC. PHOS.
**Source** *Calcarea phosphorica.*
**Uses** Helps with teething problems; aids digestion and assimilation of nutrients.
**Dosage** Take 2 tablets every 30 minutes until relief is obtained; then reduce dosage to 3 times a day.

## ❑ COMBINATION H
**Contains** *Mag. phos.*, *Natrum mur.*, and *Silica.*
**Uses** Alleviates hay fever (allergic rhinitis).
**Dosage** Adults, 4 tablets, and children, 2 tablets, taken 3 times a day; start 6 weeks before expected onset of symptoms.

## ❑ COMBINATION Q
**Contains** *Ferrum phos.*, *Kali mur.*, *Kali sulf.*, and *Natrum mur.*
**Uses** Helps alleviate phlegm and is good for sinus congestion, colds, and flu.
**Dosage** In acute attacks, adults, 4 tablets, and children, 2 tablets, taken every 30 minutes until symptoms are relieved; then reduce dosage to 3 times a day.

## ❑ COMBINATION R
**Contains** *Calc. fluor.*, *Calc. phos.*, *Ferrum phos.*, *Mag. phos.*, and *Silica.*
**Uses** Helps alleviate teething problems.
**Dosage** Take 2 tablets every 30 minutes until symptoms are relieved; then reduce dosage to 3 times a day.

## ❑ MAG. PHOS.
**Source** *Magnesia phosphorica.*
**Uses** Cramps, for example in pregnancy (it is not advisable to take tissue salts during the first 14 weeks of pregnancy).
**Dosage** Take 4 tablets every 30 minutes until symptoms are relieved; then reduce to 3 times a day.

# SPECIAL DIETS

*Healthy eating, as well as good sleeping habits and regular exercise, all help give the body the best possible chance to heal itself. Homeopathic remedies are thought to work more efficiently if the body is not overtaxed by too many toxins. A homeopath may recommend that before taking a homeopathic remedy, the body should be generally detoxified to boost the metabolism and optimize the absorption of the remedy.*

*To help detoxify the body, do not smoke or drink alcohol and reduce your intake of caffeine. Carefully scrutinize the contents of packaged foods for hidden sugar, salt, and additives, which should be avoided. Some homeopaths may also recommend a reduction in meat consumption.*

*Complaints that are aggravated by particular foods may benefit from the alkaline or liver diets. It is unlikely that these diets will lead to problems, providing you eat a variety of foods. If you are suffering from a severe illness or are taking orthodox medicine, however, consult a doctor before starting either diet.*

*The alkaline and liver diets should be followed for one month. If there is an improvement in your health, gradually introduce the foods you have avoided eating, twice a week. Take note of the effects. If symptoms reappear, try the diet for another month and then reintroduce specific foods to your diet gradually. If you still experience problems, see a homeopath or a nutritionist.*

## ALKALINE DIET

This diet is recommended for acidic conditions, such as osteoarthritis, rheumatism, and cystitis.

Acids, which come naturally from the intestines, are usually neutralized and eliminated through the liver, lungs, and kidneys. Illnesses can occur if the body produces too much acid or if the metabolic processes fail to detoxify it. The acid/alkaline balance of the body should be about 20 percent acid and 80 percent alkaline. When this is unbalanced, the metabolism becomes swamped with acid and unable to cope. When too much acid is present, small particles of it accumulate in the tissues, resulting in pain and inflammation. Individuals appear to differ as to how efficiently their detoxifying mechanisms work and how easily they can become overloaded.

The foods allowed in the alkaline diet can reduce the general levels of acidity in the body. Junk food and foods containing white flour, for example, white bread, should be avoided on a long-term basis.

### FOODS ALLOWED
• Fish, preferably fresh and white
• Goats' and sheeps' produce, such as milk, cheese, and yogurt
• Soy milk

• Legumes (peas, beans, lentils)
• Oats, brown rice, corn, whole-wheat pasta, millet, 100% rye crispbread, and gluten-free bread
• Sugarfree oat crackers, granola, tapioca, and white rice bread
• All dried fruit and fresh fruit, except tomatoes and citrus fruit, which can be eaten only twice a week
• All vegetables
• All nuts, especially hazel, almond, cashew, and walnut
• Molasses and sugarfree jam
• Grain coffee (available from health food stores), herbal tea, unsweetened fruit/vegetable juices, and miso soup
• Salt substitute and vegetarian stock cubes
• Vegetable oil and margarines made from vegetable oil or olive oil
• Carob

### FOODS ALLOWED ONLY TWICE A WEEK
• Smoked or canned fish
• White meat and poultry
• Eggs
• Tomatoes
• Butter and nonvegetable margarine (as little as possible)

### FOODS TO AVOID
• Red meat (lamb, beef, pork)
• Cows' produce, such as milk, cheese, and yogurt
• Foods containing brown flour, including bread, cakes, and pastries (Whole-wheat pasta may be eaten)
• Bran
• Any product where wheat starch, edible starch, cereal filler, or cereal protein is listed as an ingredient
• Citrus fruit and waxed fruit (Although citrus fruits are acidic initially, they become alkaline after being digested)
• Dry-roasted nuts, potato chips, and other salty snacks
• Sugar, corn syrup, and honey, and any foods containing them
• Coffee, decaffeinated coffee, cocoa, and tea
• Salt, pepper, and vinegar
• Chocolate
• Alcohol
• Spicy foods
• Fried foods
• Refined, processed foods

**Note** White flour and junk food should be avoided altogether and should not be reintroduced to the diet.

# Liver Diet

This is recommended for many ailments, including hemorrhoids, acne, eczema, and heavy or painful menstruation. The foods allowed in this diet are those that the liver finds easiest to metabolize. Foods that the liver finds difficult to process are avoided, thereby enhancing its function. This does not mean that there is liver disease, simply that the liver may not be functioning as well as it could.

## FOODS ALLOWED
- Fish, preferably fresh and white
- Legumes (peas, beans, lentils)
- Whole-grain bread, whole-grain cereals, brown rice, and whole-wheat pasta
- Molasses and unsweetened jams that are yeastfree (refrigerate after opening)
- Tofu (bean curd)
- All vegetables
- Pineapples, apples, grapes, melons, and fresh or canned fruit in natural juice
- Grain coffee, herb tea, soy milk, and unsweetened fruit juice made from the fruits listed above
- Almonds, sunflower seeds, sesame seeds, and pine nuts
- Carob
- Olive and sunflower oils, margarines made from cold-pressed vegetable oil
- Herbs and soy sauce

## FOODS ALLOWED IN MODERATION
- Berries, apricots, peaches, raisins, and dates twice a week
- Less than one-eighth of a teaspoon of salt a day
- Limit intake of canned fish (wash off oil if not in brine)

## FOODS TO AVOID
- Meat, poultry, and eggs
- Bread made from refined flour
- Sugar, corn syrup, and honey, and foods containing them
- All cows' and goats' produce, such as milk, cheese, and yogurt
- Tomatoes, citrus fruit, avocados, bananas, and all overripe fruit
- Nuts, except almonds
- Coffee, cocoa, and tea (2 cups in total of any of these a day is allowed)
- Chocolate
- Fried food
- Spices
- Alcohol

# Complex Carbohydrate & Protein-rich Foods

These are recommended for menopause, migraines, and PMS. A drop in the blood sugar level may trigger a migraine or cause a hormone imbalance. To ensure the blood sugar level is stable, eat small amounts of food when you feel hungry, rather than large meals.

Avoid refined carbohydrates, which are found in foods made with refined sugar and white flour, dairy products (except milk and yogurt), caffeine, and alcohol. Instead, eat protein-rich foods, such as chicken, tuna, sardines, and complex carbohydrates, which include potatoes, whole-grain bread, legumes, whole-wheat pasta, brown rice, and other whole-grain cereals.

Suitable snacks include raw nuts or seeds, a glass of milk or some yogurt, and unsweetened oat crackers.

# Types of Food

As well as recognizing that different types of people have individual desires and aversions in foods, homeopaths also are aware that certain foods may aggravate or upset certain people and that different constitutional types tend to have different food preferences.

## FOOD LIST CATEGORIES

### Acidic foods
- Red meat, white meat, and poultry
- Cows' produce
- Wheat
- Dry-roasted nuts
- Salt, pepper, and vinegar
- Sugar and sweet foods, chocolate
- Coffee (both caffeinated and decaffeinated), tea, cola drinks, and other caffeinated drinks.

**Note** Citrus fruit should be avoided in the first month of an alkaline diet (see p. 228). They are acidic initially, but become alkaline after being digested.

### Dairy products
- Dairy products include all products from sheep, goats and cows, including butter, cheese, milk, and yogurt.

### Fatty foods
- Fatty meat
- Butter and cheese
- Most processed and fried foods

### Salty foods
- Foods with added salt and flavor enhancers, such as monosodium glutamate
- Meat with preservatives

**Note** Use potassium chloride/sodium substitutes instead of table salt

### Spicy foods
- Curries, chilli peppers, and highly seasoned/spiced food

### Starchy foods
- Bread, potatoes, and cereals

### Sweet foods
- Sugar, honey, corn syrup, glucose, glucose syrup, dextrose and fructose, and all foods containing these, such as cakes, pies, puddings, cookies, candies, and custard

## FOODS TO AVOID FOR PARTICULAR AILMENTS

### Acne
- Seafood, seaweed, kelp, iodized salt, and fish liver oils

### Bloating & gas (flatulence)
- Legumes
- Onions and cabbage
- Nuts

### Cold sores
- Foods that contain arginine, including peanuts, chocolate, seeds, and cereals

### Migraine
- Salty and fried foods
- Food additives
- Alcohol
- Lima beans
- Chocolate
- Cheese and other dairy products
- Citrus fruit
- Coffee, cola drinks, cocoa, and tea
- Onions, sauerkraut
- Shellfish
- Wheat, yeast extract
- Meat, especially bacon, liver, pork, salami, and sausages

# CONSULTING A HOMEOPATH

*Self-prescribing homeopathic remedies is a safe and effective method of treating most minor complaints. If symptoms persist or an illness recurs, however, it may be an indication of a chronic illness. You may need constitutional treatment (see pp. 24–5) and should seek professional help from a suitably qualified homeopath. The increasing popularity of homeopathy has made choosing a practitioner much easier. If you are unable to find a homeopath in your area, contact the National Center for Homeopathy (see p. 231) for further details about homeopaths near you.*

### WHERE IS HOMEOPATHY PRACTICED?
Many countries now consider homeopathy a viable alternative.

In the US and Canada, homeopathic medications are regulated by the FDA and the Ministry of Health, and the practice of homeopathy is widespread.

Homeopathy is now officially recognized in India as a separate branch of medicine, and that country boasts the largest number of homeopathic hospitals in the world.

In Germany, where homeopathy began, it is accepted as commonplace to visit a homeopath. Many orthodox physicians also incorporate homeopathy into their practices.

In France, many doctors practice homeopathy and most pharmacies stock a wide range of remedies. Some French hospitals now have homeopathic consultants, and it is estimated that a quarter of all prescriptions are for homeopathic remedies.

In the UK, homeopathy has been included as an approved method of treatment within the National Health Service since 1950. With six homeopathic hospitals and many private practices, homeopathy is steadily growing in popularity and is supported by the royal family.

In South America, homeopathy is highly regarded and has a good standard of practice. It is also gaining popularity in Israel and Greece. In Australia and New Zealand, the number of homeopaths and of people seeking homeopathic treatment have increased steadily.

In other parts of the world, such as South Africa and the Arab states, homeopathy is not officially recognized, and in eastern Europe and such European countries as Spain, Iceland, and Denmark, it is not yet well represented.

### CHOOSING A HOMEOPATH
In the US and Canada, homeopathy is given as a postgraduate training for licensed health care practitioners. There are also individuals practicing homeopathy who are not medically qualified. Although many of these individuals are excellent homeopaths, the practice of homeopathy is considered part of the practice of medicine and technically requires a medical license. Physicians, physician assistants, nurse practitioners, nurses, naturopaths, chiropractors, and acupuncturists have access to a variety of training programs in homeopathy. These training programs may vary in sophistication from a weekend workshop to a four-year training program with some of the leading homeopaths in the US at Hahnemann College of Homeopathy in Albany, California.

There are professional bodies with standards for homeopathic training. A physician may qualify as a homeopathic specialist by taking a certifying examination, the Diplomate in Homeotherapeutics (D.Ht.) offered by the American Board of Homeotherapeutics. This examination and the resulting qualification is very similar to the MF Hom. examination offered in the UK by the Faculty of Homeopathy.

Naturopathic physicians receive an introductory training in homeopathy in the three nationally recognized naturopathic medical schools: John Bastyr University in Seattle, Washington; National College of Naturopathic Medicine in Portland, Oregon; and the Southwest Naturopathic Medical College in Phoenix, Arizona.

This historical practice of homeopathy involves the use of single remedies for a given medical condition. This is not the only way that homeopathy is practiced, and you may find licensed health care practitioners who use combination remedies, electronic testing devices, and other methods of prescribing remedies. This book is based on the classical approach to homeopathy and remedy prescription.

If you are unable to find a medically qualified homeopath in your area and the homeopath you wish to see is not medically qualified, you should remain under the continued care and observation of your general practitioner.

### WHAT HOMEOPATHS DO
The first visit to a homeopath includes an assessment of your overall condition. You will be asked a great many questions about the symptoms of your illness and what affects them, your medical history, your appetite, food likes and dislikes, and the regularity of your bodily functions. Some questions concerning your occupation, recreational activities, and emotional state are aimed at determining which constitutional type you most closely match.

The homeopath will prescribe a remedy in addition to any other medical advice he or she may offer. The remedy is likely to be dispensed by the practitioner. The initial consultation may vary in length but usually lasts for an hour.

At the second, or follow-up consultation, particularly in a constitutional rather than an acute visit, the homeopath will want to interpret your response to the remedy as a part of the homeopathic evaluation. This and subsequent visits are usually shorter and may last about one half hour.

# USEFUL ADDRESSES

## SOCIETIES & ORGANIZATIONS
### CANADA:
Canadian Foundation for Homeopathic
Research & Development
P.O. Box 8213, Station F
Edmonton, Alberta T6H 4P1

Canadian Society of Homeopathy
87 Meadowlands Drive West
Nepean, Ontario, K2G 2R9

Centre de techniques homéopathiques
7 Laurier Avenue East
Montreal, Quebec H2T 1E4

International Academy of Homeopathy
and The Toronto Homeopathic Clinic
3255 Yonge Street
Toronto, Ontario M4N 2L5

École d'homéopathique familiale
et professionelle
10727 Tanguay Street
Montreal, Quebec H3L 3H3

L'Institut Hahnemannien
795 Davaar Street
Montreal, Quebec H2V 3B3

### UNITED STATES:
Homeopathic Academy of Naturopathic
Physicians
Pres. Durr Elmore, N.D.
11231 SE Market Street,
Portland, OR 97216

Homeopathic Nurses Association
3403–17th Avenue So.,
Minneapolis, MN 55407

National Board of Homeopathy In
Dentistry, Inc.
P.O. Box 423, Marengo, IL 60152

Chiropractic Academy of Homeopathy
Daniel Towle D.C.
6536 Stadium Drive,
Zephyrhills, FL 33540

National Board of Homeopathic
Examiners
Rae Kelly D.C., Pres.
2815 South Jones,
Las Vegas, NV 89102

American Institute of Homeopathy
Pres. Edward H. Chapmen M.D.
1585 Glencoe, Denver, CO 80220

American Board of Homeotherapeutics
Pres. Henry N. Williams, M.D., D.Ht.
801 N. Fairfax Street, Suite 306,
Alexandria, VA 22314

National Center for Homeopathy
Pres. William Shevin, M.M., D.Ht.
801 N. Fairfax Sreet, Suits 306,
Alexandria, VA 22314

American Association of
Homeopathic Pharmacists
P.O. Box 11280, Albuquerque, NM 87192

American Foundation for Homeopathy
Pres. Allen C. Neiswander, M.D.
1508 S. Garfield, Alhambra, CA 91801

Homeopathic Pharmacopoeia Convention
of the United States
P.O. Box 40360, 4974 Quebec Street NW
Washington, DC 20016

American Homeopathic
Pharmacists Association
P.O. Box 60167, Los Angeles, CA 90061

## SUPPLIERS OF HOMEOPATHIC
REMEDIES

### CANADA:
Homéocan Inc.
1900 St. Catherine Street, East
Montreal, Quebec, H2K 1H5

Boiron Canada Inc.
816 Guimond Blvd.
Longueil, Quebec, J4G 1T5

Thompson's Homeopathic Supplies
844 Yonge Street
Toronto, Ontario, M4W 2H1

Dolisos Homeopathics
P.O. Box 56603
861 Warden Avenue
Markham, Ontario L3R 0M6

### UNITED STATES:
B & T
281 Circadian Way, Santa Rosa, CA 95407

BHI
11600 Cochiti SE, Albuquerque, NM 87123

Bioforce of America, Ltd.
P.O. Box 507, Kinderhook, NY 12106

Boiron
6 Campus Boulevard, Building A,
Newton Square, PA 19073, Dolisos,
NV 89102

HoboN
4594 Enterprise Avenue, Naples, FL 33942

Humphreys
63 Meadow Road, Rutherford, NJ 07070

Luyties
P.O. Box 8080, St. Louis, MO 63165-8080

Nature's Way Products
10 Mountain Springs Parkway,
Springville, UT 84663

Similisan Corp.
1321 D South Central Avenue, Kent,
WA 98003

Standard Homeopathic Co.
210 West 131 Street, Los Angeles,
CA 90061

Waleda
841 South Main Street,
Spring Valley NY 10977

Washington Homeopathic Products
4914 Del Ray Avenue, Bethesada,
MD 20814

## HOMEOPATHIC MEDICAL
JOURNALS
### UNITED STATES:
Journal of the American Institute
of Homeopathy
1585 Glencoe, Denver, CO 80220

Homeopathy Today
801 N. Fairfax Street, Suite 306
Alexandria, VA 22314

### UNITED KINGDOM:
British Homeopathic Journal
2, Powis Place
Great Ormond Street
London WC1N 3HT England

## HOMEOPATHIC SCHOOLS OF
EDUCATION
### UNITED STATES:

Hahnemann College of Homeopathy
1918 Bonita Avenue,
Berkeley, CA 94704

International Foundation for Homeopathy
2366 Eastlake Avenue E, Suite 301
Seattle, WA 98102

National Center for Homeopathy
801 N. Fairfax, Suite 306
Alexandria, VA 22314

## NATUROPATHIC SCHOOLS
### UNITED STATES:

National College of
Naturopathic Medicine
11231 SE Market Street
Portland, OR 97216

# INDEX

**Bold** page numbers: these refer to entries in the Index of Homeopathic Remedies, which include details of source and parts used, historical background, constitutional types, and ailments treated.

*Italic* page numbers: these refer to entries in Remedies for Common Ailments, which include details of ailments, appropriate homeopathic remedies, other self-help treatments, and precautions.

Remedy names: all remedies are indexed under their abbreviated homeopathic names, with their full Latin names in brackets. Cross-references to remedy names are made from the common names.

Constitutional types: information on a constitutional type includes details of personality and temperament, food preferences, fears, physical appearance, and general features that relate to that type.

# ACKNOWLEDGMENTS

**Authors' acknowledgments** Dr. Andrew Lockie would like to thank Barbara Lockie for her understanding, support, and research; David, Kirsty, Alastair, and Sandy for their help, encouragement, and patience; and Denis and Mary Thomson for their extensive input and research on herbal medicine. Dr. Nicola Geddes would like to thank her partner Donald for his ready encouragement and forbearance, and Dr. Caragh Morrish and the staff of Baillieston Homoeopathic Outpatients for their support. Both authors would like to thank the tutors and pupils of the Homeopathic Physicians Teaching Group, Oxford, especially Dr. Charles Forsyth, Dr. John English, Dr. Brian Kaplan, and Dr. Dee Ferguson for their kind assistance; all the members of Year Three who acted as guinea pigs for the questionnaire; all the doctors who read and approved clinical information; all those who kindly and generously allowed their photographs to be taken, especially Lesley Adams; Dr. David Riley for his help with the American edition; Dr. John Hughes-Games of Bristol, for his kind offer of support; David Warkentin for his kind permission to use the latest *Reference Works* in the research for the book; Michael Thomson for his help and encouragement; Minerva Books for their reference books; Dragon's Health Club, Guildford for their advice on physical fitness and exercise; the practice staff for their help and support including Pat Webb, Ann Slaymaker, and Chris Donne for their word processing skills and Chris Donne, Clare Lindsay, Lesley Holloway, and Marjorie Edmonds for keeping everything ticking over; the agents, Lutyens & Rubinstein; everyone at DK, especially Blanche Sibbald and Rosie Pearson.

**Dorling Kindersley** would like to thank Karen Ward for picture research and organizing some of the plants and minerals photography; Millie Trowbridge for picture research; Michele Walker for casting the models, styling and photo art direction; Thomas Keenes for design assistance; Helen Barnett for her specialist knowledge of complementary medicine; Antonia Cunningham, Valerie Horn, and Constance Novis for editorial help; and Sue Bosanko for the index. We are grateful to various people at homeopathic pharmacies and manufacturers for their invaluable assistance, especially Matthew Edwards at A. Nelson & Co. Ltd.; Tom Kelly, Michael Bate, and everyone at Weleda (UK) Ltd.; and Tony Pinkus and Evelyn Eglington at Ainsworths Pharmacy. We would also like to thank the following for supplying props and plants for photography: Ainsworths Pharmacy; Droopy & Browns, Covent Garden; Duncan Ross at Pointzfield Herb Nursery; Kings College Pharmacology Department; the Liverpool School of Tropical Medicine; A. Nelson & Co. Ltd., and Weleda (UK) Ltd. In addition, we would like to thank the following for their general help with the project: Elvia Bury, Cally Hall, Mark O'Shea, Mair Searle, and Enid Segul. For modeling, special thanks to Robert Clarke, Alastair Lockie, Peter Jessup, Rachel Gibson, Lesley Adams, Françoise Morgan, Peter Murphy, Christopher Nugent, Shareen Rouvray, Maddy Kaye, Steve Gorton, Eloise Morgan, Lorraine Gunnery, Susannah Marriott, Jade Lamb, Kenzo Okamoto, Leslie Sibbald, Antony Heller, Emily Gorton, and Jane Mason.

**Key to illustration positions**  t = top; b = bottom; l = left; r = right; c = center

## ILLUSTRATORS
Tracy Timson; Sarah Ponder.
## PICTURE CREDITS
All photograhy by Andy Crawford and Steve Gorton except for: Heather Angel: p.74cr; Michael Bate: p.138tl; The Bridgeman Art Library, London: p.52br / *Biblioteca Nazionale*, Turin, p.109tl; Elvira Bury (by kind permission): p.15t; Jean Loup Chatmel: p.92tl; Bruce Coleman: pp.96c, 133b / Dr. Frieder Sauer p.107c; E.T. Archive: p.95tl; Faculty of Homeopathy: pp.16t, 16b, 17r, 58r, 91c, 93tl, 103tl, 122, 125bl, 126cr, 138cr, 145tl; Garden Matthew Photographic Library © John Feltwell: p.99tl; Geoscience Features Picture Library: pp.18t, 66cl, 87c, 90cl; Gregory, Bottley & Lloyd: pp.129b, 131c, 134b, 146b; Pat Hodgeson Library: pp.50tl, 54tl, 66tr, 94cr; The Mansel Collection: pp.10tl, 11tr, 12tl, 13bl, 56tl, 58tl, 74tl, 96tl, 97br, 105tl, 109cr; Mary Evans Picture Library: pp.5, 11br, 12bl, 64tl, 68tl, 70tl, 76tl, 82tl, 83br, 84tl, 85tl, 86tl, 87tl, 88tl, 91tl, 102tl, 106tl, 107tl, 110tl, 111tl, 117b, 141cl; National History Photographic Library: © Andy Callow p.117t; Peter Newark: p.100tl: Mark O'Shea: pp.20cl, 78c, 126bl, 136b, 149tl; Oxford Scientific Films Ltd. – Scott Camazine: p.25t / Michael Fogden p.128bl; Ann Ronan at Image Select: pp.89tl, 101tl; Science Photo Library – Bill Longcore p.98tl / Vaughan Fleming p.103c / Prof. P. Motta p.104br / Arnold Fisher p.142bl; Seven Seas: p.104tl; Harry Smith Collection: pp.93cr, 110cr, 123t; South American Pictures: p.92cr; Weleda: pp.90tl, 118t, 138tl; Zefa Pictures.

# BIBLIOGRAPHY

**Blackie,** Marjorie: *The Patient Not the Cure,* MacDonald, London, 1975.
**Castro,** Miranda: *The Complete Homoeopathy Handbook,* Macmillan, London, 1990.
**Coulter,** Catherine R: *Portraits of Homoeopathic Medicines, Volume 1,* North Atlantic Books, Berkeley, California, 1986.
**Coulter,** Catherine R: *Portraits of Homoeopathic Medicines, Volume 2,* North Atlantic Books, Berkeley, California, 1988.
**Gaier,** Harold: *Thorson's Encyclopedic Dictionary of Homoeopathy,* Thorsons, Glasgow, 1991.
**Lesser,** Otto: *The Text Book of Homoeopathic Materia Medica,* B. Jain, New Delhi, 1980.
**Livingstone,** Dr. Ronald: *Evergreen Medicine,* Asher Asher, Poole, England, 1991.

**Lockie,** Dr. Andrew: *The Family Guide to Homeopathy,* Hamish Hamilton, London, 1989.
**Lockie,** Dr. Andrew and **Geddes,** Dr. Nicola: *The Women's Guide to Homoeopathy,* Hamish Hamilton, London, 1992.
**Mac Repertory** and **Reference Works,** computerized data bases, Kent Associates, California, 1986–94.
**Murphy,** Robin: *Homoeopathic Medical Repertory,* HANA, Colorado, 1993.
**Ody,** Penelope: *The Herb Society's Complete Medicinal Herbal,* Dorling Kindersley Ltd., London, 1993.
**Pelikan,** Wilhelm: *The Secrets of Metals,* Anthroposophic Press Inc., New York, 1973.

**Polunin,** Miriam and **Robbins,** Christopher: *The Natural Pharmacy,* Dorling Kindersley Ltd., London, 1992.
**Shepherd,** Dorothy: *Magic of the Minimum Dose,* C. W. Daniel, Saffron Walden, England, 1964.
**Shepherd,** Dorothy: *Physician's Posy,* C. W. Daniel, Saffron Walden, England, 1969.
**Tyler,** Dr. M. L: *Homoeopathic Drug Pictures,* C. W. Daniel, Saffron Walden, England, 1952.
**Vannier,** Leon: *Typology in Homoeopathy,* Beaconsfield Publishers Ltd., Beaconsfield, England, 1992.
**Vermeulen,** Frans: *Synoptic Materia Medica,* Merlijn Publishers, Häarlem, 1992.